AF180573

Respiratory Medicine

Series Editor:
Sharon I.S. Rounds

For further volumes:
http://www.springer.com/series/7665

Damon C. Scales • Gordon D. Rubenfeld
Editors

The Organization of Critical Care

An Evidence-Based Approach to Improving Quality

Humana Press

Editors
Damon C. Scales, MD, PhD
Interdepartmental Division of Critical Care
University of Toronto
Department of Critical Care
Sunnybrook Health Sciences Centre
Toronto, ON, Canada

Gordon D. Rubenfeld, MD, MSc
Interdepartmental Division of Critical Care
University of Toronto
Department of Critical Care
Sunnybrook Health Sciences Centre
Toronto, ON, Canada

ISSN 2197-7372 ISSN 2197-7380 (electronic)
ISBN 978-1-4939-5163-5 ISBN 978-1-4939-0811-0 (eBook)
DOI 10.1007/978-1-4939-0811-0
Springer New York Heidelberg Dordrecht London

Printed on acid-free paper

Humana Press is a brand of Springer
Springer is part of Springer Science+Business Media (www.springer.com)

Contents

List of Contributors

Neil Adhikari, MD, CM, MSc Department of Critical Care Medicine, Health Sciences and University of Toronto, Toronto, ON, Canada

Andre Carlos Kajdacsy-Balla Amaral, MD Department of Critical Care Medicine, Sunnybrook Health Sciences Centre, Toronto, ON, Canada

Interdepartmental Division of Critical Care Medicine, University of Toronto, Toronto, ON, Canada

Lee Daugherty Biddison, MD, MPH Department of Medicine, Johns Hopkins School of Medicine, Baltimore, MD, USA

Division of Pulmonary and Critical Care, Johns Hopkins School of Medicine, Baltimore, MD, USA

Timothy G. Buchman, PhD, MD, FACS, FCCP, MCCM Emory Center for Critical Care, Emory University Hospital, Atlanta, GA, USA

Surgery and Anesthesiology, Emory University School of Medicine, Atlanta, GA, USA

Shannon S. Carson, MD Division of Pulmonary and Critical Care Medicine, University of North Carolina School of Medicine, Chapel Hill, NC, USA

Jack Chen, MBBS, PhD, MBA (Exec) South West Sydney Clinical School, University of New South Wales, Liverpool, NSW, Australia

The Simpson Centre for Health Services Research, Australian Institute of Health Innovation, University of New South Wales, Kensington, NSW, Australia

J. Randall Curtis, MD, MPH Division of Pulmonary and Critical Care, Department of Medicine, University of Washington, Seattle, WA, USA

Section of Pulmonary and Critical Care, Harborview Medical Center, Seattle, WA, USA

Brian H. Cuthbertson, MD, FRCA Department of Critical Care Medicine, Sunnybrook Health Sciences Centre, Toronto, ON, Canada

Christopher Dale, MD Division of Pulmonary and Critical Care, Department of Medicine, University of Washington, Seattle, WA, USA

Kathleen Dalton, PhD Rural Health Research and Policy Analysis Center, University of North Carolina, Chapel Hill, NC, USA

Allan Garland, MD, MA Medicine and Community Health Sciences, University of Manitoba, Winnipeg, MB, Canada

Hayley B. Gershengorn, MD Albert Einstein College of Medicine, Beth Israel Medical Center, New York, NY, USA

Ken Hillman, MBBS, MD, FRCA (Eng), FCICM Intensive Care, South West Sydney Clinical School, University of New South Wales, Liverpool Hospital, Kensington, NSW, Australia

Simpson Centre for Health Services Research, Australian Institute of Health Innovation, University of New South Wales, Kensington, NSW, Australia

Michael D. Howell, MD, MPH Clinical Quality, University of Chicago Medicine, Chicago, IL, USA

Theodore J. Iwashyna, MD, PhD Division of Pulmonary and Critical Care Medicine, University of Michigan School of Medicine, Ann Arbor, MI, USA

Veterans Affairs Center for Clinical Management Research, Ann Arbor, MI, USA

Daniel B. Jamieson, MD Department of Pulmonary, Critical Care and Sleep Medicine, Medstar Georgetown University Hospital, Washington, DC, USA

Jeremy M. Kahn, MD, MS Department of Critical Care, University of Pittsburgh School of Medicine, Pittsburgh, PA, USA

Department of Health Policy and Management, University of Pittsburgh Graduate School of Public Health, Pittsburgh, PA, USA

Jason N. Katz, MD, MHS Divisions of Cardiology and Pulmonary and Critical Care Medicine, Department of Medicine, University of North Carolina, Chapel Hill, NC, USA

UNC Center for Heart and Vascular Care, 160 Dental Circle, CB# 7075, Burnett-Womack Building, Chapel Hill, NC, USA

Ruth M. Kleinpell, PhD, RN, FCCM Center for Clinical Research and Scholarship, Rush University Medical Center, Chicago, IL, USA

Rush University College of Nursing, Chicago, IL, USA

Stephen E. Lapinsky, MB, BCh, MSc, FRCPC Intensive Care Unit, Mount Sinai Hospital, Toronto, ON, Canada

Interdepartmental Division of Critical Care, University of Toronto, Toronto, ON, Canada

Omar B. Lateef, DO Rush University Medical Center, Chicago, IL, USA

Srinivas Murthy, MD, CM Department of Pediatric Critical Care Medicine, Hospital for Sick Children, Toronto, ON, Canada

Gourang Patel, PharmD, MSc Pulmonary and Critical Care, Pharmacy, and Pharmacology, RUSH Medical College, RUSH University Medical Center, Chicago, IL, USA

Michael R. Pinsky, MD, CM, Dr hc, MCCM, FCCP Critical Care Medicine, University of Pittsburgh Medical Center, Pittsburgh, PA, USA

Tom W. Reader, PhD Department of Social Psychology, London School of Economics, London, UK

Matthew Rosengart, MD, MPH Surgery and Critical Care Medicine, University of Pittsburgh Medical Center, Pittsburgh, PA, USA

Gordon D. Rubenfeld, MD, MSc Interdepartmental Division of Critical Care, University of Toronto, Toronto, ON, Canada

Sadath A. Sayeed, JD, MD Department of Global Health and Social Medicine, Boston Children's Hospital, Boston, MA, USA

Damon C. Scales, MD, PhD Interdepartmental Division of Critical Care, University of Toronto, Toronto, ON, Canada

Rachel Start, RN, MSN Magnet Program Director, Rush Oak Park Hospital, Oak Park, IL, USA

Jennifer P. Stevens, MD, MS Division of Pulmonary, Critical Care and Sleep Medicine, Beth Israel Deconess Medical Center, Boston, MA, USA

Nicole Tran, MD Division of Cardiology, Department of Medicine, University of North Carolina, Chapel Hill, NC, USA

Hannah Wunsch, MD, MSc Department of Anesthesiology, College of Physicians and Surgeons, Columbia University, New York, NY, USA

Department of Epidemiology, Mailman School of Public Health, Columbia University, New York, NY, USA

Part I
Organizing Intensive Care

Chapter 1
Organizational Change in Critical Care: The Next Magic Bullet?

Gordon D. Rubenfeld and Damon C. Scales

Abstract Unlike other fields of medicine, critical care is not defined by a unique procedure or, in some countries, even by a unique type of clinician. While often defined geographically as in, *critical care is what happens in an intensive care unit*, this definition has become increasingly untenable as critical care is frequently provided in emergency departments, on wards, and during transport. Therefore, the innovation we recognize as modern critical care is less a technologic creation and more of an organizational innovation. This book is designed to offer evidence-based solutions to important questions. How might outcomes improve without a specific targeted improvement in measurable processes? Who should deliver critical care and what sort of training should they have? How do you facilitate and enhance team communication and leadership? Can critical care be optimized by regionalizing, specializing, or outreach? How can care be organized under extreme scenarios of pandemic and limited resources? Can staff burnout be prevented or its effects mitigated? Our field has an even greater responsibility to incorporate the available information on organizing critical care and improving quality at the hospital level as we are developing more compelling evidence for patient level interventions.

Keywords Care • Treatment • Observation • Intervention • Definition

Unlike other fields of medicine, critical care is not defined by a unique procedure or, in some countries, even by a unique type of clinician. While often defined geographically as in, *critical care is what happens in an intensive care unit*, this definition has become increasingly untenable as critical care is frequently provided

G.D. Rubenfeld (✉) • D.C. Scales
Interdepartmental Division of Critical Care Medicine, Department of Critical Care, Sunnybrook Health Sciences Center, University of Toronto, Room D108, 2075 Bayview Avenue, Toronto, ON, Canada M4N 3M5
e-mail: Gordon.rubenfeld@sunnybrook.ca; damon.scales@sunnybrook.ca

D.C. Scales and G.D. Rubenfeld (eds.), *The Organization of Critical Care*, Respiratory Medicine 18, DOI 10.1007/978-1-4939-0811-0_1,

in emergency departments, on wards, and during transport. Dialysis, mechanical ventilation, intubation, noninvasive ventilation, and monitoring all occur throughout the hospital and are performed by a variety of clinicians so also cannot be used to define the field. Therefore, the innovation we recognize as modern critical care is less a technologic creation and more of an organizational innovation. Critical care is defined by the ability to focus human and technologic resources in a specific place or at a specific time to deliver monitoring and care to patients with acute clinical decompensation or who are at high risk of such a deterioration. This seems a cumbersome definition for a specialty and, in fact, it is this dynamic organizational definition that plagued the field's maturation in its early years [1].

Data from studies in the earliest years of the twenty-first century pose a difficult question for the critical care community and for advocates of evidence-based medicine. Several of these studies suggest that the outcomes for our most common diagnoses, ARDS and sepsis, are improving over time [2]. This contrasts starkly with a disappointing series of clinical trials in mechanical ventilation, pharmacotherapy, nutrition, invasive monitoring, and other treatments that have either failed to replicate early successes or to validate well-conceived hypotheses. In fact, other than the general sense that low tidal volume ventilation, protocolized weaning, less sedation, and more fluid and antibiotics early in sepsis are beneficial, intensivists are hard pressed to identify the innovations that might explain falling mortality. Of course, the studies showing improved outcomes in critical care may simply be wrong; the results of coding changes or selection bias for admission to the ICU. There may also be clinical strategies that actually work whose benefit we simply have been unable to demonstrate in clinical trials because the studies are underpowered or poorly designed. Certainly, there have been no pharmaceutical discoveries for sepsis or ARDS to explain falling mortality rates.

In this book we will explore an alternate explanation for the observation that mortality rates in critical illness are falling despite a lack of identifiable new treatments. It is possible that a field that is essentially founded on organizational innovation might exploit this fact to optimize outcomes by improving the fundamental organization of care delivery rather than delivery of a specific therapy or device. This may seem counterintuitive because mechanistically we believe that any improvements in outcome *must* be caused by a change in a therapy that we know works. Available evidence suggests this is not always the case. Two notable examples will suffice. The Surviving Sepsis Campaign using a multifaceted quality improvement strategy documented a 5 % absolute mortality reduction which translates to an impressively small number needed to treat of only 20 [3, 4]. This mortality reduction is even more remarkable when two factors are taken into account. First, most of the items on the Surviving Sepsis Campaign checklist including drotrecogin alfa, low dose steroids, and glucose control have since been shown to be either ineffective or harmful. The hemodynamic endpoints of resuscitation including a central venous pressure target and oxygenation are currently being critically evaluated and also may fall away. Second, Surviving Sepsis essentially failed as a quality improvement intervention to improve process measures. Adherence to the entire bundle of treatments increased marginally in both of the multicenter studies. How can a barely effective quality improvement project targeted at treatments that mostly do not appear to be effective reduce mortality?

A second quality improvement study evaluated the implementation of a preoperative checklist on surgical outcomes [5]. This study, carried out in 8 hospitals and evaluating nearly 4,000 patients, demonstrated a halving of mortality and complication risk. Overall, these mortality and complication reductions were associated with improvement in specific processes of care such as use of a pulse oximeter and completed sponge count. However, a careful examination of site-specific data discloses that the centers with the greatest effect on processes of care did not have the greatest change in outcomes and some centers with improved outcomes did not appreciably change their processes of care with the intervention. Again, the changes in outcome did not appear to be specifically linked to changes in specific, evidence-based, processes of care.

It is possible that the outcome improvements in both studies are simply wrong and reflect limitations in the study designs and analyses. However, perhaps the most surprising observation about this lack of association between outcome improvement and process of care is that there is nothing at all unexpected about it. There is a large body of evidence that suggests that improvements in outcome can occur without changes in targeted processes of care. In a landmark 1990 paper in JAMA, the RAND research group noted that variations in mortality in hospitalized patients with congestive heart failure and myocardial infarction could not be attributed to variations in processes of care [6]. Some hospitals were delivering effective therapy with poor outcomes, while others appeared to achieve better outcomes without using the therapies identified as high quality. This suggests that the mechanisms of outcome improvement are complex and may not work via the treatments we think we understand.

The authors in this book have tried to address these complex pathways by unpacking the organization of critical care. How might outcomes improve without a specific targeted improvement in measurable processes? Who should deliver critical care and what sort of training should they have? How do you facilitate and enhance team communication and leadership? Can critical care be optimized by regionalizing, specializing, or outreach? How can care be organized under extreme scenarios of pandemic and limited resources? Can staff burnout be prevented or its effects mitigated? These chapters do not address specific ventilator settings or resuscitation endpoints but may provide advice on improving outcome in ways that are much more effective when specific recommendations on many treatments are not yet clear. The authors have identified many possibilities by building on lessons from disparate fields including organizational psychology, behavioral economics, and crisis management. If the care of critically ill patients involves getting dozens of little things right every single day rather than delivering one or two key medications correctly, improved organization and communication can ensure reliability. Organizing information is an important part of effective communication and can allow clinicians to make more correct decisions.

There are challenges to developing evidence and recommendations about critical care organization. The unit of analysis, almost by definition, in these studies is care at the level of the hospital. This can cause confusion in interpreting research results. For example, many studies have explored the effect of trained intensivists' leadership of critical care units on outcome [7]. Almost uniformly, these studies show a benefit from this organizational approach, although this is defined in various ways across the studies. One study even appeared to demonstrate harm from intensivists' leading care [8]. However, close examination of this outlier study showed that the research question addressed was different in an important way [9]. Instead of studying the organization of the ICU, the researchers looked at the type of physician caring for an individual patient in the ICU. They found an association between care of an individual patient by an intensivist and increased harm. However, this is a fundamentally different research question than the organization and leadership of the ICU. It is also particularly susceptible to the bias introduced by the decision to admit a particular patient to one type of physician versus another. This study demonstrates how important it is to be clear about the difference between a study evaluating the *organization* of the ICU versus who is a patient's doctor.

Research on organization is also challenging because trials that randomize individual patients are usually not feasible leading to quasi-experimental and observational designs. The interventions can rarely be blinded. In an important way, the sample size of organizational studies is the number of *units* studied not the number of *patients*. Therefore, evidence is derived from cohort studies of relatively few sites compared to the number of patients where organizational characteristics are associated with outcome, and this limits the power of these studies to detect differences between sites. Other common study designs are before-after or time-series experiments where organizational changes are implemented over time. These studies are inherently susceptible to biases due to selection of patients, coding of outcomes, confounding from changes in the severity of illness, secular trends, and regression to the mean.

Because of these study design limitations, the results of studies on critical care organization need to be considered in your local context of care. For example, there is mixed, but persuasive data that patients who are discharged from an ICU during off-hours have poor outcomes with increased mortality and a greater likelihood of readmission [10]. However, a busy trauma center with limited beds might need to discharge patients at night from the ICU to maintain 24 h access to critical care beds. In the face of frequent off-hours transfers, this hospital would face a challenging decision with two potential opposing risks: discharging patients at night from the ICU or boarding critically ill patients in the emergency department until the morning when ICU beds could be made available. Depending on how this hospital uses its ICU beds and stepdown beds, nursing staffing on the floor, and the availability of an ICU outreach team, off-hours discharge might actually be safer than emergency department boarding. A reasonable approach would be for this center to look at the outcomes of the patients discharged off-hours and verify in their center the safety or harm of this practice. It is important to realize that organizational issues reflect average effects across many hospitals, and the individual effect in a given hospital might vary and may need to be specifically evaluated.

In 1908 Paul Ehrlich hypothesized that the newly discovered dyes that stained bacteria but not normal cells might be adapted to target what were increasingly realized as the causes of sepsis. He reasoned that these Zauberkugeln or magic bullets would kill bacteria but not people. Based on this hypothesis, Gerhard Domagk tested hundreds of azo dye compounds and eventually discovered that the bright red dye sulfamidochrysoidine (Prontosil) killed bacteria in mice. The initial clinical experience was indeed magical; reducing mortality in bacteremic streptococcal sepsis from 71 to 27 % [11]. Critical care continues to look for treatments with effects like the antibiotic magic bullets for sepsis with limited success. Despite this failure at finding blockbuster discoveries, outcomes appear to be improving likely through the complex organizational and quality measures described in this book. As noted, a frequent, but frustrating, lesson from these types of interventions is that the exact mechanism of their effects is not always clear. Here the magic bullet story provides some reassurances for those skeptical of the value of organizational improvement in the absence of understandable mechanisms. It turns out that the entire dye-staining hypothesis was incorrect and Prontosil's mechanism and efficacy was unrelated to its color; but was due to it serendipitously being the pro-drug for colorless sulfonalimide. The evidence that organizational change and quality improvement can improve outcome in critical care is compelling, and the fact that we don't yet fully understand their mechanisms should not prevent us from using them to improve care or from carefully studying them to better implement them.

References

1. Grenvik A, Pinsky MR. Evolution of the intensive care unit as a clinical center and critical care medicine as a discipline. Crit Care Clin. 2009;25(1):239–50, x.
2. Erickson SE, Martin GS, Davis JL, Matthay MA, Eisner MD, NIH NHLBI ARDS Network. Recent trends in acute lung injury mortality: 1996–2005. Crit Care Med. 2009;37(5):1574–9.
3. Ferrer R, Artigas A, Levy MM, et al. Improvement in process of care and outcome after a multicenter severe sepsis educational program in Spain. JAMA. 2008;299(19):2294–303.
4. Levy MM, Dellinger RP, Townsend SR, et al. The Surviving Sepsis Campaign: results of an international guideline-based performance improvement program targeting severe sepsis. Crit Care Med. 2010;38(2):367–74.
5. Haynes AB, Weiser TG, Berry WR, et al. A surgical safety checklist to reduce morbidity and mortality in a global population. N Engl J Med. 2009;360(5):491–9.
6. Park RE, Brook RH, Kosecoff J, et al. Explaining variations in hospital death rates. Randomness, severity of illness, quality of care. JAMA. 1990;264(4):484–90.
7. Wilcox ME, Chong CA, Niven DJ, et al. Do intensivist staffing patterns influence hospital mortality following ICU admission? A systematic review and meta-analyses. Crit Care Med. 2013;41(10):2253–74.
8. Levy MM, Rapoport J, Lemeshow S, Chalfin DB, Phillips G, Danis M. Association between critical care physician management and patient mortality in the intensive care unit. Ann Intern Med. 2008;148(11):801–9.

9. Rubenfeld GD, Angus DC. Are intensivists safe? Ann Intern Med. 2008;148(11):877–9.
10. Cavallazzi R, Marik PE, Hirani A, Pachinburavan M, Vasu TS, Leiby BE. Association between time of admission to the ICU and mortality: a systematic review and metaanalysis. Chest. 2010;138(1):68–75.
11. Colebrook L, Purdie AW. Treatment of 106 cases of puerperal fever by sulphanilamide (streptocide). Lancet. 1937;230(5961):1237–42.

Chapter 2
Origins of the Critically Ill: The Impetus for Critical Care Medicine

Matthew R. Rosengart and Michael R. Pinsky

Abstract The history of the organization of critical care medicine mirrors the evolution of modern medicine as it has evolved into the management of acute illness. This acute, highly specialized care is provided by anesthesiologists, surgeons, and internists, and its origins can be found within these specialties. Critical care medicine is often associated with complex life-saving treatments, and thus we can track the origins of critical care medicine to the treatment of respiratory failure with mechanical ventilation, severe infections to antiseptic treatments and antibiotics, and cardiovascular insufficiency to hemodynamic monitoring and pharmacologic support. But critical care medicine embodies more than a collection of treatments. It is a health care delivery process demanding specially skilled health care providers (physicians, nurses, respiratory therapists, pharmacists, and physical therapists) within an organizational framework that titrates often conflicting treatments, minimizes potential treatment errors, and promotes the safe and efficient application of appropriate and timely care.

Keywords Critical care medicine • Intensive care unit • Mechanical ventilation • Antisepsis • Hemodynamic monitoring • Cecil Drinker • Joseph Lister • H.J.C. Swan • William Ganz

Critical care medicine is the management of the unstable patient who needs titration of care, often life-saving, on a moment-to-moment basis. That such care is similar

M.R. Rosengart (✉)
Surgery and Critical Care Medicine, University of Pittsburgh Medical Center, 200 Lothrop Street, Pittsburgh, PA 15213, USA
e-mail: rosengartmr@upmc.edu

M.R. Pinsky
Critical Care Medicine, University of Pittsburgh Medical Center, 200 Lothrop Street, Pittsburgh, PA 15213, USA
e-mail: pinskymr@upmc.edu

D.C. Scales and G.D. Rubenfeld (eds.), *The Organization of Critical Care*, Respiratory Medicine 18, DOI 10.1007/978-1-4939-0811-0_2,

to that provided by anesthesiologists in the operating room in high-risk surgeries, surgeons in the Emergency Department treating trauma victims and internists for those with primary circulatory shock or respiratory failure defines its origins within these specialties. Furthermore, specialized expertise with life-saving treatment often requiring complex mechanical artificial life-support systems characterizes treatments. Indeed, critical care medicine is often associated with the complex life-saving treatments given as much as the close labor-intensive monitoring and management it demands. Thus, we can track the origins of critical care medicine to the treatment of respiratory failure with mechanical ventilation, severe infections to antiseptic treatments and antibiotics, and cardiovascular insufficiency to hemodynamic monitoring and pharmacologic support. But critical care medicine is more than a collection of treatments; it is a health care delivery process demanding specially skilled health care providers (physicians, nurses, respiratory therapists, pharmacist, and physical therapists) within an organizational framework that titrates often conflicting treatments, minimizes potential treatment errors, and promotes the safe and efficient application of appropriate and timely care. The history of the evolution of critical care medicine into what it is today is also the history of modern medicine as it has evolved in the management of acute illness (Fig. 2.1).

Mechanical Ventilation

The ability to artificially support failing ventilation with mechanical positive-pressure ventilation provided an initial and pivotal impetus to the development of the ICU and critical care medicine. Recording on the use of mouth-to-mouth resuscitation can be traced back to the Old Testament, in which it is described that the Prophet Elisha successfully resuscitated a dead child. In the sixteenth century, the Swiss alchemist and physician Paracelsus first provided artificial ventilation to both animals and dead humans using fireplace bellows [1, 2]. In 1543 Vesalius explored this concept and published his classical work "De Humani Corporis Fabrica," [1–3] in which he described the ability to keep animals alive by rhythmic insufflation of air into the trachea. These are the first known applications of intermittent positive-pressure ventilation (IPPV) under controlled conditions.

Subsequent advancements in positive-pressure ventilation would await means of secure tracheal cannulation through which ventilation could be reliably delivered. Matas in 1902 first described an automatic respiratory apparatus, which employed a metal laryngeal cannula, guided by extrinsic palpation into the trachea [4–7]. In the beginning he used a double pump giving intermittent positive–negative pressure ventilation (IPNPV). Continued efforts to develop the techniques of laryngoscopy and endotracheal intubation were uniformly discouraging, and emphasis shifted to the use of subatmospheric (i.e., negative pressure) devices to create the driving pressure necessary for tidal breathing.

In 1904 Sauerbruch introduced his low-pressure chamber for use in thoracic surgery, which provided continuous positive airway pressure (CPAP) ventilation

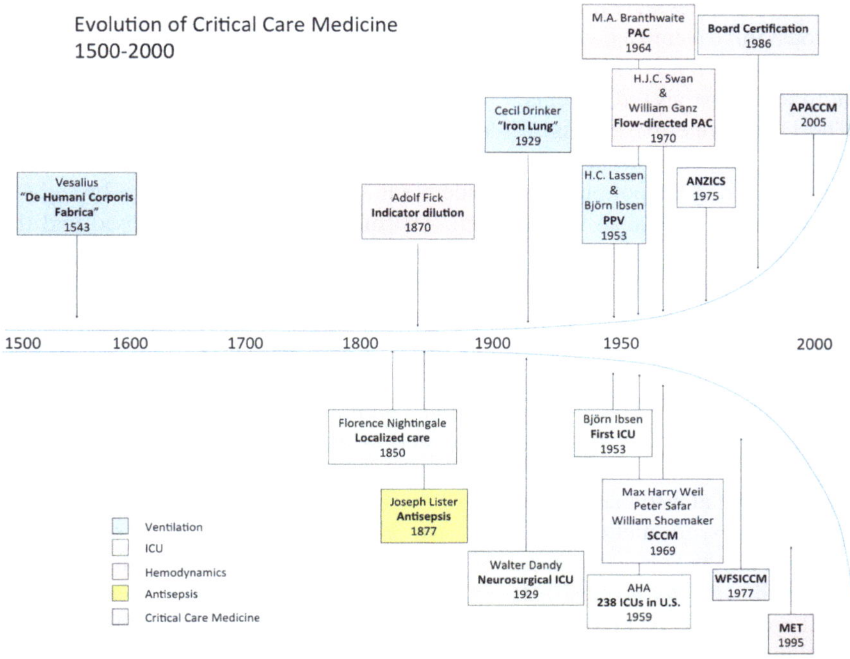

Fig. 2.1 Evolution of critical care medicine 1500–2000

[1, 8, 9]. In this initial prototype both surgeon and patient were enclosed with only the patient's head emerging through an airtight neck collar. It was soon realized that CPAP yielded ineffective ventilation, and oxygen had to be administered to prevent cyanosis [2]. Volhard [10] claimed that it was this oxygen supply, rather than the differential pressure method, that was responsible for the success of Sauerbruch's method. Thus, CPAP was correctly identified as a form of apneic diffusion oxygenation, a term introduced by Holmdahl [11].

With the emergence of the great polio epidemic, efforts to support failing ventilation were further strengthened. In 1918 Dr. Steuart constructed an airtight wooden box, which sealed the patient at the shoulders and waist and powered gas exchange by motor-driven bellows [9]. In 1929 Dr. Cecil Drinker, a Harvard University Professor of Physiology, combined efforts with his brother Philip and developed the negative-pressure tank ventilator, which subsequently became known as the "iron lung" [12, 13]. This monumental discovery was a serendipitous idea generated while observing a colleague quantify the respirations of an anesthetized cat enclosed in a metal box sealed at the neck. Recreating the experimental model, Drinker, by pumping air in and out of the box was able to sustain the paralyzed cat for hours [13]. It would be during the late 1940s, as polio ravaged both Europe and North America, that the Drinker tank ventilator would be first used to provide ventilatory support to a polio stricken child at Boston City Hospital.

The tanks became widely accepted and employed as a life-saving measure. Though numerous improvements upon the design of delivering intermittent negative-pressure ventilation (INPV) would subsequently follow, the system was not efficient in totally paralyzed patients.

The Danish anesthesiologist Ibsen [14] therefore suggested that tracheostomy and manual bag ventilation with IPPV of the patient replace the cuirass and body respirator. During the poliomyelitis epidemic in Denmark, patients were brought to the University Hospital in Copenhagen. The medical school was closed and the medical students were called upon to manually ventilate the patients in shifts. Lassen and Ibsen emphasized basic principles of airway management: protection, humidification, avoidance of elevated oxygen tension, and meticulous physiotherapy [14, 15]. This approach resulted in a drop in mortality from 80 to 25 %. The respiratory ICU was born.

The introduction of the Salk and Sabin vaccines brought eradication of polio; however, controlled airway management and positive-pressure mechanical ventilation had become established standards of practice. Giertz in 1916 [16] clearly demonstrated that artificial ventilation by rhythmic insufflation was superior to the differential pressure method of Sauerbruch. He collaborated with an otolaryngologist who had developed a series of endotracheal and endobronchial tubes and conceived the idea for an air-driven ventilator. His successor, Crafoord, a renowned cardiothoracic surgeon in Sweden, ended the dominance of Sauerbruch's method by introducing "the Spiropulsator" in thoracic surgery [1, 17]. Mörch presented his piston ventilator in 1947 primarily for use in the operating room during thoracic surgery, but it was Björk and Engström who in 1955 introduced the use of prolonged mechanical ventilation by a machine in the postoperative period after lung surgery [18, 19]. At that time, Engström had already demonstrated the advantage of his ventilator in the treatment of totally paralyzed polio victims during the Copenhagen epidemic [20]. From this time onward, mechanical positive-pressure ventilation of patients with endotracheal intubation became not only common place but also the center piece of ventilatory support in critical care medicine.

Antisepsis

Since the birth of recorded civilization, death from infection has been the most common cause, regardless of the initial problem. Women died in childbirth from either hemorrhage or sepsis. Pneumonia was aptly referred to as the "old man's friend." Surgery too was limited in its success primarily by pain, bleeding, and ultimately, infection. However, by the mid-nineteenth century, surgery had traversed the theoretical and had become a reality. The discovery of anesthetics (chloroform, nitrous oxide) eliminated the trepidation of pain, and the incidence of surgery was accelerating at an exponential pace. Now death consequent to wound sepsis remained the primary fear, and its incidence paralleled that of surgery itself.

In 1861 a new surgical facility was constructed at Glasgow with the purpose of reducing the incidence of operative sepsis and its high associated mortality. Its first director was Professor Joseph Lister [21, 22]. His initial efforts proved to be in vain, as approximately 50 % of his amputation cases died of sepsis. During this period, Louis Pasteur was demonstrating that fermentation resulted from small microbes, rather than gases of air. This information was relayed to Lister, who reasoned that fermentation mirrored the processes of wound suppuration and speculated that these same microbes were the etiology of wound sepsis. Concomitantly, an engineer named Crooks had eliminated the malodor of sewage in Glasgow by adding carbolic acid. Uniting these concepts, Lister began applying carbolic acid dressings and thereby reduced the incidence of wound sepsis. In 1877, as Chair of Clinical Surgery at King's College, Lister introduced antisepsis to surgery and simultaneously eliminated both the smell of wound sepsis and those who denounced his theories. That same year, under aseptic technique, Lister performed an open patella repair, an intervention that previously had often resulted in death. News of the operation was widely publicized, and its success was instrumental in forcing surgical opinion throughout the world to accept that his methods greatly added to the safety of operative surgery [21, 22]. A new population was thus developed that required ICU care: the postoperative patient.

Hemodynamic Monitoring

> It is astonishing that no one has arrived at the following obvious method by which the amount of blood ejected by a ventricle of the heart with each systole may be determined directly...

In 1870, with this introduction, Fick [23] described how to compute an animal's cardiac output (CO) from arterial and venous blood oxygen measurements.

$$\mathrm{CO} = \mathrm{VO}_2/(C_\mathrm{a} - C_\mathrm{v})$$

Fick's original principle was later adopted in the development of Stewarts's indicator-dilution method in 1897 [24]. Stewart injected a bolus of a sodium chloride solution into the central venous circulation of anesthetized dogs and rabbits, and then collected blood samples containing diluted sodium chloride from a femoral artery catheter. An electric transducer on the contralateral femoral artery sensed the arrival of diluted injectate. Fegler [25] first described the use of thermodilution for measuring cardiac output.

The clinic use of these techniques would not arrive until 1968. Though it is to Swan and Ganz that we attribute the pulmonary artery catheter (PAC) and the birth of clinical hemodynamic monitoring, it is in fact R.D. Bradley who first described the use of a miniature flow-directed PAC and its use in critically ill patients [26, 27]. In collaboration with M.A. Branthwaite, he described the assessment of cardiac output by thermal dilution using a thermistor mounted on the tip of the catheter [28]. However, it was adapting a balloon to the tip, as first demonstrated by M. Lategola, that enabled the development of the *flow-directed* PAC to measure pulmonary artery occlusion pressure, as we understand it today [29].

In 1951 Dr. Swan immigrated to America to work at the Mayo Clinic under the tutelage of Dr. Earl Wood, playing an integral role in the development of indicator dilution techniques, using indocyanine green [30, 31]. Dissatisfied with life in a communist system, Dr. Ganz emigrated to America in 1966, joining Dr. Swan in the Department of Cardiology of the Cedars of Lebanon Hospital [30, 31]. In 1968 they began to work together on the development of a flow-directed catheter [31]. Dr. Swan's conception of the flow-directed PAC occurred in a brief moment of enlightenment during an outing with his children in Santa Monica [31]. In the days preceding this event, he had used, to little success, a Bradley thermodilution catheter in managing an elderly patient. Dr. Swan noted that among the sedentary sailboats in the harbor, a large spinnaker was moving through the water at a reasonable speed. He contemplated that a sail or parachute anchored to the end of a highly flexible catheter might facilitate the safe passage of the device into the pulmonary artery. This original proposal triggered the concept to attach an inflatable balloon to the tip of a highly flexible catheter. Through the support of Edwards Laboratory, the company that had developed the Starr–Edwards heart valve and the Fogarty embolectomy catheter, he manufactured the first flow-directed PAC [30–32]. Dr. Ganz piloted their invention in an anesthetized dog. Upon balloon inflation, the catheter floated through the right heart into the pulmonary artery, "wedging" itself into a small arterial branch. The transduced waveform represented the pressure in the distal pulmonary artery. In the decades that ensued the catheter gained universal acceptance and widespread use in the management of all critically ill patients.

The introduction of the PAC in 1970 and its subsequent use in performing thermodilution CO measurements in humans translated the ability to measure CO from the experimental physiology laboratory to multiple clinical settings. Following the introduction of the PAC into clinical practice, the single-bolus thermodilution measurement of CO has been widely accepted as the "clinical standard" for advanced hemodynamic monitoring. The ability to monitor CO is a cornerstone of hemodynamic assessment for managing critically ill patients.

Intensive Care as an Organizational Rather Than Technologic Invention

The Unit

Nightingale [33] is considered to be the first to have utilized an intensive care unit (ICU). Serving on the British side in the Crimean War (1850–1854), she collected the worst injured and most infirmed soldiers in an area close to her nursing station, where she could maintain a constant eye on their condition and provide expeditious care when needed. However, it was the establishment in 1929 by Dr. Walter Dandy of the Johns Hopkins Hospital of a three-bed unit for postoperative neurosurgical patients that heralded the development of geographic centralization of critically ill patients, the ICU, in the USA [34].

No similar efforts involving intensive care were reported until the worldwide epidemic of poliomyelitis in the early 1950s. Many acknowledge that the world's first ICU, as defined as "a ward where physicians and nurses observe and treat 'desperately ill' patients 24 hours a day," was developed during this period by Dr. Björn Ibsen in Copenhagen [35]. The first patient admitted to that unit at 6 p.m. on December 21st, 1953 was a 43-year old man who had unsuccessfully attempted to hang himself.

Success of these new techniques in mechanical ventilation spread quickly and respiratory ICUs were established in many university medical centers especially in Europe and North America. The Danish anesthesiologists Bendixen and Pontoppidan, who had both participated in manual ventilation of polio victims in Copenhagen, immigrated to Boston and established the respiratory ICU at Massachusetts General Hospital [36]. By the late 1950s, ICUs had been established in a quarter of large community hospitals, and by the late 1960s, this proportion had expanded to a majority. Peter Safar, the Austrian anesthesiologist, who with Elam introduced mouth-to-mouth ventilation replacing outdated and inefficient traditional techniques used in emergencies, such as drowning victims with apnea, started the first round-the-clock physician covered ICU at Baltimore City Hospital [37, 38]. He later established the first fellowship training program in Critical Care Medicine at Presbyterian University Hospital in Pittsburgh after moving to this city from Baltimore in 1961. Safar is best known as "The Father of Cardiopulmonary Cerebral Resuscitation" having introduced and outlined the relevant steps of CPCR, all of special importance in CCM [39].

Parallel with the development of respiratory ICU services, advanced postoperative care centers also evolved into ICUs. This was initially the case for postoperative open-heart surgery patients where the combined issues of hemodynamic instability, volume shifts, and arrhythmias made recovery safer in a highly monitored environment.

The Nurse

The first ICU was introduced by a nurse, and critical care nurses remain one of the most important personnel categories in ICUs today. Although for decades constrained to acting only under direct physician order, it was soon realized that critically ill patients required nurses with special skills and knowledge to take action, often independent of direct physician supervision. Initially prevented from performing any medical intervention without a direct order from a physician, treatment protocols were developed and agreed upon by physicians and nurses that not only permitted, but actually required, ICU nurses to intervene in various acute situations, such as cardiac arrest. Soon, nurses developed their own insights and procedures. In the USA, in the late 1960s, groups of ICU and coronary care nurses were meeting to exchange experiences, and in 1969, the American Association of Cardiovascular Nurses (AACN) was created [40]. However in 1971, the name was changed to the American Association of Critical Care Nurses changing the acronym to ACCN. This association began holding annual meetings and the membership has grown enormously in recent years. The AACN also provides for specialty certification upon examination of qualifying nurses, who then become critical care registered nurses (CCRN).

The Respiratory Therapist

Since ventilatory support is central to the care of the critically ill, another important ICU personnel is the respiratory therapist [41]. They supervise and manage the function of mechanical ventilators and monitor the patient's respiratory function during mechanical ventilation and weaning from these devices, as well as, the spontaneously breathing patients until they can be discharged from the ICU. In Europe and in most other countries outside North America, these duties are provided by critical care nurses in addition to all other aspects of patient care in the ICU. It is unclear if the presence of registered respiratory therapists (RRTs) in North America has resulted in better respiratory care than in the rest of the world, since mortality rates for acute respiratory failure are similar across the developed world. However, the development of a strong respiratory therapy arm in critical care medicine in North America has certainly helped advance artificial ventilation development worldwide. In addition to the above categories of caregivers to the critically ill and injured patients, social workers, nutritionists, clinical pharmacologists, clergy, and others have become important for the complex management of ICU patients.

Transition from Perioperative Care to Other Diseases

Initially most ICUs were either medical (MICU), focusing upon the treatment of acute respiratory failure, sepsis or cardiovascular collapse, or surgical (SICU), primarily treating postoperative surgical patients. Nonetheless, they tended to favor certain types of patients based on the nature of the hospital patient mix and the bias of the ICU medical teams. In addition, cardiologists introduced separate coronary care units (CCU). Notably absent from this initial progress was the presence of pediatric ICUs. Pediatric intensive care became relevant in pediatric departments and major hospitals for sick children, and then separately for neonatal support. In the 1950s, newborn babies weighing less than four pounds were put in incubators and merely observed. Gradually, the knowledge and technology were developed for intubation and mechanical ventilation of smaller newborns, who were frequently premature, and the neonatal ICU was established.

In the USA, medical ICUs split off as separate units in large, particularly tertiary care hospitals and became the domain of pulmonary specialists with increasing emphasis on broader medical aspects of care of critically ill patients. However, this is not typical for the rest of the world outside North America. Because of the greater need for intensive care of surgical patients, especially postoperatively after increasingly complex procedures, large hospital facilities established separate ICUs for general surgery, cardiothoracic surgery, trauma, neurosurgery, burns, and transplantation [42]. Initially, these units were frequently directed by anesthesiologists, but increasingly, surgical specialists and internists became involved in the management of these patients. Today many ICUs in smaller centers are combined medical-surgical ICUs; this separation of care by patient diagnosis persists today. From a purely functional perspective there is very little difference between the treatments given to classic MICU and SICU patients outside those directly related to routine postoperative care.

In 1959, the American Hospital Association (AHA) began to collect statistical information on ICUs. At that time there were 238 ICUs in short-term acute care hospitals. However within 6 years, over 90 % of large American hospitals with more than 500 beds had ICUs. Today practically all acute care hospitals, not only in the USA but also throughout the world, have at least one ICU. Furthermore, with the change in health care economics, patients are being discharged sooner, increasing the average disease severity of the remaining inpatients. Furthermore, since maximal throughput of care usually requires some short-term stays in ICUs, the proportion of hospital beds being allotted to ICUs has continued to increase worldwide.

Hospital-Wide Medical Emergency Response Teams (MET)

Today the acute care center is the hospital, and the ICU only one part of this dynamic diagnosis/treatment complex. However, not all critical illness occurs within an ICU. In fact, recent studies highlight that up to 17 % of hospital inpatients suffer serious adverse events [43]. A significant proportion of these events is unexpected, being unrelated to the admission diagnosis or underlying medical condition. As such, these events commonly occur in environments ill prepared to properly address acute medical issues. Traditionally the responsibility of the medical unit or cardiac arrest team, these serious events are typically managed in a delayed fashion by personnel not specifically or sufficiently trained in acute resuscitation [44]. Of great concern is that they may result in excessive attributable morbidity and mortality [44–47].

The benefits of an expeditious and organized response and treatment team are well established in trauma and cardiology, and now the management of severe sepsis and septic shock [48–50]. A logical extension would be to apply these concepts of critical illness to the general inpatient population. The field of critical care medicine has made considerable progress in improving the outcomes of critically ill patients. Given that most acute illness develops through stages of deterioration, the logical step surely would be to bring intensive care equipment and expertise to any acutely ill patient, irrespective of location within the hospital, in what has been described as creating a "critical care system without walls." Critical care physicians and critical care nurses can theoretically deliver such expertise anywhere in the hospital within minutes.

The medical emergency team (MET) brings this expertise to the patient in a timely manner and supplies the "efferent arm" of this process of identification of at-risk patients and rapid delivery of appropriate care designated recently as the rapid response system (RRS).

RRSs have been introduced into hospitals to identify and treat at-risk ward patients in an attempt to reduce unplanned ICU admissions and cardiac arrests. The most common form of RRS is the ICU-based MET first described by Lee and colleagues in 1995 [51]. The MET differs from RRTs in that the team leader is a physician, typically with intensive care expertise. The principle of the MET is to "take critical care expertise to the patient before, rather than after, multiple organ failure or cardiac arrest occurs" [52]. Because the care of critically ill patients is their core specialty competency, intensive care doctors and nurses are ideally placed to provide immediate care to patients who are critically ill [44, 53].

The first evidence of a dose–response effect of the MET was demonstrated by DeVita. Introduction of objective MET calling criteria resulted in a significant increase in MET call rates [54, 55]. This was associated with a 17 % reduction in cardiac arrest rates [55]. Subsequently, it was demonstrated that increasing MET at a teaching hospital in Melbourne was associated with a progressive and dose-related reduction in the incidence of cardiac arrest in ward patients [56]. This study suggested that for every additional 17 MET calls, one cardiac arrest might be prevented. Other studies have come to similar conclusions [57].

Birth of the Field of Critical Care Medicine

CCM Societies and Congresses

Much of the success of critical care medicine as a recognized field integral to medicine can be attributed to the development of societies and congresses. As part of the process of maturing as a discipline, specialists from diverse origins with common interests in critical care medicine came together to form societies with the goal of defining core competencies for ICU physicians, providing relevant training and creating advocacy groups to promote the specialty. Their efforts over the years have resulted in many major milestones in the advancement of critical care medicine as a medical specialty associated with a list of core competencies and expected roles in the acute care setting.

At the 1968 FASEB Congress in Atlantic City, Drs. Max Harry Weil, Peter Safar, and William Shoemaker met and discussed the need and suitability for the creation of a society for those interested in intensive care [58]. Max Harry Weil, MD, PhD, an internist and cardiologist directing a shock research unit in Los Angeles, CA; Peter Safar, MD, the founding chairman of the Department of Anesthesiology at the University of Pittsburgh and initial director of the ICU at Presbyterian University Hospital; and William Shoemaker, MD, a trauma surgeon and director of Traumatology and Intensive Care at Cook County Hospital in Chicago, though representing three distinct medical specialties, possessed the same common interest in intensive care of the critically ill and injured patients. The following year, Dr. Weil in connection with his annual Shock Symposium arranged a meeting of selected physicians ($n = 28$) with documented interest in intensive care. And so was born the Society of Critical Care Medicine (SCCM), which was incorporated in 1971. That same year the Society published its first issue of the journal "Critical Care Medicine."

Over the past 40 years, the membership of SCCM has expanded from the initial 28 to a current membership of 15,000, representing 80 different countries and many disciplines: nursing, respiratory therapy, basic and clinic research science, technology, veterinarians, industry, social work, pharmacy that collectively now define intensive care. In 2001 the decision was made to create a separate pediatric critical care medicine journal, and Patrick Kochanek, professor of CCM and Pediatrics and director of the Safar Center for Resuscitation Research at the University of Pittsburgh, was elected founding editor of this new journal.

Over the next 10 years, almost every developed nation created its own national intensive care medicine society. The World Federation of Societies of Intensive and Critical Care Medicine (WFSICCM) was established in 1977 and from the onset involved national and regional societies as its members. In Europe and the north, intensive care was subsumed into the primary specialty of anesthesiology. Thus, in Scandinavia there is a regional Society for Anesthesiology and Intensive Care Medicine. Australia and New Zealand formed their own Australia–New Zealand Intensive Care Society (ANZICS) in 1975 [59]. The western hemisphere is represented by the Pan American Federation of Societies of Intensive Care Medicine. Similarly, the western pacific region created the Western Pacific Association of Critical Care Medicine (WPACCM), which later became the Asia Pacific Association of Critical Care Medicine (APACCM), when India joined in 2005.

The advantage of forming regional societies of like-minded intensivists with strong foci on patient advocacy, continuing medical education, ICU and practice standards, and training/certification spread. Eight European countries formed the European Society for Intensive Care Medicine (ESICM), which now boasts a membership exceeding 5,000. They have approached intensive care medicine education and credentialing head on, and their annual meeting is the third largest critical care medicine program in the world behind the International Symposium of Intensive Care and Emergency Medicine (ISICEM) and the SCCM annual meeting.

Later still, the American Thoracic Society (ATS), under pressure from its regular members, established a Critical Care Assembly in the late 1980s. The Critical Care

Assembly grew to become the second largest primary assembly in the ATS behind Structure and Function. Later, in recognition of the major role that critical care medicine was playing in its society and that a majority of the physicians certified in critical care medicine also have subspecialty boards in respiratory diseases, the ATS changed the name of its flagship journal from the *American Review of Respiratory Disease* to the *American Journal of Respiratory and Critical Care Medicine*. About the same time, the ESICM and the ATS created joint conferences to develop consensus on critical care issues. Perhaps the most successful were the three part series entitled the ATS-ESICM Consensus conferences on Acute Respiratory Distress Syndrome. The SCCM and ESICM have continued these consensus conferences in a more formal way up until the present.

Education and Board Certification

In the USA, the need for separate and advanced training in CCM became evident early. Peter Safar in Pittsburgh was the first to introduce a fellowship training program in CCM for anesthesiologists. In 1968, Dr. Ake Grenvik, a certified general and cardiac surgeon, joined Safar to support the inclusion of other specialists. Through SCCM, a recommendation was made in the late 1970s to the American Board of Medical Specialties to establish a board certification process in CCM [28]. A national committee was formed with the initial intention to have one common certification examination of qualifying physicians [60]. However, representatives of the American Boards of Anesthesiology, Internal Medicine, Pediatrics and Surgery did not agree. Therefore, each of these four specialty boards applied for separate certification examinations, starting in 1986. Within Internal Medicine the decision was made to require 2 years of training in CCM unless the individual already held certification in another subspecialty, commonly pulmonary medicine, in which case 1 year of CCM training would suffice. The common denominator was for all physicians seeking certification examination in CCM to have a minimum of 5 years of postgraduate training. With anesthesiology having a 4-year residency and general surgery 5 years, these two specialties required only 1 year of CCM fellowship. However, the American Board of Pediatrics, with 3 years of residency for ABP certification, decided not only to require 2 years of CCM fellowship, but also an additional year of research in Pediatric CCM-related topics.

Spain and most Latin American countries pursued a different tact and declared intensive care medicine a separate primary specialty, requiring 5 years of training. ESICM arranged a certification approach similar to, but different from the USA and Canada. The ESICM requirements are primary specialty certification with 2 years of training in ICM followed by first a written and then an oral exam for certification. This process is extended to anesthesiology, internal medicine, pediatrics, and surgery. Therefore, physicians with different primary specialty backgrounds in the USA may apply for and take the ESICM diploma exam.

To address the need to standardization across countries, the ESICM developed a Core Competency program for intensive care medicine called CoBaTrICE that emphasizes a define set of core skills and medical competencies: (1) the establishment of a European Forum for national Intensive Care Medicine training organizations that functions as an expert group and acquires ownership over future developments through the Division of Professional Development to the European Board of Intensive Care Medicine; (2) nationally survey current education and training provisions and needs so as to identify current challenges for trainers and trainees and develop a database for benchmarking and accreditation; (3) develop minimum training program standards for quality assurance and harmonize minimum accreditation standards across the European Union; (4) review workplace-based methods of assessment of individual competence, including case-based discussion, simulation techniques, multi-source feedback, link assessment methods to competencies and identify quality indicators within these measures; and finally (5) create a web-based tools for evaluation and testing support and life-long learning for trainers and trainee. To aid in the process of education, the ESICM created its own Patient-Centered Advance Care Training (PACT) program. PACT is a modular multidisciplinary distance-learning program, aimed at improving and harmonizing the quality of acute care medicine. The Program contains 44 modules covering the complete ICU curriculum. Although some of these objectives are uniquely European, most could be directly applied in North America as well.

Research

A fundamental aspect of the maturation of a new specialty is its development of a durable knowledge base and the growth of a robust and well-funded research arm to advance its field. In the early days of CCM, there were no comprehensive textbooks to which trainees and practitioners could refer. With its rapid growth, CCM identified an acute need for this resource. To address this issue Drs. William Shoemaker (surgery), Ake Grenvik (anesthesiology), Peter Holbrock (pediatrics), and Steven Ayers (internal medicine) edited the first *Textbook of Critical Care* in 1984, and continued to edit this textbook through subsequent editions in 1989, 1995, and 2000. Today the student of critical care medicine has an impressive array of superb comprehensive textbooks specializing in specific facets of the field of specialty, including pulmonary, nephrology, surgery, trauma, anesthesiology, and emergency medicine. Nonetheless, the *Textbook of Critical Care*, now in its sixth edition, continues to be the reference standard.

Originally, CCM evolved from a descriptive discipline that tended to categorize symptoms and disease states, describing hemodynamic and metabolic patterns linked closely to the use of the PAC, artificial ventilation, and cardiopulmonary resuscitation. The initial source of the data and evidence for practice and dissemination came from the medical field at large. From these humble roots, however, CCM has advanced into a field focused upon mechanism-based disease and therapeutics, and now generates much of the evidence that supports current practice. These scientific, outcomes, and processes of care data are yielded by CCM physician-scientists, whose publications routinely appear in major medical journals like *JAMA*, the *New England Journal of Medicine*, and *Lancet*. Furthermore, CCM basic science research often appears in *Journal of Clinical Investigation*, *Nature Medicine*, *Biochem Biophys Res Acta*, *Journal of Immunology*, *American Journal of Physiology*, *Journal of Applied Physiology*, and *Circulation*, which highlights the rigorous quality that the foundations of critical care medicine enjoy.

As managed care and cost containments force the less sick to be discharged much earlier and optimizing throughput of care becomes an economic survival practice for hospitals, CCM has become the epicenter of acute care medicine. Accordingly, process of care research, patient safety, ethics of life support, and health care economics have evolved into major areas of expertise and research for critical care physicians. In fact, CCM research interests and productivity compare as equals to any other specialty, an impressive statement considering that its first ICU was only built in 1963.

References

1. Somerson SJ, Sicilia MR. Historical perspectives on the development and use of mechanical ventilation. AANA J. 1992;60(1):83–94.
2. Grenvik A, Eross B, Powner D. Historical survey of mechanical ventilation. Int Anesthesiol Clin. 1980;18(2):1–10 (Summer).
3. Vesalius A. De Humani Corporis Fabrica. 1543:659.
4. Matas R. The history and methods of intralaryngeal insufflation for the relief of acute surgical pneumothorax with a description of the latest devices for the purpose. Trans Southern Surg Gynecol Assoc. 1899;12:52–84.
5. Matas R. Intralaryngeal insufflation for the relief of acute surgical pneumothorax. Its history and methods with a description of the latest devices for this purpose. JAMA. 1900;34:1468–73.
6. O'Dwyer J. Intubation of the larynx. N Y Med J. 1885;42:145–7.
7. O'Dwyer J. Fifty cases of croup in private practice treated by intubation of the larynx, with a description of the method and the dangers incident thereto. Med Rec. 1887;32:557–61.
8. Sauerbruch F. Pathologie des offenen Pneumothorax und de Grundlagen meines verfahrens zur seiner Ausehalturg. Mitt Greuzgeb Med Chir. 1904;8:399–411.
9. Dunphy LM. "The steel cocoon". Tales of the nurses and patients of the iron lung, 1929–1955. Nurs Hist Rev. 2001;9:3–33.
10. Volhard F. Ueber Kunstliche Atmung durch Ventiltion der Trachea und eine einfache Vorrichtung zur rhytmischen kunstlichen Atmung. Munchen Med Wchnschr. 1908;55:209.
11. Holmdahl MH. Pulmonary uptake of oxygen, acid-base metabolism, and circulation during prolonged apnoea. Acta Chir Scand Suppl. 1956;212:1–128.
12. Drinker P, McKhann C. The use of a new apparatus for prolonged administration of artificial respiration. JAMA. 1929;92:1658.
13. Drinker P, Shaw L. An apparatus for the prolonged administration of artificial respiration. J Clin Invest. 1929;7:229–47.
14. Ibsen B. Treatment of respiratory complications in poliomyelitis; the anesthetist's viewpoint. Dan Med Bull. 1954;1(1):9–12.
15. Lassen HC. A preliminary report on the 1952 epidemic of poliomyelitis in Copenhagen with special reference to the treatment of acute respiratory insufficiency. Lancet. 1953;1(1):37–41.
16. Giertz KH. Studier over tryckdifferensandning enlight Sauerbruch och over konstgjord andning (rytmisk luftinblasning) vid intrathoracala operationer. Upsala Lkarefor forhandl 1915;22.

17. Crafoord C. On the technique of pneumonectomy in man, vol. 86. Stockholm: Tryckiri Aktiebolaget Thule; 1938.
18. Morch ET. Controlled respiration by means of special automatic machines as used in Sweden and Denmark. Proc R Soc Med. 1947;40(10):603–7.
19. Björk VO, Engström CG. The treatment of ventilatory insufficiency after pulmonary resection with tracheostomy and prolonged artificial ventilation. J Thorac Surg. 1955;30(3):356–67.
20. Engstrom CG. The clinical application of prolonged controlled ventilation. Acta Anaesthesiol Scand. 1963;13(Supplementum):50.
21. Parker S. Joseph Lister (1827–1912). 1997. http://www.surgical-tutor.org.uk/default-home.htm?surgeons/lister.htm~right. Accessed 31 July 2006.
22. Francoeur JR. Joseph Lister: surgeon scientist (1827–1912). J Invest Surg. 2000;13(3):129–32.
23. Fick A. Uber die Messung des Blutguantums in der Herzventrikeln. Verh Phys Med Ges Wurzburg. 1870;2:16–28.
24. Stewart GN. Researches on the circulation time and on the influences which affect it. J Physiol. 1897;22(3):159–83.
25. Fegler G. Measurement of cardiac output in anaesthetized animals by a thermodilution method. Q J Exp Physiol Cogn Med Sci. 1954;39(3):153–64.
26. Achan V. Another European view: the origin of pulmonary artery catheterization. Crit Care Med. 1999;27(12):2850–1.
27. Bradley RD. Diagnostic right-heart catheterisation with miniature catheters in severely ill patients. Lancet. 1964;67:941–2.
28. Branthwaite MA, Bradley RD. Measurement of cardiac output by thermal dilution in man. J Appl Physiol. 1968;24(3):434–8.
29. Lategola M, Rahn H. A self-guiding catheter for cardiac and pulmonary arterial catheterization and occlusion. Proc Soc Exp Biol Med. 1953;84(3):667–8.
30. Swan HJ, Ganz W. Hemodynamic monitoring: a personal and historical perspective. Can Med Assoc J. 1979;121(7):868–71.
31. Palmieri TL. The inventors of the Swan–Ganz catheter: H.J.C. Swan and William Ganz. Curr Surg. 2003;60(3):351–2.
32. Swan HJ, Ganz W, Forrester J, Marcus H, Diamond G, Chonette D. Catheterization of the heart in man with use of a flow-directed balloon-tipped catheter. N Engl J Med. 1970;283(9):447–51.
33. Nightingale F. In: Longman G, editor. Notes on hospitals, vol. 89. London: Longman; 1863.
34. Hanson 3rd CW, Durbin Jr CG, Maccioli GA, et al. The anesthesiologist in critical care medicine: past, present, and future. Anesthesiology. 2001;95(3):781–8.
35. Berthelsen PG, Cronqvist M. The first intensive care unit in the world: Copenhagen 1953. Acta Anaesthesiol Scand. 2003;47(10):1190–5.
36. Bendixen HH, Egbert LD, Hedley-Whyte J, Laver MB, Pontoppidian H. Respiratory care. Saint Louis: The CV Mosby; 1965.
37. Safar P, Dekornfeld TJ, Pearson JW, Redding JS. The intensive care unit. A three year experience at Baltimore city hospitals. Anaesthesia. 1961;16:275–84.
38. Safar P, Escarraga LA, Elam JO. A comparison of the mouth-to-mouth and mouth-to-airway methods of artificial respiration with the chest-pressure arm-lift methods. N Engl J Med. 1958;258(14):671–7.
39. Safar P. Cerebral resuscitation after cardiac arrest: a review. Circulation. 1986;74(6 Pt 2):IV138–53.
40. Fairman J, Lynaugh JE. Critical care nursing: a history. Philadelphia: University of Pennsylvania Press; 1998.
41. Grenvik A. Role of allied health professionals in critical care medicine. Crit Care Med. 1974;2(1):6–10.
42. Safar P, Grenvik A. Critical care medicine. Organizing and staffing intensive care units. Chest. 1971;59(5):535–47.

43. Vincent C, Neale G, Woloshynowych M. Adverse events in British hospitals: preliminary retrospective record review. BMJ. 2001;322(7285):517–9.
44. Tee A, Calzavacca P, Licari E, Goldsmith D, Bellomo R. Bench-to-bedside review: The MET syndrome—the challenges of researching and adopting medical emergency teams. Crit Care. 2008;12(1):205.
45. Jones D, Bellomo R, DeVita MA. Effectiveness of the medical emergency team: the importance of dose. Crit Care. 2009;13(5):313.
46. Brennan TA, Leape LL, Laird NM, et al. Incidence of adverse events and negligence in hospitalized patients. Results of the Harvard Medical Practice Study I. N Engl J Med. 1991; 324(6):370–6.
47. Baker GR, Norton PG, Flintoft V, et al. The Canadian Adverse Events Study: the incidence of adverse events among hospital patients in Canada. CMAJ. 2004;170(11):1678–86.
48. Rivers E, Nguyen B, Havstad S, et al. Early goal-directed therapy in the treatment of severe sepsis and septic shock. N Engl J Med. 2001;345(19):1368–77.
49. Nardi G, Riccioni L, Cerchiari E, et al. Impact of an integrated treatment approach of the severely injured patients (ISS =/> 16) on hospital mortality and quality of care. Minerva Anestesiol. 2002;68(1–2):25–35.
50. Fresco C, Carinci F, Maggioni AP, et al. Very early assessment of risk for in-hospital death among 11,483 patients with acute myocardial infarction. GISSI investigators. Am Heart J. 1999; 138(6 Pt 1):1058–64.
51. Lee A, Bishop G, Hillman KM, Daffurn K. The medical emergency team. Anaesth Intensive Care. 1995;23(2):183–6.
52. England K, Bion JF. Introduction of medical emergency teams in Australia and New Zealand: a multicentre study. Crit Care. 2008;12(3):151.
53. Jones D, Duke G, Green J, et al. Medical emergency team syndromes and an approach to their management. Crit Care. 2006;10(1):R30.
54. Iyengar A, Baxter A, Forster AJ. Using medical emergency teams to detect preventable adverse events. Crit Care. 2009;13(4):R126.
55. DeVita MA, Braithwaite RS, Mahidhara R, Stuart S, Foraida M, Simmons RL. Use of medical emergency team responses to reduce hospital cardiopulmonary arrests. Qual Saf Health Care. 2004;13(4):251–4.
56. Jones D, Bellomo R, Bates S, et al. Long term effect of a medical emergency team on cardiac arrests in a teaching hospital. Crit Care. 2005;9(6):R808–15.
57. Buist MD, Moore GE, Bernard SA, Waxman BP, Anderson JN, Nguyen TV. Effects of a medical emergency team on reduction of incidence of and mortality from unexpected cardiac arrests in hospital: preliminary study. BMJ. 2002;324(7334):387–90.
58. Weil MH. The Society of Critical Care Medicine, its history and its destiny. Crit Care Med. 1973;1(1):1–4.
59. Trubuhovich RV, Judson JA. Intensive care in New Zealand – a history of the New Zealand region of ANZICS: with notes on the development of intensive care in New Zealand. In: Judson T, editor. History of the New Zealand region of ANZICS. Auckland: Department of Critical Care Medicine, Auckland Hospital; 2001. p. 1–4.
60. Grenvik A, Leonard JJ, Arens JF, Carey LC, Disney FA. Critical care medicine. Certification as a multidisciplinary subspecialty. Crit Care Med. 1981;9(2):117–25.

Chapter 3
Intensivist and Alternative Models of ICU Staffing

Hayley B. Gershengorn and Allan Garland

Abstract In many ways, the leader of a critical care team is the senior physician—the intensivist. In considering the organization of intensive care, it is important to understand the roles and responsibilities of this person as well as how best to utilize him/her. In this chapter we will first consider the definition of the intensivist and then explore strategies for staffing and scheduling a physician of this type. Finally, we will discuss alternatives to the traditional intensivist role.

Keywords Intensivist • Intensivist workload • Intensivist scheduling • ICU staffing • Non-physician providers • Nighttime intensivist/nocturnalist • Rapid response/medical emergency teams • Nurse practitioner • Physician assistant

The Intensivist

Critical care can no longer be considered in its infancy—in the USA the first intensive care unit (ICU) was created in Boston in 1926. More than a quarter-century ago, board certification for a physician with subspecialty training in critical care, an intensivist, was made available around the world [1–4]. Despite this longevity, however, the description of the intensivist has remained fairly amorphous.

H.B. Gershengorn (✉)
Division of Critical Care Medicine, Albert Einstein College of Medicine, Montefiore Medical Center, 111 East 210th Street, Gold Zone, Main Floor, Bronx, NY 10467, USA
e-mail: hgershen@montefiore.org

A. Garland
Medicine and Community Health Sciences, University of Manitoba, Room GF-222, 820 Sherbrook Street, Winnipeg, MB, Canada R3R 0A1
e-mail: agarland@hsc.mb.ca

D.C. Scales and G.D. Rubenfeld (eds.), *The Organization of Critical Care*, Respiratory Medicine 18, DOI 10.1007/978-1-4939-0811-0_3,

A 1992 article entitled "Guidelines for the definition of an intensivist and the practice of critical care medicine" is the sole reference we could find detailing the roles and responsibilities of a critical care physician [5]. In this document, an intensivist is described as having both patient care responsibilities—proficiency in managing complex, often multiorgan dysfunction and procedural competencies—and unit management duties which include facilitation of appropriate resource allocation, quality improvement, and effective communication with other specialties. Additionally, he/she is required to spend more than 50 % of his/her time devoted to the practice of critical care medicine, must willingly participate in a clinical coverage scheme which provides care by intensivists 24 h per day, and should function as either the attending physician or a consultant for all patients in his/her ICU.

This definition is detailed and may be appealing. Yet, it is inconsistent with the description of most currently practicing physicians who would consider themselves intensivists. In the USA, the average intensivist spends only 26.1 % of his/her time providing clinical ICU-based critical care [6]. In only 27 % of hospitals with "high intensity" staffing (where at least 80 % of ICU patients are cared for by or in conjunction with an intensivist) was the intensivist exclusively dedicated to the care of ICU patients [7]. Finally, 87 % of hospitals with high intensity ICU staffing had no in-hospital intensivist coverage for these patients during nighttime hours [7]. While the 1992 guidelines define one view of what an intensivist *should be*, therefore, these data show that this definition is not consistent with the majority of current practice.

Major critical care medicine professional societies are either vague or silent on the topic of defining an intensivist. The Society of Critical Care Medicine (SCCM) states only that intensivists receive board certification in critical care [8]. The websites for the European [9], Australian [10], and Canadian [11] societies do not provide definitions at all. The Leapfrog Group, a for-profit USA organization aimed at improving transparency in healthcare, describes intensivists similar to SCCM as having obtained board certification in critical care or its equivalent [12]. Board certification in critical care, however, is also somewhat difficult to define. In the USA alone, five different organizations (the American Board of Internal Medicine, the American Board of Anesthesiology, the American Board of Surgery, the American Board of Emergency Medicine, and the American Board of Pediatrics) provide certification in critical care medicine. In each case, the prerequisite training as well as the content and duration of critical care education is unique [13].

While an intensivist, therefore, may be simply "known when he/she is seen" [14], we propose the following six-part definition of an intensivist as a clinician who: (1) has subspecialty training focused on the care of critically ill patients and who is (2) knowledgeable about the diagnosis and treatment of acute organ dysfunctions, (3) proficient in procedures related to the care of the critically ill, (4) comfortable liaising with colleagues and assuming care for and/or adding to the care of others' patients, and (5) at ease in emergency situations as well as with end-of-life discussions and decisions. Lastly, intensivists must be more than subspecialty clinicians; they (6) should be advocates for quality assessment and improvement, a culture of safety, multidisciplinary team collaboration, and optimal resource allocation.

How to Best Utilize the Intensivist

Almost as difficult as defining an intensivist is figuring out how best to employ him/her. In the USA, in 1997 only 36.8 % of ICU patients received care by an intensivist and several years later, surveys revealed 53 % of hospitals had no critical care physician in their ICUs at all [6, 7]. As such, our supply of intensivists may lag behind our demand for them. Consequently, as a healthcare community, we must carefully consider how to best deploy this scarce resource. In the following sections, areas of discussion in the realm of intensivist staffing are explored.

The Intensivist "Dose"

Intuitively, it is reasonable to assert that "more intensivist care" may be better than less. How much more is best and whether there is a threshold over which no additional benefit is garnered is unclear.

Early exploration of this question took the form of "closed" versus "open" ICUs. "Closed" ICUs are those in which the primary responsibility for the care of all patients in the ICU is transferred to an attending physician specializing in critical care assigned to the ICU. In contrast, an "open" ICU model allows for multiple physicians (usually, but not always, without specialty training in critical care) to assume/maintain primary responsibility for patients. Open models are more common in some parts of the world (e.g., the USA) [15–17], while closed models are more the norm elsewhere [18, 19]. Over 30 studies have been published exploring the impact of one staffing structure versus the other. Most were single center studies with a historical control design (pre- versus post-change from an open to a closed structure). Results are inconsistent. Moreover, closed ICUs are more likely to be found in academic institutions in which physicians-in-training (residents and fellows) are a constant presence in the ICU [15, 17]. As such, studies comparing open and closed staffing models may be significantly confounded.

The dichotomous characterization of ICUs as open versus closed is an oversimplification. Many ICUs take on an intermediate structure—where consultation with an intensivist is available and, sometimes, mandatory [17, 20]. A more inclusive nomenclature has developed in which ICUs are referred to as "high intensity" versus "low intensity." A meta-analysis of 27,000 patients in 27 ICUs used this framework, defining high intensity ICUs as having either a closed structure or an open structure but with mandatory consultation by an intensivist [21, 22]. This study found lower mortality (hospital and ICU), shorter lengths of stay (hospital and ICU), and lower cost associated with high intensity staffing. Wallace et al. found that the addition of a nighttime in-hospital intensivist to an ICU in which daytime staffing was of lower intensity improved rates of survival to hospital discharge [23]—again suggesting that providing intensivist care to patients who do not otherwise receive it is associated with improved outcomes.

Not all studies support the belief that an intensivist improves care delivery. In fact, one controversial study using the Project IMPACT database of over 100,000 patients in 123 ICUs found an odds ratio (OR) for hospital mortality of 1.42 associated with having an intensivist involved in a patient's care [24]. As the accompanying editorial detailed, there are many plausible explanations for this finding (other than that intensivists truly worsen outcomes of their patients) [25]. How much weight to give this study when faced with a robust literature supporting the beneficial effects of intensivist involvement is unclear; at the least, however, we should consider the notion that more intensivist involvement may not, in all situations, produce better outcomes.

Nighttime In-hospital Intensivists

Recently, significant attention has been paid to nighttime intensivist staffing. Patients develop critical illnesses outside of regular business hours and the impact of interventions in the face of such illness is often time-sensitive [26–28]. In addition, there is concern that the quality of care provided at night is less than that delivered during the daytime hours; while several studies have supported this notion [29–35], others refute it [36–42]. Having intensivists in the hospital 24 h per day is common in some European countries [19] while it has been more rare in North American ICUs [7, 15, 43, 44].

Data on the impact of 24/7 in-hospital intensivist coverage are inconsistent. A single ICU, historically controlled study in the UK found a reduction in the standardized mortality ratio (1.11 to 0.81) following the introduction of a 24/7 intensivist program [45]. A similarly designed study at the Mayo Clinic demonstrated shorter hospital lengths of stay, fewer complications, greater adherence to evidence-based guidelines, and better staff satisfaction following the addition of on-site intensivists throughout the day and night [46]. Neither ICU-, hospital-, nor long-term survival was affected by the change in staffing in this study, however [46, 47]. The largest study addressing the impact of nocturnal intensivist coverage included over 65,000 admissions in 49 ICUs across 25 hospitals and combined clinical information from the APACHE database with surveys regarding staffing patterns [23]. In this analysis, when a nighttime intensivist was added to an ICU with "high intensity" staffing (either a closed unit or one with mandatory intensivist consultation) there was no impact on hospital mortality. However, the addition of a nighttime intensivist to ICUs without high intensity daytime staffing resulted in a lower likelihood of in-hospital death (OR 0.38). The only prospective, non-historically controlled evaluation of the impact of 24-h intensivist staffing was a crossover study conducted in two Canadian ICUs, one academic and one in a community hospital [48]. In this study, neither patient outcomes nor family satisfaction improved with nighttime intensivists. Interestingly, however, the shift work model used to implement 24/7 coverage was associated with lower job and life stresses for the intensivists themselves. An interpretation of this data may be that nighttime in-hospital intensivist coverage is beneficial in some, but not all, ICU environments.

Recruiting intensivists to work at night may be costly. First, critical care manpower is in short supply [6, 49]; asking intensivists to work more hours will further strain the resources of the healthcare system. Second, there is significant cost in salary support to staff an ICU 24/7 with intensivists. One study suggested that nighttime intensivists may reduce the total cost of caring for the sickest ICU patients [50]. A second study, however, demonstrated that replacing 24-h intensivists with a 16-h per day model (with robotic assistance overnight) reduced total hospital costs by 29 % [51]. These costs—in both resource strain and financial investment—must be carefully weighed against the potential benefit of nighttime intensivist staffing.

Intensivist Workload

Many factors combine to determine the workload of an intensivist. The staffing model is one of these, and one of the easiest to modify. Workload, and therefore staffing, is important because job burnout is common among critical care providers and has been linked to desires to find other lines of work [52–55]. Physicians-in-training perceive workload in critical care to be high and cite this as a reason to pursue other fields of medicine [56]. And though there has been great concern that patient care may suffer when physicians-in-training work long hours [57], little attention has focused on the impact of overworked or overtired intensivists [58]. Few investigators have studied these issues.

The European Society of Intensive Care Medicine states that the optimal size for an ICU is 8–12 beds [59]. A survey of academic ICUs in the USA found that the median number of patients cared for by an intensivist was 13 (interquartile range 10–16) [60]. Intensivists practicing in ICUs with higher patient-to-intensivist ratios reported more time constraints, stress, and problems with education of trainees than did those in lower census units. A study performed at the Mayo Clinic explored the impact of increasing the size of their medical ICU, and the patient-to-intensivist ratio, from 7.5 to 15 patients per intensivist [61]. ICU length of stay increased with more patients per physician, but neither ICU nor hospital mortality were affected.

A preliminary study of academic intensivists found that job burnout and job distress were not related to measures of workload [55]. However, other studies have found that scheduling does affect the lives of intensivists. A cluster-randomized study in five USA medical ICUs found that providing intensivists with weekend cross-coverage (and, hence, "breaks") resulted in less burnout and stress for the intensivist without compromising either length of stay or mortality

[62]. Two studies that compared around-the-clock, in-hospital shift work with the historical paradigm of a single intensivist taking call from home at night found that shift work reduced physician burnout without affecting patient outcomes [46, 48].

While intensivists are increasingly working in shifts, the ideal structure of these shifts is unknown. An observational study in surgical ICUs in Germany suggested that having intensivists work 12-h shifts was associated with better patient outcomes than having them work 8-h shifts [63].

Extending the Reach of the Intensivist

Traditionally, we think of the intensivist's interaction with the critically ill patient occurring within the physical confines of an ICU. Over time, however, there has been more focus on the impact of intensivist intervention when either the patient or the physician is outside of the unit. As the American College of Critical Care Medicine stated, "the geographic location of the patient in the hospital does not limit the need for critical care, but rather, it is the nature of the illness that defines the care needed." [15] Similarly, the emergence of telemedicine has suggested that the intensivist can provide care when physically removed from the ICU.

Teams of critical care providers—often called rapid response teams or medical emergency teams (METs)—reaching out of the ICU to care for critically ill patients elsewhere in the hospital have been promoted by the Joint Commission National Safety Goals [64] and the Institute for Healthcare Improvement [65] in the USA. The enthusiasm for the implementation of these teams, however, is not matched by data supporting their efficacy. A large, multicenter, cluster-randomized study of 23 Australian hospitals (the MERIT study) demonstrated a reduction in out-of-ICU cardiac arrests, but no difference in hospital mortality or the need for unplanned ICU transfer associated with the implementation of METs [66]. Interestingly, a post-hoc analysis which evaluated patients "as treated" instead of according to "intention to treat" did suggest a mortality benefit of MET teams, however [67]. Two meta-analyses have been published on the topic of METs. In the first [68], only two studies met criteria to be included and consisted of the MERIT study and a multi-ward study in a single English hospital in which METs were sequentially introduced into different wards [69]. In this second study, hospital mortality was decreased with the introduction of METs [OR (95 % CI): 0.52 (0.32–0.85)]. In light of this conflicting data, the authors were unable to draw a conclusion regarding the efficacy of METs. The second meta-analysis which included 1.3 million hospital admissions across 18 studies found a 33.8 % reduction in the risk of out-of-ICU cardiac arrests with the introduction of METs, but, again, no difference in hospital mortality [70]. Taken together, therefore, current literature does not support a benefit for patients to the implementation of METs. Such teams, however, may have indirect benefits which should be considered; improvements in ward nursing morale [71], access to immediate expert care providers [71], and education of non-ICU providers regarding care of the critically ill [72–74] have been reported.

Telemedicine for the ICU (eICU or teleICU) allows the critical care provider to be external to the ICU and, yet, provide care to the patients therein. Critical care providers are offsite and can electronically access information about the patients (e.g., telemetry, diagnostic tests, information from ventilators and other devices, electronic medical records, and computer orders). In some circumstances, software can help identify worrisome trends in clinical data. Additionally, teleICU clinicians can sometimes view patients via live video feeds or through a robotic presence in the ICU. Hundreds of ICUs in the USA have invested in and implemented this technology. As with METs, however, the data for the impact of these services on outcomes (ICU length of stay [75–78], hospital length of stay [77, 78], ICU mortality [76, 78], hospital mortality [75–78], and cost [75, 76, 79]) is inconsistent. A meta-analysis by Young et al. [80] including 41,374 patients across 35 ICUs in 13 studies found teleICU involvement was associated with lower ICU length of stay and mortality, but no change in hospital length of stay or mortality.

In both METs and teleICU services, there is wide variety in the engagement of intensivists. In Australia and New Zealand, only 12.8 % of METs include intensivists at least some of the time [81]. In two studies comparing intensivist-led METs to those led by other providers (a nurse practitioner [82] or a senior resident physician [83]), no difference in rates of cardiac arrest outside of the ICU, unplanned ICU transfer, or hospital mortality were seen. And, in a provocative single center study, the implementation of a rapid response system which summoned a patient's usual care providers urgently to the bedside resulted in a 5 % relative risk reduction in hospital death suggesting that it may be the rapid response and not the specific responders that influences outcomes [84]. Telemedicine programs have been staffed in similarly variable ways. We could find no data comparing the relative effectiveness of different approaches.

Non-intensivist Care Providers in the Critical Care Setting

Given the shortage of intensivists and concerns for growing unmatchable demand [6, 49, 85–87], it is important to consider what part non-intensivist clinicians can play in caring for the critically ill. In the late 1990s, only 36.8 % of USA ICU patients received care by an intensivist and in Michigan in 2005, in only 20 % of ICUs were all physicians board-certified intensivists [6, 43]. In many ICUs the providers being asked to assume roles previously believed to be the exclusive purview of the intensivist are non-intensivist physicians (those either without critical care training or with nontraditional backgrounds) and non-physician providers.

Non-intensivist Physicians in the ICU

Hospitalists are often asked to assume care of critically ill patients in the ICU [43]. Hospitalists are physicians who, once finished with training, have focused on the care of hospitalized patients [88]. While a relatively new field within medicine, these providers are quickly growing in number [89] and have provided a solution for many hospitals to the intensivist shortage [90]. Two studies have addressed the impact of hospitalists in the ICU. An observational study compared outcomes in two adult medical ICUs—one staffed by intensivists and the other by hospitalists with intensivist consultation available as needed [91]. After adjustment for large differences in case mix, the hospitalist-based ICU had similar hospital mortality (OR $= 0.80$, $p = 0.22$), ICU mortality (OR $= 0.80$, $p = 0.41$), and ICU length of stay (mean difference -0.3 days, $p = 0.32$). The second was a before/after study comparing outcomes when night coverage provided by residents was replaced with hospitalists in an intensivist-led pediatric ICU [92]. ICU mortality (OR $= 0.36$, $p = 0.01$) and ICU length of stay (mean difference -21 h, $p = 0.01$) were lower when care was provided by hospitalists; hospital mortality and length of stay were not evaluated. There are ongoing discussions about how to better train hospitalists to provide care to the critically ill [13].

Acute care surgeons are a newly conceived group of surgeons with combined subspecialty training in emergency care, trauma, and critical care [93]. Brought about by the recognition that surgical capacity is decreasing (due to more retirements relative to new entrants into the field, as well as reductions in workload by active practitioners), the field was born in 2003 to address inadequate manpower available to perform emergency surgery [94]. Currently, there are seven acute care surgery fellowship programs in the USA. No data exist on the impact of this new type of practitioner on the care of ICU patients; however, surveyed members of the surgical section of SCCM believe there will be no negative impact associated with redefining the model of surgical critical care providers in this manner [95].

In 2011, board certification in critical care medicine was opened to emergency medicine physicians [96]. Even prior to this, however, these providers were often assuming critical care responsibilities outside of the emergency department [97]. No data exist on the impact that this new certification mechanism will have on intensivist numbers in the USA or on the impact these providers will have on patient outcomes.

Non-physician Providers in the ICU

Nurse practitioners (NPs) and physician assistants (PAs) are increasingly involved in the care of ICU patients [43, 98, 99]. Although different in background and training, these providers often assume similar roles in the ICU [100]. The literature describes their utilization in several ways: (1) integrated into housestaff-based ICU teams [101–103], (2) as primary care providers with intensivist support in separate ICUs [104, 105], (3) as members of specialty-based teams that remain involved in care of patients who enter the ICU [106–109], and (4) as ICU-based outcomes managers [110–112].

Studies support the use of a non-physician provider as an additional, novel component of the care team. Hospital mortality, hospital and ICU length of stay, duration of mechanical ventilation, complications, and costs were reduced when an NP was employed as an outcomes manager [110, 112]. Clinical practice guidelines were more frequently adhered to when an NP was added to an open-model surgical ICU [111].

Several studies attest to the comparability of non-physician providers and physicians-in-training in adult ICUs. An older historically controlled study found mortality rates to be similar for medical ICU patients cared for by physicians-in-training as compared with PAs [113]. Two more recent studies comparing a medical ICU staffed by medical residents to another staffed by NPs/PAs operating simultaneously in a single academic institution found lengths of stay, mortality, and hospital discharge destination to be similar [104, 105]. Finally, patients cared for by ICU fellows or NPs in a subacute ICU had similar mortality rates, lengths of stay, duration of mechanical ventilation, and ICU readmissions [102, 114].

Although studied primarily as ICU overseers and as alternatives to physicians-in-training in academic hospitals, there are other possible roles and benefits related to these providers. They may fit nicely into a staffing model in combination with non-intensivist physicians and/or teleICU technology. Given their consistency and enthusiasm for critical care, they may improve communication among ICU care providers, foster a safer ICU culture, and achieve high procedural proficiency [115–119]. We must be wary, however, that their implementation may require on-the-job education [101, 103], an initial financial investment will be needed, and they are likely to be subject to the same propensity for burnout as are other permanent ICU providers [53].

Conclusions

Intensivists are more than clinicians schooled in the care of the critically ill. Their responsibilities include ongoing quality assessment and improvement, management of ICU resources, and leadership of a multidisciplinary team. How to best staff our ICUs and schedule these physicians such that their value is maximized—in light of both their clinical and non-clinical duties—is not clear. Arguments are often made for the use of closed-model ICUs [59], but the data on their impact on care are inconsistent [21, 24]. Similarly, significant attention has been focused recently on studying and advocating for the presence of round-the-clock in-hospital intensivists. Data supporting this strategy are also not convincing [23, 45, 46, 48]. Perhaps the facet of ICU staffing with the largest literature is the use of non-physician providers in which studies repeatedly demonstrate comparable care provided by these clinicians [100].

As we aspire to provide appropriate critical care coverage to more patients in more locations at more times of the day, understanding how to best deploy intensivists is becoming ever more pressing. Additionally, both non-intensivist physicians and non-physician providers play a significant role in the care of the critically ill—in some instances by design and, in others, out of necessity. As we move forward, we must continue to evaluate the relative impact of different staffing strategies in an effort to maximize the impact of our critical care workforce.

These types of evaluations can be daunting. First, there is unlikely to be one optimal ICU staffing model; instead, the success of each model will likely depend on ICU characteristics such as size, type, and case-mix. Second, it is difficult to conduct statistically powerful studies. Observational and historical-controlled trials are inherently confounded. Cluster-randomized trials are more robust, yet obtaining funding and buy-in for them is challenging. Third, there are numerous stakeholders (e.g., the patient, the healthcare providers, and/or society) for whom different outcomes may be most relevant (e.g., hospital mortality, staff stress level, financial cost). If one staffing model is best for maximizing patient survival but is financially unsustainable and leads to high levels of burnout among care providers, is it really best? Finally, staffing models are complex and comparing among them is more complicated than assessing the impact of a single, identifiable intervention. If one staffing model appears superior, it will be important to investigate which of its components (e.g., which care providers are utilized, what schedule they keep, etc.) are responsible for its success.

As such, the task of understanding and optimizing ICU staffing is difficult. We cannot let the enormity of this challenge stymie us, however. The manner in which we provide critical care is changing. We must embrace this change and the opportunity to study and learn from it.

References

1. Society of Critical Care Medicine: History of critical care. http://www.sccm.org/AboutSCCM/History_of_Critical_Care/Pages/default.aspx (2012). Accessed 10 Aug 2012.
2. Sibbald WJ, Singh T. Critical care in Canada. The North American difference. Crit Care Clin. 1997;13:347–62.
3. College of Intensive Care Medicine of Australia and New Zealand: About us—history. http://www.cicm.org.au/history.php (2012). Accessed 10 Aug 2012.
4. Menon D, Nightingale P, The Intensive Care Society. An Intensive Care Society (ICS) introduction to UK adult critical care services. Crit Insight. 2006:1–14.
5. Guidelines Committee; Society of Critical Care Medicine: Guidelines for the definition of an intensivist and the practice of critical care medicine. Crit Care Med. 1992;20:540–2.
6. Angus D, Kelley M, Schmitz R, White A, Popovich JJ. Caring for the critically ill patient. Current and projected workforce requirements for care of the critically ill and patients with pulmonary disease: can we meet the requirements of an aging population? JAMA. 2000;284:2762–70.

7. Angus DC, Shorr AF, White A, et al. Critical care delivery in the United States: distribution of services and compliance with Leapfrog recommendations. Crit Care Med. 2006;34:1016–24.
8. Society of Critical Care Medicine: Our members: intensivists. http://www.sccm.org/AboutSCCM/Pages/default.aspx (2012). Accessed 30 July 2012.
9. European Society of intensive Care Medicine: Who we are. http://www.esicm.org/Data/ModuleGestionDeContenu/PagesGenerees/01-about/0A-whoweare/12.asp (2012). Accessed 30 July 2012.
10. Australian and New Zealand Intensive Care Society: About us. http://www.anzics.com.au/about-us (2012). Accessed 30 July 2012.
11. Canadian Critical Care Society: History, vision, values. http://www.canadiancriticalcare.org/aboutcccs_hmv.htm (2012). Accessed 30 July 2012.
12. ICU Physician Staffing Factsheet. http://www.leapfroggroup.org/media/file/FactSheet_IPS.pdf (2009). Accessed 17 Dec 2009.
13. Siegal EM, Dressler DD, Dichter JR, Gorman MJ, Lipsett PA. Training a hospitalist workforce to address the intensivist shortage in American hospitals: a position paper from the Society of Hospital Medicine and the Society of Critical Care Medicine. Crit Care Med. 2012;40:1952–6.
14. Jacobellis v. Ohio. US Supreme Court Center: Supreme Court of the United States; 1964:184.
15. Brilli RJ, Spevetz A, Branson RD, et al. Critical care delivery in the intensive care unit: defining clinical roles and the best practice model. Crit Care Med. 2001;29:2007–19.
16. Scribante J, Bhagwanjee S. National audit of critical care resources in South Africa – open versus closed intensive and high care units. S Afr Med J. 2007;97:1319–22.
17. Bell R, Robinson L. Final Report of the Ontario Critical Care Steering Committee March 2005. Toronto 2005.
18. Bellomo R, Stow PJ, Hart GK. Why is there such a difference in outcome between Australian intensive care units and others? Curr Opin Anaesthesiol. 2007;20:100–5.
19. Graf J, Reinhold A, Brunkhorst FM, et al. Variability of structures in German intensive care units – a representative, nationwide analysis. Wien Klin Wochenschr. 2010;122:572–8.
20. Rubenfeld GD. The structure of intensive care: if you've seen one ICU, you've seen one ICU. Critical care alert. Atlanta: Thomson American Health Consultants; 2000.
21. Pronovost P, Angus D, Dorman T, Robinson K, Dremsizov T, Young T. Physician staffing patterns and clinical outcomes in critically ill patients: a systematic review. JAMA. 2002; 288:2151–62.
22. Pronovost PJ, Needham DM, Waters H, et al. Intensive care unit physician staffing: financial modeling of the Leapfrog standard. Crit Care Med. 2004;32:1247–53.
23. Wallace DJ, Angus DC, Barnato AE, Kramer AA, Kahn JM. Nighttime intensivist staffing and mortality among critically ill patients. N Engl J Med. 2012;366:2093–101.
24. Levy MM, Rapoport J, Lemeshow S, Chalfin DB, Phillips G, Danis M. Association between critical care physician management and patient mortality in the intensive care unit. Ann Intern Med. 2008;148:801–9.
25. Rubenfeld GD, Angus DC. Are intensivists safe? Ann Intern Med. 2008;148:877–9.
26. Kumar A, Roberts D, Wood KE, et al. Duration of hypotension before initiation of effective antimicrobial therapy is the critical determinant of survival in human septic shock. Crit Care Med. 2006;34:1589–96.
27. De Luca G, Suryapranata H, Zijlstra F, et al. Symptom-onset-to-balloon time and mortality in patients with acute myocardial infarction treated by primary angioplasty. J Am Coll Cardiol. 2003;42:991–7.
28. Clark WM, Wissman S, Albers GW, Jhamandas JH, Madden KP, Hamilton S. Recombinant tissue-type plasminogen activator (Alteplase) for ischemic stroke 3 to 5 hours after symptom onset. The ATLANTIS Study: a randomized controlled trial. Alteplase Thrombolysis for Acute Noninterventional Therapy in Ischemic Stroke. JAMA. 1999;282:2019–26.
29. Peberdy M, Ornato J, Larkin G, et al. Survival from in-hospital cardiac arrest during nights and weekends. JAMA. 2008;299:785–92.

30. Merrer J, De Jonghe B, Golliot F, et al. Complications of femoral and subclavian venous catheterization in critically ill patients: a randomized controlled trial. JAMA. 2001;286:700–7.
31. Goldfrad C, Rowan K. Consequences of discharges from intensive care at night. Lancet. 2000;355:1138–42.
32. Beck DH, McQuillan P, Smith GB. Waiting for the break of dawn? The effects of discharge time, discharge TISS scores and discharge facility on hospital mortality after intensive care. Intensive Care Med. 2002;28:1287–93.
33. Priestap FA, Martin CM. Impact of intensive care unit discharge time on patient outcome. Crit Care Med. 2006;34:2946–51.
34. Duke GJ, Green JV, Briedis JH. Night-shift discharge from intensive care unit increases the mortality-risk of ICU survivors. Anaesth Intensive Care. 2004;32:697–701.
35. Singh MY, Nayyar V, Clark PT, Kim C. Does after-hours discharge of ICU patients influence outcome? Crit Care Resusc. 2010;12:156–61.
36. Wunsch H, Mapstone J, Brady T, Hanks R, Rowan K. Hospital mortality associated with day and time of admission to intensive care units. Intensive Care Med. 2004;30:895–901.
37. Uusaro A, Kari A, Ruokonen E. The effects of ICU admission and discharge times on mortality in Finland. Intensive Care Med. 2003;29:2144–8.
38. Morales I, Peters S, Afessa B. Hospital mortality rate and length of stay in patients admitted at night to the intensive care unit. Crit Care Med. 2003;31:858–63.
39. Arabi Y, Alshimemeri A, Taher S. Weekend and weeknight admissions have the same outcome of weekday admissions to an intensive care unit with onsite intensivist coverage. Crit Care Med. 2006;34:605–11.
40. Luyt C, Combes A, Aegerter P, et al. Mortality among patients admitted to intensive care units during weekday day shifts compared with "off" hours. Crit Care Med. 2007;35:3–11.
41. Giraud T, Dhainaut JF, Vaxelaire JF, et al. Iatrogenic complications in adult intensive care units: a prospective two-center study. Crit Care Med. 1993;21:40–51.
42. Sheu CC, Tsai JR, Hung JY, et al. Admission time and outcomes of patients in a medical intensive care unit. Kaohsiung J Med Sci. 2007;23:395–404.
43. Hyzy RC, Flanders SA, Pronovost PJ, et al. Characteristics of intensive care units in Michigan: not an open and closed case. J Hosp Med. 2010;5:4–9.
44. Parshuram CS, Kirpalani H, Mehta S, Granton J, Cook D, Canadian Critical Care Trials Group. In-house, overnight physician staffing: a cross-sectional survey of Canadian adult and pediatric intensive care units. Crit Care Med. 2006;34:1674–8.
45. Blunt MC, Burchett KR. Out-of-hours consultant cover and case-mix-adjusted mortality in intensive care. Lancet. 2000;356:735–6.
46. Gajic O, Afessa B, Hanson A, et al. Effect of 24-hour mandatory versus on-demand critical care specialist presence on quality of care and family and provider satisfaction in the intensive care unit of a teaching hospital. Crit Care Med. 2008;36:36–44.
47. Reriani M, Biehl M, Sloan JA, Malinchoc M, Gajic O. Effect of 24-hour mandatory vs on-demand critical care specialist presence on long-term survival and quality of life of critically ill patients in the intensive care unit of a teaching hospital. J Crit Care. 2012;27: 421.e1–7.
48. Garland A, Roberts D, Graff L. Twenty-four-hour intensivist presence: a pilot study of effects on intensive care unit patients, families, doctors, and nurses. Am J Respir Crit Care Med. 2012;185:738–43.
49. Ewart GW, Marcus L, Gaba MM, Bradner RH, Medina JL, Chandler EB. The critical care medicine crisis: a call for federal action: a white paper from the critical care professional societies. Chest. 2004;125:1518–21.
50. Banerjee R, Naessens JM, Seferian EG, et al. Economic implications of nighttime attending intensivist coverage in a medical intensive care unit. Crit Care Med. 2011;39:1257–62.
51. Barrera R, Bily T, Ritter G, Goldberg M. Economic implications of a novel intensivist coverage in a surgical intensive care unit. American Thoracic Society International Conference. San Francisco, 2012, A1627.

52. Embriaco N, Azoulay E, Barrau K, et al. High level of burnout in intensivists: prevalence and associated factors. Am J Respir Crit Care Med. 2007;175:686–92.
53. Embriaco N, Papazian L, Kentish-Barnes N, Pochard F, Azoulay E. Burnout syndrome among critical care healthcare workers. Curr Opin Crit Care. 2007;13:482–8.
54. Guntupalli KK, Fromm RE. Burnout in the internist–intensivist. Intensive Care Med. 1996; 22:625–30.
55. Shaman Z, Roach M, Marik P, Carson S, Garland A. Job stress and workload among intensivists. Proc Am Thorac Soc. 2005;2:A597.
56. Lorin S, Heffner J, Carson S. Attitudes and perceptions of internal medicine residents regarding pulmonary and critical care subspecialty training. Chest. 2005;127:630–6.
57. Pastores SM, O'Connor MF, Kleinpell RM, et al. The Accreditation Council for Graduate Medical Education resident duty hour new standards: history, changes, and impact on staffing of intensive care units. Crit Care Med. 2011;39:2540–9.
58. Mercurio MR, Peterec SM. Attending physician work hours: ethical considerations and the last doctor standing. Pediatrics. 2009;124:758–62.
59. Valentin A, Ferdinande P, ESICM Working Group on Quality Improvement. Recommendations on basic requirements for intensive care units: structural and organizational aspects. Intensive Care Med. 2011;37:1575–87.
60. Ward NS, Read R, Afessa B, Kahn JM. Perceived effects of attending physician workload in academic medical intensive care units: a national survey of training program directors. Crit Care Med. 2012;40:400–5.
61. Dara SI, Afessa B. Intensivist-to-bed ratio: association with outcomes in the medical ICU. Chest. 2005;128:567–72.
62. Ali NA, Wolf KM, Hammersley J, et al. Continuity of care in intensive care units: a cluster-randomized trial of intensivist staffing. Am J Respir Crit Care Med. 2011;184:803–8.
63. Bollschweiler E, Krings A, Fuchs KH, et al. Alternative shift models and the quality of patient care. An empirical study in surgical intensive care units. Langenbecks Arch Surg. 2001;386:104–9.
64. Revere A, Eldridge N. Joint Commission National Patient Safety Goals for 2008. Top Patient Saf. 2008;12(1):1–4.
65. Berwick DM, Calkins DR, McCannon CJ, Hackbarth AD. The 100,000 lives campaign: setting a goal and a deadline for improving health care quality. JAMA. 2006;295:324–7.
66. Hillman K, Chen J, Cretikos M, et al. Introduction of the medical emergency team (MET) system: a cluster-randomised controlled trial. Lancet. 2005;365:2091–7.
67. Chen J, Bellomo R, Flabouris A, et al. The relationship between early emergency team calls and serious adverse events. Crit Care Med. 2009;37:148–53.
68. McGaughey J, Alderdice F, Fowler R, Kapila A, Mayhew A, Moutray M. Outreach and Early Warning Systems (EWS) for the prevention of intensive care admission and death of critically ill adult patients on general hospital wards (Review). Cochrane Database Syst Rev. 2007;(3):CD005529.
69. Priestley G, Watson W, Rashidian A, et al. Introducing critical care outreach: a ward-randomised trial of phased introduction in a general hospital. Intensive Care Med. 2004;30: 1398–404.
70. Chan PS, Jain R, Nallmothu BK, Berg RA, Sasson C. Rapid response teams: a systematic review and meta-analysis. Arch Intern Med. 2010;170:18–26.
71. Benin AL, Borgstrom CP, Jenq GY, Roumanis SA, Horwitz LI. Defining impact of a rapid response team: qualitative study with nurses, physicians and hospital administrators. BMJ Qual Saf. 2012;21:391–8.
72. Buist M, Bellomo R. MET: the emergency medical team or the medical education team? Crit Care Resusc. 2004;6:88–91.
73. Jones D, Baldwin I, McIntyre T, et al. Nurses' attitudes to a medical emergency team service in a teaching hospital. Qual Saf Health Care. 2006;15:427–32.

74. Bagshaw SM, Mondor EE, Scouten C, et al. A survey of nurses' beliefs about the medical emergency team system in a Canadian tertiary hospital. Am J Crit Care. 2010;19:74–83.
75. Breslow MJ, Rosenfeld BA, Doerfler M, et al. Effect of a multiple-site intensive care unit telemedicine program on clinical and economic outcomes: an alternative paradigm for intensivist staffing. Crit Care Med. 2004;32:31–8.
76. Rosenfeld BA, Dorman T, Breslow MJ, et al. Intensive care unit telemedicine: alternate paradigm for providing continuous intensivist care. Crit Care Med. 2000;28:3925–31.
77. Thomas EJ, Lucke JF, Wueste L, Weavind L, Patel B. Association of telemedicine for remote monitoring of intensive care patients with mortality, complications, and length of stay. JAMA. 2009;302:2671–8.
78. Morrison JL, Cai Q, Davis N, et al. Clinical and economic outcomes of the electronic intensive care unit: results from two community hospitals. Crit Care Med. 2010;38:2–8.
79. Franzini L, Sail KR, Thomas EJ, Wueste L. Costs and cost-effectiveness of a telemedicine intensive care unit program in 6 intensive care units in a large health care system. J Crit Care. 2011;26:329.e1–6.
80. Young LB, Chan PS, Lu X, Nallamothu BK, Sasson C, Cram PM. Impact of telemedicine intensive care unit coverage on patient outcomes: a systematic review and meta-analysis. Arch Intern Med. 2011;171:498–506.
81. ANZICS-CORE MET Dose Investigators, Jones D, Drennan K, Hart GK, Bellomo R, Web SA. Rapid response team composition, resourcing and calling criteria in Australia. Resuscitation. 2012;83:563–7.
82. Scherr K, Wilson DM, Wagner J, Haughian M. Evaluating a new rapid response team: NP-led versus intensivist-led comparisons. AACN Adv Crit Care. 2012;23:32–42.
83. Morris DS, Schweickert W, Holena D, et al. Differences in outcomes between ICU attending and senior resident physician led medical emergency team responses. Resuscitation. 2012;83: 1434–7.
84. Howell MD, Ngo L, Folcarelli P, et al. Sustained effectiveness of a primary-team-based rapid response system. Crit Care Med. 2012;40:2562–8.
85. Kelley MA, Angus D, Chalfin DB, et al. The critical care crisis in the United States: a report from the profession. Chest. 2004;125:1514–7.
86. Krell K. Critical care workforce. Crit Care Med. 2008;36:1350–3.
87. Barnato AE, Kahn JM, Rubenfeld GD, et al. Prioritizing the organization and management of intensive care services in the United States: the PrOMIS conference. Crit Care Med. 2007;35: 1003–11.
88. Wachter RM, Goldman L. The emerging role of "hospitalists" in the American health care system. N Engl J Med. 1996;335:514–7.
89. Wachter RM, Goldman L. The hospitalist movement 5 years later. JAMA. 2002;287:487–94.
90. Heisler M. Hospitalists and intensivists: partners in caring for the critically ill – the time has come. J Hosp Med. 2010;5:1–3.
91. Wise KR, Akopov VA, Williams BR, Ido MS, Leeper KV, Dressler DD. Hospitalists and intensivists in the medical ICU: a prospective observational study comparing mortality and length of stay between two staffing models. J Hosp Med. 2012;7:183–9.
92. Tenner PA, Dibrell H, Taylor RP. Improved survival with hospitalists in a pediatric intensive care unit. Crit Care Med. 2003;31:847–52.
93. The American Association for the Surgery of Trauma: Acute care surgery. http://www.aast.org/AcuteCareSurgery.aspx (2012). Accessed 1 Aug 2012.
94. Napolitano LM, Fulda GJ, Davis KA, et al. Challenging issues in surgical critical care, trauma, and acute care surgery: a report from the Critical Care Committee of the American Association for the Surgery of Trauma. J Trauma. 2010;69:1619–33.
95. Tisherman SA, Ivy ME, Frangos SG, Kirton OC. Acute care surgery survey: opinions of surgeons about a new training paradigm. Arch Surg. 2011;146:101–6.

96. American Board of Emergency Medicine: Internal medicine-critical care medicine announcement. http://www.abem.org/PUBLIC/portal/alias__rainbow/lang__en-US/tabID__4264/DesktopDefault.aspx (2011). Accessed 1 Aug 2012.
97. Sherwin RL, Garcia AJ, Bilkovski R. Quantifying off-hour emergency physician coverage of in-hospital codes: a survey of community emergency departments. J Emerg Med. 2011;41:381–5.
98. Moote M, Krsek C, Kleinpell R, Todd B. Physician assistant and nurse practitioner utilization in academic medical centers. Am J Med Qual. 2011;26:452–60.
99. Riportella-Muller R, Libby D, Kindig D. The substitution of physician assistants and nurse practitioners for physician residents in teaching hospitals. Health Aff (Millwood). 1995;14:181–91.
100. Gershengorn HB, Johnson MP, Factor P. The use of nonphysician providers in adult intensive care units. Am J Respir Crit Care Med. 2012;185:600–5.
101. D'Agostino R, Halpern N. Acute care nurse practitioners in oncologic critical care: the memorial Sloan–Kettering cancer center experience. Crit Care Clin. 2010;26:207–17.
102. Hoffman LA, Tasota FJ, Zullo TG, Scharfenberg C, Donahoe MP. Outcomes of care managed by an acute care nurse practitioner/attending physician team in a subacute medical intensive care unit. Am J Crit Care. 2005;14:121–30. quiz 31–2.
103. Landsperger JS, Williams KJ, Hellervik SM, et al. Implementation of a medical intensive care unit acute-care nurse practitioner service. Hosp Pract. 2011;39:32–9.
104. Gershengorn HB, Wunsch H, Wahab R, et al. Impact of nonphysician staffing on outcomes in a medical ICU. Chest. 2011;139:1347–53.
105. Kawar E, DiGiovine B. MICU care delivered by PAs versus residents: do PAs measure up? JAAPA. 2011;24:36–41.
106. McNatt GE, Easom A. The role of the advanced practice nurse in the care of organ transplant recipients. Adv Ren Replace Ther. 2000;7:172–6.
107. Dahle KL, Smith JS, Ingersoll GL, Wilson JR. Impact of a nurse practitioner on the cost of managing inpatients with heart failure. Am J Cardiol. 1998;82:686–8. A8.
108. Haan JM, Dutton RP, Willis M, Leone S, Kramer ME, Scalea TM. Discharge rounds in the 80-hour workweek: importance of the trauma nurse practitioner. J Trauma. 2007;63:339–43.
109. Jarrett LA, Emmett M. Utilizing trauma nurse practitioners to decrease length of stay. J Trauma Nurs. 2009;16:68–72.
110. Burns SM, Earven S, Fisher C, et al. Implementation of an institutional program to improve clinical and financial outcomes of mechanically ventilated patients: one-year outcomes and lessons learned. Crit Care Med. 2003;31:2752–63.
111. Gracias VH, Sicoutris CP, Stawicki SP, et al. Critical care nurse practitioners improve compliance with clinical practice guidelines in "semiclosed" surgical intensive care unit. J Nurs Care Qual. 2008;23:338–44.
112. Russell D, VorderBruegge M, Burns SM. Effect of an outcomes-managed approach to care of neuroscience patients by acute care nurse practitioners. Am J Crit Care. 2002;11:353–62.
113. Dubaybo BA, Samson MK, Carlson RW. The role of physician-assistants in critical care units. Chest. 1991;99:89–91.
114. Hoffman LA, Miller TH, Zullo TG, Donahoe MP. Comparison of 2 models for managing tracheotomized patients in a subacute medical intensive care unit. Respir Care. 2006;51:1230–6.
115. Petersen LA, Brennan TA, O'Neil AC, Cook EF, Lee TH. Does housestaff discontinuity of care increase the risk for preventable adverse events? Ann Intern Med. 1994;121:866–72.
116. Huang DT, Clermont G, Kong L, et al. Intensive care unit safety culture and outcomes: a US multicenter study. Int J Qual Health Care. 2010;22:151–61.
117. Dong Y, Suri HS, Cook DA, et al. Simulation-based objective assessment discerns clinical proficiency in central line placement: a construct validation. Chest. 2010;137:1050–6.

118. Loukas C, Nikiteas N, Kanakis M, Moutsatsos A, Leandros E, Georgiou E. A virtual reality simulation curriculum for intravenous cannulation training. Acad Emerg Med. 2010;17: 1142–5.
119. Mulcaster JT, Mills J, Hung OR, et al. Laryngoscopic intubation: learning and performance. Anesthesiology. 2003;98:23–7.

Chapter 4
Health Professionals in Critical Care

Timothy G. Buchman

Abstract Critical care is commonly delivered by an integrated multiprofessional team. Clinical operations that attain peak performance depend on familiarity with the training, professional scope, and capabilities of each team member. This chapter focuses on non-physician team roles and reviews evidence supporting their collective contributions to better health, better care, and lower costs. While every ICU is likely to have a division of labor reflecting local skill sets and historic work flows, the data suggest that evidence-based, need-driven reallocation of tasks across the professional team can improve outcomes without incurring additional expense.

Keywords Critical care • Nurse • Nurse practitioner • Physician assistant • Respiratory therapist • Dietitian • Pharmacist • Value • Cost of care

The prior chapter in this book focused on the physician staffing—particularly intensivists—of critical care units. Effective intensive care generally requires a team of caregivers each contributing a focus and set of competencies that constitute their profession. Our purpose in this chapter is to discuss their professional roles and their contributions to a high-functioning critical care team, and further to discuss how their selection and deployment affects quality of care, value of care, and access to care. Optimizing quality, value, and access should produce better health, better care, and lower costs.

T.G. Buchman (✉)
Emory Center for Critical Care, Emory University Hospital, Woodruff Health Science Center Administration Building (WHSCAB), 1440 Clifton Road NE, Suite 313A, Atlanta, GA 30322, USA

Surgery and Anesthesiology, Emory University School of Medicine, Atlanta, GA 30322, USA
e-mail: tbuchma@emory.edu

D.C. Scales and G.D. Rubenfeld (eds.), *The Organization of Critical Care*,
Respiratory Medicine 18, DOI 10.1007/978-1-4939-0811-0_4,

Nurses

The foundation of every intensive care unit is its nursing staff. No other ICU professional is required to be present continuously at the bedside throughout the unit stay. Indeed, the first intensive care unit—Walter Dandy's three-bed neurosurgical postoperative unit at Johns Hopkins in the 1920s—differed from the ordinary ward only by virtue of cohorting patients with specific needs and nurses with specific skills. Such *ad hoc* arrangements met clinical needs until the poliomyelitis epidemic of the early 1950s, which brought both administrative and operational challenges of simultaneously caring for dozens of patients who required negative pressure ventilation ("iron lungs") to sustain life. The unprecedented survival of so many patients with severe respiratory failure prompted hospitals and their nurses to design patient care areas dedicated to complex care. In 1958, the Baltimore City Hospital established the nation's first ICU that featured dedicated nursing and physician staff. Early reports of that unit are notable for a 25-module curriculum designed for ICU nurses taught by physicians from four specialties. This was clear evidence that professions were working as partners (vs. a strict superior-subordinate arrangement) [1].

Several advances fueled the nationwide expansion of ICUs during the 1960s. One was the development of mechanical ventilators that could be used in assistive/supportive modes without need for pharmacologic neuromuscular blockade. Another was the rapid expansion of "open heart" surgery following the first commercial production of the heart–lung (cardiopulmonary bypass) machine. A specialized body of knowledge had developed, and in 1967 Nashville's Baptist Hospital thought to ask about the formation of a national organization focused on coronary care. A year later, 400 nurses convened to propose the formation of such an organization: the American Association of Cardiovascular Nurses was launched in 1969. Within 2 years it was apparent that the breadth of critical care was expanding far beyond the cardiovascular system or service, and in 1971 the association adopted its current name: the American Association of Critical Care Nurses. Although AACN membership exceeds 516,000, only a fraction of nurses (around 58,000) delivering critical care services have achieved the advanced credential of critical care registered nurse (CCRN) [2].

Hospitals were soon faced with staffing challenges: how many staff were required, and what training was necessary to ensure that staff could safely accomplish the necessary work? In 1974, Cullen and colleagues reported a method for quantitatively estimating the complexity and intensity of nursing care: the therapeutic intervention scoring system (TISS) [3]. The TISS score was adopted, revised, simplified, and generally accepted nationwide as a method for estimating how much work—and therefore how much staff was needed to care for ICU patients.

The problem, of course, is that patient need varies from hour to hour and day to day: redeployment of staff in response to changing need is difficult. While TISS was arguably the first successful risk-stratification tool—patients who needed more care were more likely to die—most ICUs came to a common conclusion: either staffing followed a standard 1:1 model in which nurses did more or less everything for their patients or else staffing followed a 1 nurse:2 patient model in which the nurse was supported by additional professionals with focused expertise such as respiratory therapists and pharmacists as well as the ability to "flex up" to 1:1 when confronted by an especially sick patient.

There is an abundance of literature suggesting that nurse staffing ratios approaching 1:1 improve job satisfaction as well as objective outcomes [4]. Yet availability and cost of qualified and competent critical care nurses often dictate less than that ratio. The challenge then changes to engineering safety into a more sparse staffing pattern [5]. In addition to adding other professionals to the primary on-site safety strategy, tele-ICU has emerged as a secondary strategy in which seasoned critical care professionals leverage electronic tools. Advanced alerts and two-way audio-visual monitoring towards identifying and mitigating threats to safety and well-being [6].

Given the aging of the nursing workforce, the paucity of critical care nurses with advanced credentials, and the burgeoning demand for critical care services, a reference staffing ratio of 1 nurse:2 critically ill patients seems reasonable. As patients emerge from the critical state and require fewer interventions, even thinner coverage will be proposed. The problem is that such low-acuity patients are inevitably shuttled to a lower-intensity area when a high-intensity patient requires admission to the ICU.

Respiratory Therapists

Point prevalence studies suggest that approximately 40 % of patients are mechanically ventilated [7]. It is therefore fitting that a separate profession focuses on enabling this life-saving therapy. In most modern ICUs, however, the respiratory therapist has several roles. In addition to maintenance, preparation, connection and monitoring of the mechanical ventilator, the respiratory therapist often is the nurse's closest care partner. The therapist may commonly participate and lead oral care protocols; perform spontaneous breathing trials; intubate, adjust the endotracheal tube and extubate; offer and provide noninvasive positive pressure ventilatory support; recommend and supervise inhalational treatments ranging from bronchodilators, prostanoids, antimicrobials and special gases (such as NO); and participate in extracorporeal oxygenation treatments.

Yet as exhaustive as the preceding list may appear, it reflects only one of the several dimensions of respiratory care. In other roles, respiratory therapists commonly obtain, analyze, and report the composition of arterial and mixed venous blood specimens ("blood gas analysis"). Those results drive not only ventilator but just as often cardiovascular and renal therapies since modern analyses often include measurement of lactate and electrolytes.

Respiratory therapists often lead the ICU outreach efforts as part of the response team attending medical emergencies ("Code METs") and cardio-respiratory arrests. They are equally integral to transport of critically ill patients on and off-unit, such as may be required for advanced imaging procedures. In this sense, respiratory therapists are often the "face" of the ICU to other parts of the hospital.

Respiratory therapists often play key roles in strategic planning and quality and financial management of the ICU. For example, respiratory therapist leadership is commonly a cornerstone of quality programs that reduce ventilator-associated pneumonias because those programs require more frequent spontaneous breathing trials (to accelerate extubation); systematic oral care; and perfect maintenance of the mechanical equipment.

A 2006 review of respiratory care manpower allocation suggested that each increment of 9–11 ICU beds creates a need for an additional respiratory therapist [8]. Arithmetic suggests that during a typical shift (40/168 h) a therapist may be responsible for around 40–50 ICU beds, of which 16–20 (40 % prevalence) are receiving mechanical ventilator support. In smaller hospitals with fewer critical care beds, it is common for respiratory therapists to have duties outside the ICU.

There is an important paradox to consider when indexing therapist work hours to the number of ventilated patients or ventilated hours: substantial amounts of therapist time are devoted to weaning patients from ventilator support, performance of spontaneous breathing trials and support of patients who are extubated on the cusp of readiness. Thus reduction in ventilator hours typically signal an increase in respiratory therapist effort. Since the cost of treatment of a ventilator-associated pneumonia is estimated in the range of $11,000–57,000 the appropriate response to reduced ventilator hours and reduced VAP rates should include consideration of increasing—not cutting—respiratory therapist staff [9–11].

Pharmacists

Different from physicians, nurses, and respiratory therapists who typically provide hands-on treatments, the role of the critical care pharmacist is mostly that of a knowledge worker. The pharmacist serves as a critical care safety officer (such as detecting and preventing errors in infusions and exposing potential adverse drug effects); as a pharmacokinetic consultant (recommending and adjusting doses of medications as the patient's clinical status changes); and as a steward of resources. Such stewardship may be required owing to safety concerns (some drugs such as anti-cancer drugs have a very narrow margin of safety); owing to direct cost (including biologicals such as immune globulins); or owing to population considerations (such as management of the antimicrobial formulary to preserve effectiveness).

A landmark study reported in 1999 showed that the presence of a critical care pharmacist reduced adverse drug events by two-thirds [12]. Interestingly, a European study performed more than a decade later showed a reduction in preventable ADEs of similar magnitude [13]. Recent estimates of the cost of adverse drug events in critical care are in the range of $6,000–9,000 per event [14]. Prevention of only a few adverse drug events will save sufficient money to justify the employment of a dedicated critical care pharmacist.

Critical care pharmacists are in high demand. There is a supply limitation. Two years of training following the Pharm.D. degree is required to qualify, the first year as a Residency in Pharmacy Practice followed by a second year in Critical Care Pharmacy Practice. Only 104 programs in Critical Care Pharmacy exist in the USA, and most train a single critical care resident each year. This production rate cannot and will not meet the demands of thousands of critical care units in the USA.

Affiliate Providers

The appellation "Affiliate Provider" is used to aggregate advanced practice nurses and physician assistants who have acquired special competencies to practice in intensive care units. These non-physician professionals (sometimes referred to as "midlevel providers" or "associate providers") are emerging in many communities as pivotal to the delivery of critical care services. While a few units have enjoyed affiliate provider services for decades, the recent expansion in demand and employment of affiliate providers seems linked to two secular workforce issues in critical care. First, teaching hospitals that traditionally depended on trainees to fill in gaps in attending physician coverage have had to sharply limit trainee duty hours in the wake of regulations issued by government and by the Accreditation Council on Graduate Medical Education. Second, the numbers of physicians qualified to care for intensive care patients have not kept pace with the expansion of patient numbers or acuity: anemic increases in trainee numbers are met with accelerating departures and retirements as America emerges from the economic downturn of 2007. Together, the decline in trainee hours and the failure to expand intensivist numbers has accelerated growth the provider workforce gap.

Integration of affiliate providers into critical care depends on at least three factors. First, these providers must acquire, demonstrate, and retain a set of special competencies. Although traditionally acquired through apprenticeship to a seasoned critical care provider as "on-the-job-training," newer approaches include formal training programs and even post-graduate "residencies" that include lectures, simulations, computer-based learning, and supervised bedside experience. Second, the roles of affiliate providers must be established and embraced by the existing community of professionals serving critically ill patients. Retention and job satisfaction appears to depend on progressive challenges that culminate in increasing the affiliate providers' responsibilities and authorities within the team. Yet, these affiliate providers must work collaboratively with supervising physicians. Third, a mechanism to collect revenues to offset the costs of training and employing affiliate providers must be established early in the business plan.

According to published studies, the care delivered by affiliate providers equals (and often exceeds) the care provided by supervised medical trainees with respect to completion of evidence-based processes as well as with respect to meaningful and measurable outcomes [15–19]. The benefit to patients, families, and hospitals therefore includes not only the revenue stream but also cost-avoidance through prevention and mitigation of adverse events and through reduction in random process variance.

In general, affiliate providers working in critical care units will command a salary premium (~15 %) and additional compensation for taking shifts in unsocial hours. That premium may rise somewhat as national nursing policy will restrict critical care practice to nurses who have achieved acute care (ACNP) certification (and thereby restricting supply) beginning 2015.

Affiliate providers provide both billable and essential but non-billable services. Tracking and self-reporting suggests that about half of paid hours are associated with activities that result in a fair charge for professional services, including evaluation and management, procedures, and direct critical care [20]. Calculations suggest that affiliate providers who are practicing to the limit of their license, training, and credentialing are high-value providers even though the federal government pays 85 % for their services versus physician reimbursement.

Nutrition Support Specialists (Dietitians)

Admission to critical care units carries substantial risk of malnutrition. The predecessors of ICU nutritional failure are numerous. Nutritional defects are common at the time of ICU admission: the underlying disease may cause defects in deglutition, transit, digestion, absorption, metabolism, and elimination. Common treatments such as mechanical ventilation may preclude eating. Widely used medications such as opiates slow transit while vasopressors compromise absorption. Even corrective therapies such as enteral supplementation via tube are commonly interrupted for tests and procedures. Yet failure to restore and sustain metabolic balance can significantly prolong critical illness and ICU lengths of stay.

For all of these reasons, nutrition support specialists (dietitians with advanced competencies in critical care) have emerged as key members of the critical care team. Their roles include assurance that every patient has a nutritional plan tailored to their specific illness. This includes prescriptions for macro as well as micronutrients delivered via enteral, parenteral, and combination routes. It also includes leadership of enteral feeding tube placement and maintenance, tasks that are essential to achieving continuity of nutritional support.

Most importantly, dietitians' support and advocacy for early appropriate feeding translates into reduced infection rates and lower mortality [21]. Yet despite strong evidence, patients go underfed as gaps remain between actual practice and evidence-based guidelines [22]. This creates a compelling rationale for the consistent inclusion of a nutrition support specialist as a member of the critical care team.

Physiotherapists

Critical illness carries risk of polymyopathy and polyneuropathy that translates into prolonged reduction of functional status and diminished quality of life [23, 24]. Until recently, however, many ICUs did not realize the great benefit of early physiotherapy [25]. Over the past decade, it has become standard care to mobilize patients in the ICU to the maximum extent possible, including routinely walking patients who are dependent on life support devices such as mechanical ventilators, artificial hearts, and ventricular assist devices.

These mobilization programs, which are commonly led by physiotherapists, have several positive effects [26]. Patients lose less muscle mass and less muscle function. They have improved pulmonary toilet. They fatigue naturally and therefore require less sedative medication. They can perceive progress.

The institutional return on investment from such an early mobilization program is typically measured in shortened lengths of stay which create space into which additional patients can be admitted. Given the rapid expansion of demand for critical care services as the baby-boomers become the world's elderly, early mobilization programs become a cost-effective strategy to sustain and grow access to critical care services.

Perfusionists

Perfusionists are underrepresented in critical care. Their primary role is in service of patients who require cardiopulmonary extracorporeal life support (ECLS) via ventricular assist devices and extracorporeal membrane oxygenation. Since ECLS remains an uncommon treatment mode in many ICUs, perfusionists must serve both as providers and as just-in-time educators [27]. Thus perfusionists are rarely employed by the ICU but rather are shared between the ICU and the cardiac surgical operating rooms on a scheduled (where an ECLS program is established) or ad hoc basis.

When called into critical care services, perfusionists are logically assigned only to the most critically ill patients, namely those requiring ECLS. Their presence and activity are focused on maintaining perfusion of oxygenated blood to the tissues. Their practical knowledge both of circulatory physiology and of the engineering of their equipment can be essential, since neural tissue can be compromised within 4 min of cessation of effective circulation. Monitoring of systems and patient parameters (such as activated clotting time) become central tasks.

The hourly bedside cost of perfusionists is typically higher than that of critical care nurses. As a consequence in recent years—particularly as a result of the 2009 Influenza pandemic—there have been attempts to improve and simplify extracorporeal support technologies to the point that a specially trained critical care nurse can manage all of the common bedside problems safely. This should not, must not,

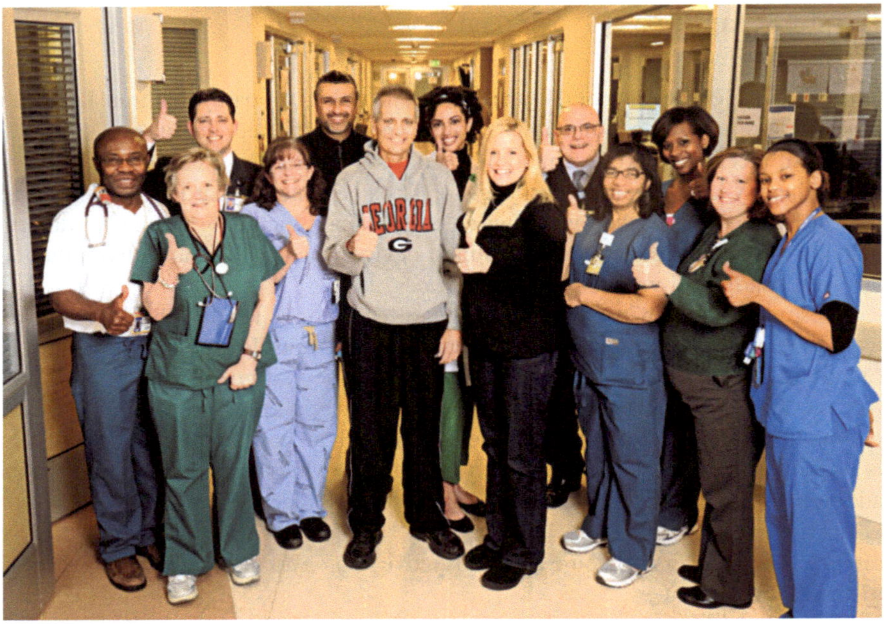

Fig. 4.1 Example of successful multiprofessional team effort. Patient survived ARDS that required 10 days of extracorporeal life support. Left-to-right: Nurse, Respiratory Therapist, Administrator, Perfusionist, Physician's Assistant, Patient, Pharmacist, Patient's Wife, Intensivist, Charge Nurse, Nurse, Nurse Unit Director, Patient Care Assistant

and does not exclude perfusionists from being members of the critical care team—their collaboration and physical presence is essential for initiating and stopping the support. However, it may relieve perfusionists and ICUs from a considerable low productivity time at the bedside. Such shifts in responsibility for ECLS must be jointly planned and embraced by nurses, physicians, and perfusionists.

Evidence for Value

Mortality is reduced through the use of multidisciplinary team care [28] (Fig. 4.1). Costs are reduced through the use of intensivist-led multiprofessional teams [29]. Improvement in quality with simultaneous reduction in cost can only augment value in critical care.

Nevertheless, the value of the intensivist-led multiprofessional team has been challenged. In 2008, Levy and colleagues used an administrative database to retrospectively evaluate mortality among ICU patients managed by intensivist-led teams, finding an *increase* in mortality when intensivists were involved [30]. Subsequent studies using curated databases have found the expected outcome, i.e. that the presence of an intensivist decreases mortality [31, 32]. Still other studies question the incremental value of having an on-site intensivist at night [33].

What appears likely is that even high-functioning ICUs can improve performance through restructuring and reallocation of critical care roles across professions [34].

In an era of shrinking resources, this alone is sufficient to prompt careful examination of the division of labor in the ICU towards better health, better care, and lower cost.

Cost and Business Model

If the multiprofessional team represents such great value, why has it not been more widely adopted? Most generally, the value can only be realized in a well-designed business model that has three characteristics. First, each professional must practice to the limit of his/her license. Often this means designing protocols that can be executed by multiple team members working in parallel versus depending on a single highly trained expert. Second, each professional must practice to the limit of his/her duty hours. While it is inevitable that there will be some unaccounted time owing to the ebb and flow of patients and acuities, staffing strategies that keep professionals busy with direct patient care activities for at least 80 % of their duty hours are readily achievable [20, 35]. Third, those professionals must have the knowledge and skill to identify appropriate and legal charges for their services [15]. Fourth, those professionals who can charge and collect fees for their services must have the means, opportunity, and motivation to do so. By "means," we intend an electronic charge capture system that is easily accessible and provides immediate feedback. By opportunity, we mean sufficient tools and opportunity during the schedule to document and create charges immediately as services are delivered, and to review those activities at end-of-shift during handover. By motivation, we suggest that the timely and accurate recording of activity and charges must be recognized and acknowledged if that practice is to become a social norm.

References

1. Safar P, et al. The intensive care unit. A three year experience at Baltimore city hospitals. Anaesthesia. 1961;16:275–84.
2. AACN: CCRN credential position statement. http://www.aacn.org/WD/Certifications/Docs/CCRNCredentialPositionStatement.pdf (2013). Cited 15 April 2013.
3. Cullen DJ, et al. Therapeutic intervention scoring system: a method for quantitative comparison of patient care. Crit Care Med. 1974;2(2):57–60.
4. Penoyer DA. Nurse staffing and patient outcomes in critical care: a concise review. Crit Care Med. 2010;38(7):1521–8. quiz 1529.

5. Zolnierek CD, Steckel CM. Negotiating safety when staffing falls short. Crit Care Nurs Clin North Am. 2010;22(2):261–9.
6. Goran SF. Measuring tele-ICU impact: does it optimize quality outcomes for the critically ill patient? J Nurs Manag. 2012;20(3):414–28.
7. Esteban A, et al. How is mechanical ventilation employed in the intensive care unit? An international utilization review. Am J Respir Crit Care Med. 2000;161(5):1450–8.
8. Mathews P, Drumheller L, Carlow JJ. Respiratory care manpower issues. Crit Care Med. 2006;34(3 Suppl):S32–45.
9. Warren DK, et al. Outcome and attributable cost of ventilator-associated pneumonia among intensive care unit patients in a suburban medical center. Crit Care Med. 2003;31(5):1312–7.
10. Rello J, et al. Epidemiology and outcomes of ventilator-associated pneumonia in a large US database. Chest. 2002;122(6):2115–21.
11. Cocanour CS, et al. Cost of a ventilator-associated pneumonia in a shock trauma intensive care unit. Surg Infect (Larchmt). 2005;6(1):65–72.
12. Leape LL, et al. Pharmacist participation on physician rounds and adverse drug events in the intensive care unit. JAMA. 1999;282(3):267–70.
13. Klopotowska JE, et al. On-ward participation of a hospital pharmacist in a Dutch intensive care unit reduces prescribing errors and related patient harm: an intervention study. Crit Care. 2010;14(5):R174.
14. Kane-Gill SL, Jacobi J, Rothschild JM. Adverse drug events in intensive care units: risk factors, impact, and the role of team care. Crit Care Med. 2010;38(6 Suppl):S83–9.
15. McCarthy C, O'Rourke NC, Madison JM. Integrating advanced practice providers into medical critical care teams. Chest. 2013;143(3):847–50.
16. Garland A, Gershengorn HB. Staffing in ICUs: physicians and alternative staffing models. Chest. 2013;143(1):214–21.
17. Gershengorn HB, et al. Impact of nonphysician staffing on outcomes in a medical ICU. Chest. 2011;139(6):1347–53.
18. Cramer CL, Orlowski JP, DeNicola LK. Pediatric intensivist extenders in the pediatric ICU. Pediatr Clin North Am. 2008;55(3):687–708. xi–xii.
19. Kleinpell RM, Ely EW, Grabenkort R. Nurse practitioners and physician assistants in the intensive care unit: an evidence-based review. Crit Care Med. 2008;36(10):2888–97.
20. Carpenter DL, et al. Patient-care time allocation by nurse practitioners and physician assistants in the intensive care unit. Crit Care. 2012;16(1):R27.
21. Doig GS, et al. Early enteral nutrition, provided within 24 h of injury or intensive care unit admission, significantly reduces mortality in critically ill patients: a meta-analysis of randomised controlled trials. Intensive Care Med. 2009;35(12):2018–27.
22. Cahill NE, et al. Nutrition therapy in the critical care setting: what is "best achievable" practice? An international multicenter observational study. Crit Care Med. 2010;38 (2):395–401.
23. Herridge MS, et al. One-year outcomes in survivors of the acute respiratory distress syndrome. N Engl J Med. 2003;348(8):683–93.
24. de Jonghe B, et al. Intensive care unit-acquired weakness: risk factors and prevention. Crit Care Med. 2009;37(10 Suppl):S309–15.
25. Needham DM. Mobilizing patients in the intensive care unit: improving neuromuscular weakness and physical function. JAMA. 2008;300(14):1685–90.
26. Truong AD, et al. Bench-to-bedside review: mobilizing patients in the intensive care unit–from pathophysiology to clinical trials. Crit Care. 2009;13(4):216.
27. McCoach RM, et al. The new role of the perfusionist in adult extracorporeal life support. Perfusion. 2010;25(1):21–4.
28. Kim MM, et al. The effect of multidisciplinary care teams on intensive care unit mortality. Arch Intern Med. 2010;170(4):369–76.
29. Pronovost PJ, et al. Team care: beyond open and closed intensive care units. Curr Opin Crit Care. 2006;12(6):604–8.

30. Levy MM, et al. Association between critical care physician management and patient mortality in the intensive care unit. Ann Intern Med. 2008;148(11):801–9.
31. Petitti D, Bennett V, Chao Hu CK. Association of changes in the use of board-certified critical care intensivists with mortality outcomes for trauma patients at a well-established level I urban trauma center. J Trauma Manag Outcomes. 2012;6:3.
32. Hackner D, et al. Do faculty intensivists have better outcomes when caring for patients directly in a closed ICU versus consulting in an open ICU? Hosp Pract (1995). 2009;37(1):40–50.
33. Wallace DJ, et al. Nighttime intensivist staffing and mortality among critically ill patients. N Engl J Med. 2012;366(22):2093–101.
34. Netzer G, et al. Decreased mortality resulting from a multicomponent intervention in a tertiary care medical intensive care unit. Crit Care Med. 2011;39(2):284–93.
35. Butler KL, et al. Optimizing advanced practitioner charge capture in high-acuity surgical intensive care units. Arch Surg. 2011;146(5):552–5.

Chapter 5
Computers in Intensive Care

Stephen E. Lapinsky

Abstract The intensive care unit is a data-rich environment where the physician may have difficulty accessing and processing the large amount of data generated by each patient. Incomplete access to all clinical information can result in suboptimal clinical decision making. A computerized clinical information systems (CIS) can enhance ICU management in a number of ways. These include the provision of complete but appropriately filtered information at the bedside, reduction in drug errors and the use of intelligent alarms for the early identification of deteriorating patients. Electronic reminders can improve compliance with guidelines, and more sophisticated decision support systems may provide patient-specific management guidance. An easily accessible and usable interface with the CIS is essential, and various mobile and context-aware systems are being developed. Several barriers to implementation exist, including financial constraints and poor acceptance among clinicians for this cultural change.

Keywords Critical care • Health services • Computer systems • Decision support systems • Quality improvement • Telemedicine

Background

The intensive care unit (ICU) is a data-rich environment—a physician may encounter more than 200 variables per patient on daily rounds [1]—and even the most experienced physician will have difficulty processing information from more than

S.E. Lapinsky (✉)
Intensive Care Unit, Mount Sinai Hospital, # 18-214, 600 University Avenue, Toronto, ON, Canada M5G 1X5

Interdepartmental Division of Critical Care, Department of Medicine, and Institute of Biomaterials and Biomedical Engineering, University of Toronto, Toronto, ON, Canada M5R 0A3
e-mail: stephen.lapinsky@utoronto.ca

D.C. Scales and G.D. Rubenfeld (eds.), *The Organization of Critical Care*, Respiratory Medicine 18, DOI 10.1007/978-1-4939-0811-0_5,

seven variables. Furthermore, the amount of clinical information documented on ICU patients is increasing, by 26 % over 6 years in one study [2]. Poor documentation and incomplete access to all clinical information can result in clinical decision making without the full clinical picture. A computerized system can be used to capture and store clinical data and provide complete, appropriate information at the bedside. Computerized order entry will reduce errors due to incorrect dosing, drug interactions and illegible handwriting. Other roles for computing technology in a critical care environment include keeping track of the exponentially growing scientific literature and the use of "intelligent" alarms for the early identification of deteriorating patients. While current utilization of computing technology in Critical Care is widespread, its use is generally limited to the most basic technology, such as access to laboratory data or medical imaging [3].

Information technology can contribute to the organization and planning in an ICU by facilitating a more rapid response after an adverse event has occurred and by tracking and providing feedback about the frequency of errors. The strategies for preventing errors using information technology include improving communication, making knowledge readily accessible, mandating key pieces of information (e.g. drug dose units of measure, administration route), assisting with calculations, performing real-time checks, assisting with monitoring, and providing decision support [4]. Electronic reminders can improve physicians' compliance with guidelines and reduce errors of omission. Compliance with best practices can be tracked and optimized. As an example, a higher level of sophistication of information technology in an institution has been shown to correlate with a reduction in catheter-related blood stream infections [5].

Definitions

A number of terms are used when discussing information technology in healthcare, sometimes with different meanings and implications. For clarity, some terms are defined as used in this chapter.

Clinical Information System (CIS): A hospital-based information system designed to collect, organize and present data relating exclusively to clinical information about the care of a patient.

Electronic Medical Record (EMR): This term usually refers to a computer-based record of healthcare information of a patient, which includes laboratory results, diagnostic imaging reports, vital signs, medication administration records and clinical reports. The term EMR is sometimes used to refer to an "EMR system" or CIS.

Electronic Health Record (EHR): This term refers to a longitudinal, secure and private lifetime record of a patient's key health history and care within the health system. The record is available in a virtual form to authorized health care providers. The personal health information in this report is generated from the various encounters an individual has with health care systems. The EHR therefore comprises an aggregate of information in hospital EMRs and outpatient practitioner EMRs.

Clinical Information Systems

The CIS is a database storing and providing clinical information about patients to caregivers. In a hospital, the CIS might be the clinical portion of a larger hospital information system. Within each hospital department, the CIS may be named according to the departmental function, for example Laboratory Information System (LIS), Pharmacy System, Radiology Information System (RIS), etc. In a hospital's ICU, the CIS will encompass all of the above, plus the system that captures and stores information unique to critical care (e.g. hemodynamic data, drug infusions, ventilation parameters). Having complete and accurate clinical and patient information available to a physician in real time will improve the likelihood that the clinical decision made is the best one for the circumstances.

To gain the full potential of a CIS, clinical data, pharmacy information, and laboratory and imaging results need to be integrated into a single interface. The Healthcare Information and Management Systems Society (HIMSS) has developed an EMR Adoption Model using an eight-step scale, to document the level of EMR integration in a hospital [6]. As of mid-2012, only about 8 % of hospitals had reached stage 6 or higher (implying integration of physician documentation and full decision support), with one-third of hospitals at stage 4 or higher (electronic order entry and clinical protocols).

There are some potential disadvantages to a computerized CIS. All such systems are operator dependent and rely on the accuracy of the data entered. Automated input of data from the bedside monitor, from infusion pumps and from the ventilator is optimal. However, as large quantities of data can be acquired from these devices, these data need to be appropriately sampled and filtered, to document representative recordings. Computer malfunctions need to be anticipated, with provision of emergency backup power and real-time data backup. Planning and documentation of downtime procedures is essential [7].

The ICU CIS

In the data-rich ICU environment, errors may occur due to the sheer volume of data available to be evaluated. The Institute of Medicine report "To Err is Human" documented that the risk for any adverse event in the ICU is nearly 46 % [8]. The most active use of sophisticated biomedical equipment is found in a hospital's ICU, with devices that monitor the patient's vital signs and control the application of therapy. These devices provide a rich source of information, which if made available to the clinicians in the right circumstances has the potential to improve patient outcomes. Although there are information systems designed for use in ICUs that make use of data output from biomedical devices (monitors, infusion pumps, ventilators), they are not yet widely used [3]. Cost may be a barrier to implementation of the Critical Care CIS. Systems designed for critical care are generally more expensive than other departmental systems. Proprietary networks and special hardware are sometimes necessary.

The ICU CIS should provide a number of functions, including patients lists and an electronic "whiteboard," vital signs flow sheets, laboratory results, fluid and medication administration records, structured notes and assessments, computerized provider order entry (CPOE), decision support and transfer and discharge summary reports.

A number of commercial CIS systems are available, with varying functionality. These may integrate data from vital signs monitors, ventilators, infusion pumps, EEG, ECG, PACS systems, laboratory and hospital EMR, into a single interface. Examples of Critical Care CIS currently available include iNet (Cerner, Kansas City, MO), Infinity (Draeger, Lübeck, Germany), GE Healthcare (Bucks, U.K.), Intellivue (Philips Medical Systems, Amsterdam, Netherlands), AXIOM Sensis (Siemens Healthcare, Erlangen, Germany), CareSuite (Picis, Wakefield, MA) and Ultraview (Spacelabs Healthcare, Issaquah, WA) as well as several others [9].

Using the ICU CIS

Results access

ICUs are serviced by other departments in a hospital, such as laboratory, radiology and pharmacy, all of which may generate information about the patient during their ICU stay. This information needs to be made available to the clinicians caring for the critically ill patient in a timely manner. Electronic access to laboratory results is one of the most commonly available CIS functions, but results need to be appropriately authorized for release by the laboratory in a timely manner. As access to laboratory information is required several times daily, the computer interface needs to be user friendly, and mobile computing access may be beneficial [10, 11]. Picture Archiving and Communication System (PACS) is technology that permits storage and rapid access to radiological images. Images are stored in a Digital Imaging and Communication in Medicine (DICOM) format and are accessible via the CIS or through a dedicated high-fidelity viewing system. Client side applications may be web-based or may utilize proprietary software. Radiologist reports may be accessible through a Radiology Information System, integrated in the PACS system or via the CIS [12].

Computerized Provider Order Entry

In addition to using the CIS to access patient information, clinician orders may be entered via the system and transmitted to the staff responsible for fulfilling the orders. This may include requests for laboratory and imaging studies, dietary orders, consultations and medication administration. CPOE provides several advantages over paper systems, including overcoming handwriting and transcription errors, more rapid communication of orders, ability to enter orders at the point-of-care or offsite, audit tracking, and incorporating decision support. Decision support (see below) may include checks for duplicate orders, drug dosing (corrected for renal function) and alerts regarding drug interactions. CPOE has a potentially very important role in the ICU, due to the complex workflow, and may provide the biggest benefit of a CIS [13].

In order to simplify and standardize the ordering process for a common clinical scenario, groups of orders or order sets are utilized. These can be developed to incorporate current evidence-based guidelines and customized for local conditions or formularies. Order sets act as checklists and reduce errors of omission and may increase patient safety and quality of care. Order sets may be complex to develop, and collaborative systems are available to share order sets between hospitals (e.g. www.patientordersets.com).

The benefits of CPOE are predominantly the ability to reduce medication errors and adverse drug events. CPOE avoids many of the pitfalls of handwritten prescriptions, including poor penmanship, ambiguous abbreviations and trailing zeros. Orders are rapidly transmitted to the pharmacy, with a full audit trail. Integrated decision support will allow allergy checks and drug interaction evaluation. Systematic reviews of CPOE in hospitalized patients suggest a reduction in medication errors and adverse drug events [14, 15]. Fewer studies are available specific to the ICU situation, but there are some data to suggest a similar benefit. Improved antibiotic prescribing [16] and reduction in prescription errors [17] have been demonstrated. Although prescription errors may be reduced, these may be errors that would have been intercepted by routine procedures in the paper environment, and the effect on actual adverse events may not be large [18]. Furthermore, although specific types of errors are clearly reduced by CPOE, this technology has the potential to increase other types of errors, such as failure of renewing or reordering medications, incorrect dosing and ordering on the incorrect patient [19]. Drug errors still occur with CPOE, although of a different type, but there does appear to be a learning curve with a reduction in errors over time [20].

Implementation of CPOE is fraught with problems. In 2002, implementation of a CIS with CPOE in the Cedars-Sinai hospital in Los Angeles was met with resistance by physicians, to the point that the CPOE was abandoned, with a return to a paper system [21]. Lessons learned include the importance of system speed, that the computers system must fit into the clinician's workflow and not vice versa, and implementation should be closely monitored with the ability to respond and make changes immediately, amongst others [22]. Similar problems have been encountered elsewhere, one report describing the implementation of a commercial CPOE system [23]. In this case, problems were resolved by comprehensively revising the system and customizing it for local workflow requirements. The implementation of a CPOE can have an adverse effect on patient outcome. Two studies report the outcome of the same CPOE product deployed in two different paediatric ICUs. In the first situation, a statistically significant increase in mortality occurred after implementation [24]. In the other setting, mortality rates fell after introduction of the same CPOE system [25]. The second implementation had, however, learned from the first group and were able to anticipate and overcome the sociological and organizational factors involved in CPOE implementation.

Decision Support

Decision support as a tool for improving the quality of health care has various components. At its simplest, decision support is a passive tool, where high quality information is simply available and facilitates the clinician making an informed decision. An example would be a link on the medication ordering screen to a pharmacopoeia, or a link on the EMR to a resource such as Up-To-Date (www.uptodate.com). Decision support can be an active tool when it interacts with the workflow of the clinician and intervenes at opportune times to inform and advise, preventing errors of both commission and omission. An example of preventing an error of commission is an alert preventing the incorrect administration of a drug. Preventing the error is triggered by the act of electronically checking, at the time of medication administration, that the drug is in is the correct dose, the correct route, and not contraindicated by a drug interaction or drug allergy.

The opportunity to prevent an error of omission occurs when an intervention that should have taken place, but has not, is detected. Prevention of errors of omission may be synchronous or asynchronous. An example of a synchronous rule is the following. The physician has opened the patient's electronic chart and is preparing to enter medication orders; the rules engine can advise that allergies have not yet been entered to the system and thus potentially prevent an allergic reaction. An example of an asynchronous rule is the detection of a failure to prescribe thromboembolism prophylaxis in a sedated, ventilated ICU patient. Preventing the error requires surveillance of the patient and notification to a caregiver that administration of an anticoagulant may be indicated. Information systems have been designed for the critical care environment that provide asynchronous decision support. They continuously monitor a patient's vital signs using algorithms to detect changes that signal a problem and alert clinicians to the fact. The key to good decision support is that it is useful in the care of the patient. Trivial alerts that are perceived as a nuisance by clinicians are to be avoided. All rules should be specifically approved by local clinicians before implementation.

Several other examples of specific decision support tools in the ICU have been described. From the LDS Hospital in Salt Lake City, an algorithm for ventilator management [26] and antibiotic prescribing based on epidemiological tracking of resistance patterns within the hospital [16]. From the Netherlands, a system prompting use of a low tidal volume ventilation was found to change clinical practice [27].

Another approach to decision support with a CIS involves utilization of the data warehouse (see below) generated by the clinical data from the CIS, to overcome the lack of evidence-based guidelines for a particular patient problem. With appropriate software, a search can be generated for the outcome of a particular intervention, filtered for similar patients (e.g. gender, age, diagnosis, co-morbidity) [28]. In the absence of published data on a topic, this individualized approach using a local clinical database likely provides a better result than the memory and/or cumulative experience of several physicians.

Interfaces

The interface with the CIS plays an important role in the usability and efficacy of the product. Most ICU-CIS allow a flowsheet-type interface, with variability in the degree of local customization. This offers an interface modelled on the paper versions of the ICU flow sheet in an attempt to parallel the paper-based workflow, but this may not be the most effective way of providing information to the clinician. The increased amount of information available can produce information overload, with few benefits over a paper system. This large amount of data requires multiple screens to review completely, which can make pattern recognition difficult. Various approaches have been used to improve the clinician–CIS interface.

Task-specific or context-aware user interfaces can prioritize the display of a limited number of high-value data elements [29]. A human-centred approach to the organization and display of data has been used to develop a novel, single-screen ICU user interface, presenting a subset of CIS data organized in a systems-based format, familiar to ICU clinicians [30]. Using simulated clinical scenarios, this approach was shown to improve errors, task load and time to completion of tasks.

Mobile interfaces include the use of smartphones, handheld computers or tablets, for retrieving data from the CIS. These have the advantage of portability and access at the point-of-care, but the potential disadvantages of small screen size and need for a customized interface. Mobile computing is discussed further below.

The computer interface may also have an impact on ICU team interactions during daily rounds. An ethnographic study of ward rounds during implementation of an ICU-CIS demonstrated that the technology impeded the ability of the team-leader to lead rounds, and affected the ability of individual team members to contribute, until various technological and social solutions were instituted [31]. A large, interactive surface computing platform such as Microsoft Pixelsense (previously called Microsoft Surface) (Microsoft Corp, Redmond, WA) may provide a team interface for ICU rounds.

Ecological interface design focuses on the work environment rather than the end-user or the specific task. This has application in complex systems, and by making constraints perceptually evident, more cognitive resources can be devoted to problem solving. However, the benefits of this approach in a critical care situation are variable [32]. Novel interface approaches include a vibro–tactile interface [33] or a head-mounted display [34] which have been used for physiological data monitoring during anaesthesia.

Data Warehousing

An ICU CIS generates a large database of clinical information that may be used for a variety of purposes, including patient safety and quality improvement initiatives, administration planning, decision support and clinical research. Patient data, including demographic, diagnostic, clinical and laboratory information can be stored in an anonymized fashion in a data warehouse, for subsequent analysis. This analytical processing information system comprises a copy of data collected by the transaction processing system or CIS, and is built to facilitate queries and analysis [35]. Standardized data dictionaries are essential and EHRs must be developed with consideration to the utilization of data for future analysis. Data to be collected and aggregated needs to be collected in a coded and computable format, using a nomenclature system such as Systemized Nomenclature of Medicine—Clinical Terms (SNOMED CT) [36]. Data may be extracted from multiple source systems requiring matching between patient identifiers and mapping data to standardized nomenclature. Data queries and analysis may be through command line structured query language (SQL), desktop database tools (e.g. Microsoft Access), web applications or customized business intelligence software. These data analyses can be used to support quality improvement initiatives, by identifying areas of concern and tracking improvement with implementation of changes. Other uses include healthcare planning and benchmarking. Clinical decision support, as described in a previous section, can be supported by data warehousing, as can clinical research projects.

CIS: Drivers and Barriers

Quality Improvement, particularly in regard to improving patient safety, is an important driver for adoption of a CIS. The Leapfrog Group, a consortium of large corporations and public agencies that buy health benefits on behalf of their enrollees, was developed to obtain the best value for health care expenditure. They have recommended computerized physician order entry with decision support capabilities as an essential safety practice (Leapfrog Group Safety Practices) [37].

The health care industry has been significantly underspending on information technology compared with other industries (e.g. banking and media), but there is growing evidence that investments in information technology can provide a financial return. These financial benefits arise from the elimination of unnecessary tests and procedures, improved revenue collection, and productivity gains. A major issue is the question of who will reap the financial benefits. Benefits do not necessarily accrue to the providers who make the investment; rather, profits may become apparent only when the health care system is considered as a whole. Financial limitations remain a major barrier to the implementation of IT, largely due to these imbalances between the funding source and the recipient of benefits. Furthermore, most commercially available products are not ready-made and require significant time investment by IT specialists and clinicians during implementation.

Interoperability is a significant barrier, due to a lack of standards for representation of clinical data and the variety of technological solutions available. The costs of interfaces between applications within an organization and between organizations may limit implementation. The expectation and benefit of information systems is that they save time [38], and this expectation is certainly the case for ICU CISs. Less time spent by the nurse documenting vital signs should translate to more time for direct patient care. However, some studies have demonstrated an increased documentation time following the introduction of an ICU CIS [39].

The change in culture produced by implementation of information technology is a potentially important barrier. The critical care environment is traditionally technology-rich, and clinicians in this area should be less reluctant to embrace this new technology. User acceptance requires detailed usability testing with emphasis on speed and ease of use. While data security is essential, there needs to be a balance between security and making data rapidly available to authorized users. The technology can, however, still be blamed for the additional workload in correcting previously unsafe work practices (e.g. verbal orders or mandating clear and complete prescriptions). Computerized systems may also be perceived to require a standardization of care and abandonment of personal style. Computer Order Entry introduces an element of process control, an important element of quality improvement. It is essential that complex medical information systems fit into clinician's current workflow.

Ubiquitous Computing in the ICU

Ubiquitous or pervasive computing implies the availability of computing systems and interfaces integrated into everyday objects and activities—"anywhere, anytime computing" [40]. In other words, computers that fit the human environment, rather than staff being required to enter a computing environment. Another term used is Ambient Intelligence, a combination of ubiquitous computing and artificial intelligence [41]. A software-agent-based paradigm enables such a system, an agent being "an entity within a computer system environment that is capable of flexible, autonomous actions with the aim of complying with its design objectives" [41].

Context-Aware Services

A context-aware network is a network that is designed to allow for customization and application operation that is compatible with both the preferences of the individual user and also the expressed preferences of the enterprise which owns the network. In a critical care environment, context awareness may support the delivery of services, where “context” incorporates a number of attributes such as location, time of day, staff profile, etc. Staff location may be provided by RFID tags on ID cards or by smartphones, allowing the system to provide immediate access to a specific patient’s electronic record, to an appropriately authorized clinician who is in proximity of the patient [42]. This would facilitate information access by automating the login and authorization procedures. Such a system requires software architecture and design that incorporates location identification, user verification, security and privacy. Similar systems may be utilized, for example, to generate “ad hoc” cardiac arrest teams by identifying a team made up of appropriately qualified personnel closest to the cardiac arrest event.

Mobile Computing

With the rapid evolution in mobile technology, including screen resolution, improved memory capability, processing power and wireless connectivity, handheld devices have the potential to become an important component of an integrated CIS [43, 44]. They offer a portable platform for point-of-care clinical reference and patient management in the ICU. Handheld computers have several benefits distinguishing them from desktop and laptop computers [45]. They are easily portable and turn on immediately without the delay of a booting process. Potential disadvantages include the small screen size and difficulty experienced by some users with data entry using small keyboards. The concept of “enterprise digital assistants” has been proposed, with the handheld device becoming an extension of the hospital CIS [46]. There is an increasing push by clinicians for hospital IT departments to support their personal devices [bring your own device (BYOD)] but this requires clear privacy and security policies to be implemented [47]. Tablet computers are an alternative mobile solution and provide a larger computer interface, at the expense of significantly larger size and weight. The iPad has been implemented successfully as a CIS interface [48]. Mobile desktop computers have been used effectively for computer access on physicians’ rounds, mounted on a mobile cart [computer on wheels (CoW)]. These computers provide a large screen to access patient information and to view radiological images, using wireless technology to connect to the hospital system and internet.

Wireless connectivity such as Bluetooth, WiFi (802.11) and cellular provides real-time access to critical data. Although the risk of electromagnetic interference with ICU equipment by cellular devices is real [49], the accumulating evidence has provided us with a better understanding of the risks. Wireless devices can be implemented in the critical care environment with appropriate precautions, particularly by ensuring a minimum distance of 1 m between the device and susceptible equipment [50].

Mobile devices may be used for a variety of roles in the ICU. They can be used to interface with a CIS or electronic patient record, to review patient information as well as to enter orders [51]. The benefit of mobility must be weighed against potential disadvantages in this role. The small screen size allows only a limited portion of the clinical record to be viewed and using a larger screen to access simultaneous data is often preferable. Data entry on the handheld carries the risk of numerical and typographical errors. Data security and patient confidentiality need to be addressed, using encryption and password protection. Systems in which the handheld acts as a browser or client to access a central database have the advantage of not storing confidential information on the peripheral device, reducing the security risk. The handheld computer also offers the ability to access drug information, management guidelines and protocols at the point-of-care, either as a component of a CIS or via stand-alone software [52]. Handheld devices are well suited to provide drug information using electronic pharmacopoeias. Their major advantages over paper-based references include the ability to update regularly, perform drug interaction checks and integrate customized formularies [53, 54]. The best known example of the many handheld pharmacopoeias currently available is ePocrates (www.epocrates.com), which is used by over 1 million healthcare professionals (including 50 % of U.S. physicians) and provides a comprehensive drug list, dosing guidelines, common side effects and a drug interaction application. Handheld devices offer the ability to provide bedside access to evidence-based information, supporting a "just-in-time" education process [55]. A number of Medline search apps are available for the various handheld device platforms. Handheld devices have been used for data collection for clinical research, taking advantage of small size and ability to turn on immediately, to collect data at the bedside. A project in Ontario, Canada, used a wirelessly connected mobile device to track adherence with quality improvement standards [56]. Handheld decision support systems may prove to be of value in the management of mass casualty events, providing guidelines and triage tools to mobile healthcare workers [57].

Transmission of infection in the ICU by contact with computer keyboards has been demonstrated [58] and the possibility of transmission by handheld devices clearly needs to be considered. Colonization of handheld computers with skin organisms is very common [59], and some pathogens may survive for days or weeks on plastic surfaces, increasing the risk of disease transmission [60]. Handheld devices can be effectively disinfected by cleaning with alcohol [61] but an awareness of the potential problem, with strict attention to handwashing, is essential.

Remote ICU Care and Telemedicine

The need to provide continuous support by trained ICU physicians in the face of a shortfall of ICU physicians has prompted the introduction of remote ICU care programs [62]. Despite literature suggesting improved outcomes with a dedicated intensive care physician model, not all ICUs have this model in place during the daytime and extremely few at night. Telemedicine offers the technology to bring the knowledge of specialized practitioners to a variety of locations, at all times of the day and night. Early studies demonstrated the feasibility of such a system as well as a reduction in ICU length of stay and hospital mortality [63], the mortality benefits being confirmed in a recent meta-analysis of 11 observational studies [64]. There has recently been a significant increase in the number of health systems adopting this care model.

In the USA, the company VISICU Inc. (now Philips eICU) initiated the implementation of remote ICU care programs [65], and now provides support to over 350 hospitals. Most are in multihospital health systems, with a flagship institution, usually an academic centre or large tertiary care facility, where the remote team is usually based.

Management Models

The remote team is responsible for (1) continuous monitoring of each patient, (2) titration of therapy, (3) identification and management of new problems, (4) facilitation of communication and (5) best practice compliance [65]. The division of responsibilities may vary between sites, depending on the presence of onsite intensivists, with the goal of providing 24 $\times$ 7 seamless oversight of all ICU patients. This model requires a restructuring of the organization and delivery of ICU services. There needs to be clear delineation of the responsibilities of each team member with excellent communication between all team members. This necessitates effective clinical information technology, to make data available to the remote teams, to flag emerging problems, and to provide active decision support. In hospitals with an open ICU, the large number of physicians admitting patients to the ICU may make buy-in to a collaborative care model difficult. Physician "category levels" have been used whereby the remote team are granted varying privileges in patient management (e.g. emergencies only, execution of daily care plan, etc.) for each individual physician's patients.

The remote care staff consists of physicians, nurses and clerical personnel, usually with one nurse and one physician covering about 70 remote beds, a second nurse for 70–90 beds and a third nurse to cover up to 120 beds. Coverage is often from noon to 7 a.m., with a gap during which time morning rounds take place on site in the remote ICU.

There are several core requirements to achieve quality goals:

1. Each patient requires a comprehensive daily care plan that addresses all clinical issues (from ventilator weaning through nutrition to social issues). This is developed by the onsite team and communicated to all onsite staff as well as to the remote team.
2. Patients require frequent assessment throughout the day by an intensivist, for titration of therapy and to detect emerging problems.
3. Specific individuals are charged with the implementation of quality improvement initiatives. It is commonplace that this is assigned to the remote team.
4. Efforts must be made to standardize therapies across the entire health system to ensure adoption of best practices.

Technology

The technological requirements for remote ICU care include:

Audio-visual equipment: Allowing the remote team to see patients and equipment and interact with onsite staff. The A-V system is off most of the time, but can be activated by the remote team, who control camera direction and magnification, or by the onsite staff (in-room call buttons). The camera resolution allows remote care providers to observe breathing patterns and equipment settings.

Bedside monitor data: Real-time waveforms are available to the remote care team.

Clinical data: The remote team need access to all relevant patient data, including progress notes, bedside flow sheets, medication lists and laboratory data, via an electronic CIS. This CIS is designed to maximize efficiency in managing the entire ICU population and prioritize activities.

Imaging studies: Access to X-rays and ECGs is achieved through the use of digital systems.

Alerting systems: Although periodic review of each individual patient is a core activity of the remote team, automated surveillance tools can ensure prompt identification of emerging problems. These tools use sophisticated rules engines, evaluating monitor data, laboratory results, medication and charted data, as they enter the CIS.

Reports: The data in the CIS is used to generate detailed system-wide reports on ICU outcomes and compliance with best practices.

Networks: The ICU beds and remote site are connected by local area and wide area networks to ensure seamless and secure transmission of data. Adequate bandwidth and data encryption are essential.

Remote Intensivist Interventions

Many sites track the interventions performed by remote site staff. The interventions with the highest probability of impacting on outcome include urgent administration of blood products, supervision of cardiac arrest management, management of mechanical ventilation, treatment of agitation, management of severe hypertension, initiation of culture-directed antibiotics, supervision of procedures, management of shock (fluid administration, inotropes), management of arrhythmias and end-of-life issues.

Outcomes Data

Several hospitals utilizing the VISICU system reported improved outcomes, including reduced ICU length of stay by 17 %, and a decrease in severity-adjusted mortality by 13–38 %, with larger improvements where admitting physicians authorized the remote site to actively manage their patients [65]. No difference in outcome can be demonstrated between technologically advanced systems (with continuous patient-data monitoring) and those providing remote intensivist consultation only [64]. Nurse satisfaction is high with reduced rates of nurse turnover in sites utilizing a remote ICU monitoring system. House staff have generated positive feedback, due in part to the active effort by the remote teams to include them in decision making and providing educational support.

Conclusions

Information technology is essential to enhance the efficacy and reliability of healthcare provision in the Critical Care situation. The technology now exists to integrate multiple databases of information in a healthcare situation to provide a comprehensive but filtered overview of the patient. This can be enhanced by decision support tools, remote access to information and mobile, point-of-need technology. The remaining barriers to implementation include financial constraints and developing acceptance among clinicians for this cultural change.

References

1. Morris AH. Computerized protocols and bedside decision support. Crit Care Clin. 1999;15:523–45.
2. Manor-Shulman O, Beyene J, Frndova H, et al. Quantifying the volume of documented clinical information in critical illness. J Crit Care. 2008;23:245–50.
3. Lapinsky SE, Holt D, Hallett D, Abdolell M, Adhikari NKJ. Survey of information technology use in Ontario intensive care units. BMC Med Inform Decis Mak. 2008;8:5.
4. Bates DW, Gawande AA. Improving safety with information technology. N Engl J Med. 2003;348:2526–34.
5. Amarasingham R, Pronovost PJ, Diener-West M, et al. Measuring clinical information technology in the ICU setting: application in a quality improvement collaborative. J Am Med Inform Assoc. 2007;14:288–94.

6. HIMSS Analytics: EMR adoption model. http://www.himssanalytics.org/home/index.aspx. Accessed 21 Apr 2014.
7. Nelson NC. Downtime procedures for a clinical information system: a critical issue. J Crit Care. 2007;22(1):45–50.
8. Kohn LT, Corrigan JM, Donaldson MS, Committee on Quality of Health Care in America, Institute of Medicine, editors. To err is human: building a safer health system. Washington, DC: National Academy Press; 1999.
9. Varon J, Marik PE. Clinical information systems and the electronic medical record in the intensive care unit. Curr Opin Crit Care. 2002;8:616–24.
10. Strain JJ, Felciano RM, Seiver A, Acuff R, Fagan L. Optimizing physician access to surgical intensive care unit laboratory information through mobile computing. Proc AMIA Annu Fall Symp. 1996:812–6.
11. Duncan RG, Shabot MM. Secure remote access to a clinical data repository using a wireless personal digital assistant (PDA). Proc AMIA Symp. 2000:210–4.
12. Nanni M, Carnassale R, Napoli M, Campioni P, Marano P. Information systems in the management of the radiology department. Rays. 2003;28:63–72.
13. Maslove DM, Rizk N, Lowe HJ. Computerized physician order entry in the critical care environment: a review of current literature. J Intensive Care Med. 2011;26:165–71.
14. Eslami S, de Keizer NF, Abu-Hanna A. The impact of computerized physician medication order entry in hospitalized patients – a systematic review. Int J Med Inform. 2008;77:365–76.
15. Ammenwerth E, Schnell-Inderst P, Machan C, Siebert U. The effect of electronic prescribing on medication errors and adverse drug events: a systematic review. J Am Med Inform Assoc. 2008;15:585–600.
16. Evans RS, Pestotnik SL, Classen DC, Clemmer TP, Weaver LK, Orme Jr JF, Lloyd JF, Burke JP. A computer-assisted management program for antibiotics and other antiinfective agents. N Engl J Med. 1998;338:232–8.
17. Colpaert K, Claus B, Somers A, Vandewoude K, Robays H, Decruyenaere J. Impact of computerized physician order entry on medication prescription errors in the intensive care unit: a controlled cross-sectional trial. Crit Care. 2006;10:R21.
18. Koppel R. What do we know about medication errors made via a CPOE system versus those made via handwritten orders? Crit Care. 2005;9:427–8.
19. Koppel R, Metlay JP, Cohen A, Abaluck B, Localio AR, Kimmel SE, Strom BL. Role of computerized physician order entry systems in facilitating medication errors. JAMA. 2005;293:1197–203.
20. Shulman R, Singer M, Goldstone J, Bellingan G. Medication errors: a prospective cohort study of hand-written and computerised physician order entry in the intensive care unit. Crit Care. 2005;9:R516–21.
21. Connolly C. Cedars-Sinai Doctors cling to pen and paper. Washington Post, 21 March 2005. http://www.washingtonpost.com/wp-dyn/articles/A52384-2005Mar20.html.
22. Shabot MM. Ten commandments for implementing clinical information systems. Proc (Bayl Univ Med Cent). 2004;17:265–9.
23. Ali NA, Mekhjian HS, Kuehn PL, Bentley TD, Kumar R, Ferketich AK, Hoffmann SP. Specificity of computerized physician order entry has a significant effect on the efficiency of workflow for critically ill patients. Crit Care Med. 2005;33:110–4.
24. Han YY, Carcillo JA, Venkataraman ST, Clark RS, Watson RS, Nguyen TC, Bayir H, Orr RA. Unexpected increased mortality after implementation of a commercially sold computerized physician order entry system. Pediatrics. 2005;116:1506–12.
25. Del Beccaro MA, Jeffries HE, Eisenberg MA, Harry ED. Computerized provider order entry implementation: no association with increased mortality rates in an intensive care unit. Pediatrics. 2006;118:290–5.
26. McKinley BA, Moore FA, Sailors RM, et al. Computerized decision support for mechanical ventilation of trauma induced ARDS: results of a randomized clinical trial. J Trauma. 2001;50:415–24.

27. Eslami S, de Keizer NF, Abu-Hanna A, de Jonge E, Schultz MJ. Effect of a clinical decision support system on adherence to a lower tidal volume mechanical ventilation strategy. J Crit Care. 2009;24:523–9.
28. Frankovich J, Longhurst CA, Sutherland SM. Evidence-based medicine in the EMR era. N Engl J Med. 2011;365:1758–9.
29. Zhu X, Lord W. Using a context-aware medical application to address information needs for extubation decisions. AMIA Annu Symp Proc. 2005:1169.
30. Ahmed A, Chandra S, Herasevich V, Gajic O, Pickering BW. The effect of two different electronic health record user interfaces on intensive care provider task load, errors of cognition, and performance. Crit Care Med. 2011;39:1626–34.
31. Morrison C, Jones M, Vuylsteke A. Electronic patient record use during ward rounds: a qualitative study of interaction between medical staff. Crit Care. 2008;12:R148.
32. Effken JA, Loeb RG, Kang Y, Lin ZC. Clinical information displays to improve ICU outcomes. Int J Med Inform. 2008;77:765–77.
33. Dosani M, Hunc K, Dumont GA, Dunsmuir D, Barralon P, Schwarz SK, Lim J, Ansermino JM. A vibro-tactile display for clinical monitoring: real-time evaluation. Anesth Analg. 2012;115:588–94.
34. Liu D, Jenkins SA, Sanderson PM, Watson MO, Leane T, Kruys A, Russell WJ. Monitoring with head-mounted displays: performance and safety in a full-scale simulator and part-task trainer. Anesth Analg. 2009;109:1135–46.
35. Sanders D, Protti D. Data warehouses in healthcare: fundamental principles. ElectronicHealthcare. 2008;6(3):1–16.
36. Lieberman MI, Ricciardi TN, Masarie FE, Spackman KA. The use of SNOMED CT simplifies querying of a clinical data warehouse. AMIA Annu Symp Proc. 2003:910.
37. Eikel C, Delbanco S, John M. Eisenberg Patient Safety Awards. The Leapfrog Group for Patient Safety: rewarding higher standards. Jt Comm J Qual Saf. 2003;29:634–9
38. Bosman RJ, Rood E, Oudemans-van Straaten HM, et al. Intensive care information system reduces documentation time of the nurses after cardiothoracic surgery. Intensive Care Med. 2003;29:83–90.
39. Saarinen K, Aho M. Does the implementation of a clinical information system decrease the time intensive care nurses spend on documentation of care? Acta Anaesthesiol Scand. 2005;49:62–5.
40. Orwat C, Graefe A, Faulwasser T. Towards pervasive computing in health care – a literature review. BMC Med Inform Decis Mak. 2008;8:26.
41. August J, O'Donoghue J. Context-aware agents (the 6Ws architecture). In: Proceedings of the international conference on agents and artificial intelligence, 2009. http://citeseerx.ist.psu.edu/viewdoc/download?doi=10.1.1.158.1502&rep=rep1&type=pdf.
42. Jandhyala S, Jhoney A, Jhoney A, Muppidi S, Nagaratnam N, Saxena A (inventors), IBM Corp (assignee), Context aware data protection. US Patent 20,110,296,430, 2011.
43. Baumgart DC. Personal digital assistants in health care: experienced clinicians in the palm of your hand? Lancet. 2005;366:1210–22.
44. Craft RL. Trends in technology and the future intensive care unit. Crit Care Med. 2001;29 (Suppl):N151–8.
45. Adatia FA, Bedard PL. "Palm reading": 1. Handheld hardware and operating systems. CMAJ. 2002;167:775–80.
46. Bergeron BP. Enterprise digital assistants: the progression of wireless clinical computing. J Med Pract Manage. 2002;17:229–33.
47. Raths D. The BYOD revolution. Healthc Inform. 2012;29:28. 30.
48. Anonymous. Ottawa Hospital surges ahead on wireless waves. Canadian Healthcare Technology, April 2012. http://www.canhealth.com/apr12.html#12aprstory1.
49. Shaw CI, Kacmarek RM, Hampton RL, et al. Cellular phone interference with the operation of mechanical ventilators. Crit Care Med. 2004;32:928–31.

50. Lapinsky SE, Easty AC. Electromagnetic interference in critical care. J Crit Care. 2006;21:267–70.
51. Ammenwerth E, Buchauer A, Bludau B, Haux R. Mobile information and communication tools in the hospital. Int J Med Inform. 2000;57:21–40.
52. Lapinsky SE, Wax R, Showalter R, et al. Prospective evaluation of an internet-linked handheld computer critical care knowledge access system. Crit Care. 2004;8:R414–21.
53. Enders SJ, Enders JM, Holstad SG. Drug-information software for Palm operating system personal digital assistants: breadth, clinical dependability, and ease of use. Pharmacotherapy. 2002;22:1036–40.
54. Robinson RL, Burk MS. Identification of drug–drug interactions with personal digital assistant-based software. Am J Med. 2004;116:357–8.
55. Bergeron BP. Technology-enabled education. Postgrad Med. 1998;103:31–4.
56. Scales DC, Dainty K, Hales B, Pinto R, Fowler RA, Adhikari NK, Zwarenstein M. A multifaceted intervention for quality improvement in a network of intensive care units: a cluster randomized trial. JAMA. 2011;305:363–72.
57. Chang P, Hsu YS, Tzeng YM, et al. Development and pilot evaluation of user acceptance of advanced mass-gathering emergency medical services PDA support systems. Medinfo. 2004;11:1421–5.
58. Bures S, Fishbain JT, Uyehara CFT, et al. Computer keyboards and faucet handles as reservoirs of nosocomial pathogens in the intensive care unit. Am J Infect Control. 2000;28:465–70.
59. Braddy CM, Blair JE. Colonization of personal digital assistants used in a health care setting. Am J Infect Control. 2005;33:230–2.
60. Neely AN, Sittig DF. Basic microbiologic and infection control information to reduce the potential transmission of pathogens to patients via computer hardware. J Am Med Inform Assoc. 2002;9:500–8.
61. Hassoun A, Vellozzi EM, Smith MA. Colonization of personal digital assistants carried by healthcare professionals. Infect Control Hosp Epidemiol. 2004;25:1000–1.
62. Rosenfeld BA, Dorman T, Breslow MJ, Pronovost P, Jenckes M, Zhang N, Anderson G, Rubin H. Intensive care unit telemedicine: alternate paradigm for providing continuous intensivist care. Crit Care Med. 2000;28:3925–31.
63. Breslow MJ, Rosenfeld BA, Doerfler M, et al. Effect of a multiple-site intensive care unit telemedicine program on clinical and economic outcomes: an alternative paradigm for intensivist staffing. Crit Care Med. 2004;32:31–8.
64. Wilcox ME, Adhikari NKJ. The effect of telemedicine in critically ill patients: systematic review and meta-analysis. Crit Care. 2012;16:R127.
65. Breslow MJ. Remote ICU, care programs: current status. J Crit Care. 2007;22:66–76.

Chapter 6
Integrating Subspecialty Expertise in the Intensive Care Unit

Nicole Tran and Jason N. Katz

Abstract The integration of subspecialty expertise in the management of critically ill patients has become an area of both great interest and controversy. The past several decades have seen the emergence and rapid implementation of such subspecialty intensive care settings as the cardiac intensive care unit (ICU) and the neuroscience ICU. By pooling individuals with similar disease processes, and capitalizing on the expertise of specially trained nurses and physicians, many believe these units can provide more efficient and effective critical care delivery. Despite limited evidence to either support or refute their significance, these ICUs have become more commonplace, and their proliferation has brought to light important questions regarding optimal structure, staffing, and training. At the same time, the role of subspecialty consultants for an increasingly complex critical care population remains an important and evolving process.

Keywords Intensive care unit • Subspecialty • Staffing • Training • Consultation • Intensivist • Critical Care • Cardiac ICU • Neuroscience ICU

The care of the critically ill has evolved considerably over time. This evolution has not only been driven by the development of novel pharmacotherapies and emerging

N. Tran
Division of Cardiology, Department of Medicine, University of North Carolina, Chapel Hill, NC, USA

J.N. Katz (✉)
Divisions of Cardiology and Pulmonary and Critical Care Medicine, Department of Medicine, University of North Carolina, Chapel Hill, NC, USA

UNC Center for Heart and Vascular Care, 160 Dental Circle, CB# 7075, Burnett-Womack Building, 6th Floor, Chapel Hill, NC 27599-7075, USA
e-mail: katzj@med.unc.edu

D.C. Scales and G.D. Rubenfeld (eds.), *The Organization of Critical Care*, Respiratory Medicine 18, DOI 10.1007/978-1-4939-0811-0_6,

technologies, but has also been influenced by significant changes in patient demographics, comorbid illness, and disease severity. At the same time, there has been substantial innovation in the structure and staffing of the intensive care units (ICUs) where these high-risk, hospitalized individuals reside.

While this chapter will focus on the contemporary integration of subspecialty ICUs for an increasingly complex patient population, it is important that we first reflect upon historical aspects of critical care that have shaped this evolution. Prior to the more recent diversification and subspecialization of intensive care, it was the general medical and surgical ICUs that were the cornerstones of care delivery.

Defining the Contemporary ICU

In response to the rapid proliferation of ICUs and the increasing utilization of critical care resources, several studies in the mid-1990s helped to define the contemporary ICU environment. A single-day "snapshot" of over 2,800 ICUs in the USA found that these units were predominantly medical, surgical, or mixed in nature [1]. While certainly not as numerous, coronary care units (CCUs) were also found to be an important mechanism for providing critical care. The most common admission diagnoses in US ICUs at the time were respiratory failure and ischemic heart disease. Subspecialty ICUs, like the CCU, were more commonplace among larger hospital systems. Intensive care occupancy and the number of critical care interventions also increased in parallel with hospital size [1].

In a similar study, Knaus et al. [2] analyzed over 17,000 ICU admissions to 40 US hospitals. These investigators found that the majority of units were combined medical/surgical ICUs, while a minority were exclusive to one of the two populations. The most common reason for admission to a surgical ICU was for post-operative care following vascular interventions. On the other hand, the most common medical ICU admitting diagnoses were congestive heart failure, gastrointestinal hemorrhage, drug overdose, and pneumonia. Across the entire ICU spectrum, the mean mortality rate was found to be approximately 16 % [2].

The transition from the 1990s to the early 2000s was associated with a total decline in the number of US hospital beds, but a seemingly paradoxical 6.5 % increase in ICU bed availability [3]. With this changing allocation came a nearly 45 % increase in overall critical care costs [3]. General medical and surgical ICUs still accounted for the majority of beds during this time period, although the CCU continued to emerge as one of the more pervasive subspecialty settings.

The Subspecialty ICU: Examples of Novel Care

The Cardiac ICU

The origins of the CCU date back to the early 1960s when Julian [4] first described a post-myocardial infarction (MI) unit for monitoring and treating cardiac arrhythmias. In 1967, Killip and Kimball [5] reported their outcomes from 250 patients at New York Hospital/Cornell Medical Center. These pioneers in cardiac critical care described a marked decrease in hospital mortality, from 27 to 6 %, after the introduction of their CCU. Following closely on the heels of this seminal investigation, others began reporting similar successes. Lown et al. [6], for example, described a reduction in ICU mortality of 11.5 % and overall hospital mortality of 16.9 % using a paradigm of arrhythmia suppression in the CCU of the Peter Bent Brigham Hospital. Goldman and Cook [7] extended the benefits of CCU care, suggesting that these units may have been epidemiologically responsible for a nearly 135 % decrease in overall cardiovascular mortality.

Like the general medical and surgical ICUs, the CCU has continued to evolve since its inception. As therapies for coronary disease have advanced, the population has aged, and the burden of heart failure has increased, the clinical scope of the CCU has broadened over time. It is not uncommon now for patients with a diverse spectrum of cardiac critical illnesses to occupy these units. Technological advances have most certainly driven a significant portion of this evolution. Early mechanical reperfusion, for instance, has become the standard of care for the management of patients with ST-segment elevation myocardial infarction (STEMI). Implantable and percutaneous ventricular assist devices have become increasingly utilized therapies for the emergent management of patients with cardiogenic shock and end-stage heart failure. In light of these and other trends, the contemporary CCU is now often heavily occupied by patients that require invasive hemodynamic monitoring, complex arrhythmia management, and multidisciplinary collaborative care.

Along with the growing diversity of advanced cardiovascular diseases, today's CCU patients have also become increasingly complex from a non-cardiac critical care perspective. In a longitudinal, descriptive analysis of nearly 30,000 patients admitted to a single, academic cardiac intensive care unit (CICU), a group of investigators recently reported both a marked increase in case-mix and a greater burden of non-cardiac critical illness over time [8]. The increasing influence of sepsis, acute and chronic renal failure, and acute respiratory failure were also matched by greater utilization of non-cardiac critical care procedures, including central venous catheterization, renal replacement therapy, mechanical ventilation, and flexible bronchoscopy, to name a few. Despite the fact that therapies for acutely managing patients with cardiac ischemia have now favorably altered the natural history of diseases once considered universally fatal, it was striking that these investigators found no changes in overall CICU mortality during their nearly two decades worth of study [8]. These compelling results raise several important questions related to the optimal staffing and structure of subspecialty ICUs, and hence their roles in an increasingly complex healthcare environment.

The Neuroscience ICU

Though a more recent addition to the critical care vernacular, the neuroscience ICU is perhaps the most well validated of all the subspecialty units. Studies have consistently shown improvements in stroke and intracranial hemorrhage outcomes for patients treated in these ICUs compared with those treated in more general critical care settings [9–12]. In addition, it has been suggested that neuroscience ICUs may substantially reduce complications, resource consumption, and costs-of-care [13].

These important findings have also informed contemporary practice. In a recent survey of critical care practitioners, there was broad consensus agreement that the creation and implementation of neuroscience ICUs, staffed by practitioners well-versed in the practice of neurologic intensive care, can improve healthcare quality for neurological and neurosurgical patients with critical illness [14].

Other Examples of Subspecialty Critical Care

By pooling individuals with similar disease processes, and capitalizing on the expertise of specially trained nurses and physicians, there has been continued interest in expanding the subspecialty model of critical care delivery to other populations. In several academic centers, for instance, ICUs dedicated to the care of the burn patient now exist. In addition, recent studies have documented improved outcomes in centers where dedicated cardiothoracic surgical ICUs have been created [15–17].

Table 6.1 highlights selected evidence supporting several of the aforementioned subspecialty models of ICU care.

Questions Essential to the Subspecialty ICU

Do Subspecialty ICUs Improve Patient Outcomes?

It is clear that subspecialty ICUs have become increasingly more commonplace, particularly within larger, academic settings. While several important studies extolling the benefits of specialized critical care have already been discussed, the true impact of these units on patient outcomes remains a topic of considerable

Table 6.1 Selected evidence in support of subspecialty ICU models

Subspecialty unit	Investigators	Study details	Outcomes
Cardiac	Killip and Kimball [5]	Evaluated first 250 patients with acute MI in new four-bed CCU	CCU care reduced in-hospital mortality from 26 to 7 %
	Lown et al. [6]	Detailed outcomes of CCU patients with a protocol emphasizing arrhythmia suppression after MI	Found reduction in CCU mortality of 11.5 % and in-hospital mortality of 16.9 %
	Goldman and Cook [7]	Modeled changing epidemiology of cardiovascular death in the USA from 1968 to 1976	Described nearly 13.5 % decline in mortality rates from ischemic heart disease due to the CCU
	Reader [47]	Studied changes in coronary heart disease mortality in Australia	Surmised that steady decline in mortality over time may have been direct effect of specialized CCU care
Neuroscience	Mirski et al. [13]	Compared patients with intracranial hemorrhage managed in NSICU versus general ICU settings	Found significant decrease in mortality favoring the NSICU, and reduced LOS and costs-of-care compared with national benchmarks
	Diringer and Edwards [12]	Queried national ICU database to assess influence of NSICU on patient outcomes after hemorrhagic stroke	Significantly reduced mortality seen in NSICU patients compared with general ICU patients
	Suarez et al. [11]	Retrospective analysis of critically ill neurologic patients admitted before and after the implementation of a neurocritical care team	Neurocritical care was associated with a significant decrease in mortality, along with ICU and hospital LOS
Cardiothoracic	Stamou et al. [15]	Evaluated impact of single-institution, multidisciplinary, quality improvement program on mortality after cardiac surgery	Found significant reduction in cardiac surgical mortality after multidisciplinary team (including intensivist care) was implemented
	Kumar et al. [16]	Retrospective, propensity-matched, cohort study of cardiac surgical patients at single center to evaluate impact of 24-h, in-house intensivist care	Intensivist care was associated with significant reductions in blood transfusion, need for mechanical ventilation, and hospital LOS

Abbreviations: *ICU* intensive care unit, *MI* myocardial infarction, *CCU* coronary care unit, *NSICU* neuroscience intensive care unit, *LOS* length of stay controversy. Among a diverse group of US hospitals, for instance, several recent investigators found that admission to a subspecialty ICU was not associated with improved risk-adjusted survival [18]. Furthermore, they found no substantial benefits in terms of resource utilization. These findings have major implications when considered within a healthcare environment keenly focused on cost containment and care efficiency.

Why then might a subspecialty ICU fail to improve outcomes? By bringing experts to the bedside to care for patients with unique disease processes, it seems only logical that specialized care should be beneficial. However, there is more and more reason to suspect that the patients within these units are not as unique as once suspected [19]. Critical illness is the tie that binds these groups together, and it is not uncommon to see multiorgan system failure, acute lung injury, and delirium within each of these ICU settings. As a result, the distinction between various units becomes blurred, and may in fact attenuate the benefits of specialization. There are also likely other confounding features of care delivery—including standardization of ICU protocols and multidisciplinary collaboration—which together may influence patient outcomes. What is most concerning, perhaps, is that there is now some evidence to suggest that inappropriately triaging critically ill patients to the wrong subspecialty unit may actually result in increased mortality [18]. While observational only, these findings warrant immediate prospective validation.

How Should the Subspecialty ICU Be Staffed?

While the influence of subspecialty ICU care on patient outcomes needs further study, the widespread implementation of specialized critical care is unlikely to be stifled. In light of this, there are several key features of care delivery that must be addressed. In particular, an understanding of how best to staff these units is paramount.

The evidence-based literature would suggest that patient outcomes are markedly improved when critical care-trained practitioners—or intensivists—lead the ICU team. In a retrospective analysis comparing risk-adjusted ICU patients treated by either a critical care specialist or a generalist, Brown and Sullivan [20] found a significant reduction in ICU mortality of 52 % and overall hospital mortality of 31 % favoring an intensivist model of care. Similarly, Reynolds et al. [21] showed that intensivist staffing improved mortality among ICU patients admitted with septic shock. Similar findings have been replicated and reported in a variety of pediatric [22] and surgical ICU cohorts [23]. These data were ultimately substantiated by a landmark meta-analysis that recently highlighted significant improvements in mortality and resource consumption associated with intensivist care—either in a primary or consultative role [24].

Despite increasing support for intensivists, only one quarter of all ICUs are currently staffed by a practitioner trained in critical care medicine [25]. Larger hospitals, academic institutions, and surgical/trauma units were most likely to employ a dedicated, intensivist-staffing model. There are many reasons which underscore this disparity, but are thought to predominantly reflect resource limitations and financial constraints. Given the well-documented projections of intensivist shortages that are expected to plague the healthcare environment over the next several decades [26], this trend in under-utilization of intensivist care is likely to continue. There are frankly not enough critical care providers available to staff every ICU setting. As a result, novel solutions must be entertained.

How Should the Subspecialty Intensivist Be Trained?

One such solution to the intensivist shortage is to simply train more providers. However, it is unclear how best to train these providers, and what requisite skills they would need to function best in each individual care setting. For instance, the evidence seems to support intensivist-led care in general medical and surgical ICUs, but little is known about how these practitioners would fare in a subspecialty unit. At the same time, the goal of specialization is to pair critically ill patients with providers who have disease-specific expertise. How then can we optimally reconcile these issues in order to provide the best and most efficient care to evolving critically ill cohorts? The answer to this question will be a key component to creating a roadmap for the future of critical care delivery.

One potential model would include joint care of critically ill patients with both a subspecialist and intensivist collaboratively guiding care. There is limited data to either support or refute such an approach. Regardless, this model does little to address the burgeoning critical care crisis whereby the projected shortage of intensivists will fail to meet the demand of nearly 35 % of affected patients within the next 15 years [26].

An alternative model would be to equip subspecialists with the requisite skills necessary to deliver high-quality critical care to their patients. Neurology training programs have already been quite proactive in this regard. The United Council of Neurologic Subspecialties (UCNS) has now officially recognized the field of "critical care neurology" [27]. There are currently 40 accredited neurocritical care fellowship programs, graduating nearly 400 trained physicians from 2007 to 2010 [28].

A similar approach has been considered by cardiologists, and was formally addressed in a recent scientific statement supported by the American Heart Association (AHA) [29]. In this document, the writing group proposed an innovative plan to keep pace with the evolving demands of patients within the CICU. In particular, they focused on developing optimal training models for CICU providers. By adapting existing training pathways within the context of current American Board of Internal Medicine (ABIM) guidelines, and tailoring them to provide more substantial critical care education, it is possible that dedicated trainees within cardiovascular medicine fellowship programs will soon be better prepared to handle the increasingly complex demands of critically ill cardiac patients. Similar

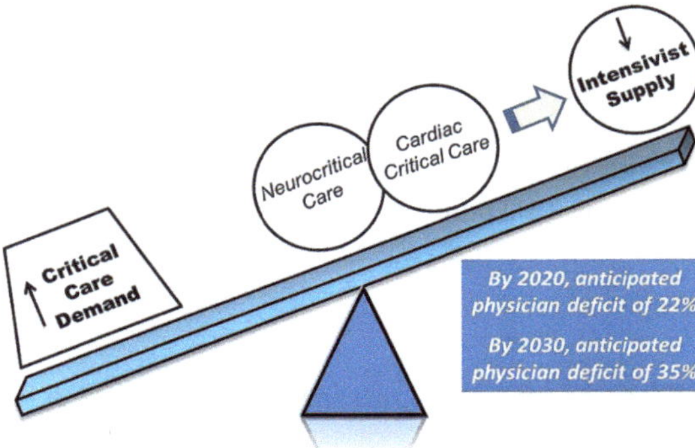

Fig. 6.1 The potential influence of subspecialty intensivists on the impending critical care crisis (Adapted from [26])

approaches for acute cardiac care accreditation have already been implemented by the European cardiovascular community [30]. At the same time, by enriching the critical care workforce through the creation of new subspecialty intensivists, novel training paradigms can be important mechanisms for averting the impending critical care crisis (Fig. 6.1).

How to Incorporate Nursing and Multidisciplinary Care Within the Subspecialty ICU?

While there is great interest in novel training approaches for enhancing physician care within the subspecialty ICU, it is important not to forget the influence of multidisciplinary collaboration. The very foundation of the contemporary CICU, for instance, began with having specially trained nurses at the bedside—capable of recognizing fatal arrhythmias and independently delivering life-saving defibrillation [31]. Neurologists and general critical care providers, when polled, suggested that it was the expected improvement in nursing quality that was their greatest motivator for supporting the implementation and rapid dissemination of neuroscience ICUs [14]. There are, in fact, many examples where nursing expertise and leadership have led to improvements in care—supported by better patient outcomes [32] and superior quality metrics [33].

The roles and benefits of other care team members, including pharmacists, case managers, dieticians, and social workers, may be less well defined within the subspecialty ICU setting, but are no less important. Pharmacy collaboration in the CICU, for instance, has been shown to improve care efficiency and to reduce costs [34]. The influence of social workers in the ICU has been shown to reliably improve continuity of care and promote better physician–nursing collaboration [35]. Future analyses of these and other components of the care team should be conducted in order to facilitate the effective growth of subspecialty critical care.

Bringing Specialty Physicians to the Patients: ICU Consultations

As we continue to address optimal subspecialty ICU models, it is important to remember that provision of care is not isolated to the clinicians who staff these units, but rather must also include the specialists who are often called upon to provide critical consultation. Palliative care providers, infectious disease specialists, and neurologists, to name a few, can all be important contributors to the subspecialty ICU team.

There is certainly data to support a more formal palliative care presence in the ICU. The Study to Understand Prognoses and Preference for Outcomes and Risks of Treatments (SUPPORT) investigators conducted a 2-year study of over 9,100 patients with one or more life-threatening diagnoses [36]. The 6-month mortality of this group was 47 %, and results suggested that existing care models were inadequate for addressing end-of-life issues among the critically ill. The investigators went so far as to propose mandatory palliative care consultation as a way to address these deficits. Bradley and Brasel [37], in an effort to understand current patterns of palliative care support, identified the most common "triggers" for palliative care consultation in the surgical ICU. They found that patient/family request, medical futility, prolonged lengths-of-stay (>1 month), and disagreement between family and providers were the most likely reasons to get the palliative care team involved. Whether these and other "triggers" should form the basis of consultative guidelines, or whether palliative care team members should more formally be introduced as members of the critical care team, is uncertain. What is clear from a burgeoning evidence-base is that better collaboration of the ICU and palliative care teams is warranted.

Given the marked prevalence of both community-acquired and nosocomial infections in the ICU, an infectious disease (ID) specialist can also serve a pivotal role as part of the critical care team. It is widely acknowledged that the presence of infection is an important predictor of patient outcomes, and there is well-documented risk associated with inappropriate initial antimicrobial strategies for hospitalized individuals [38, 39]. Collaborative ID consultation can improve antibiotic selection, can facilitate timely de-escalation of therapy, and can promote a culture of more effective infection surveillance [40]. While there is conflicting data regarding the influence of ID consultation on patient mortality, lengths-of-stay, and expenditures [41], greater collaboration between ICU physicians and ID experts will continue to be an important part of multidisciplinary care for the critically ill. In addition, with growing rates of organ transplantation, the availability of experts knowledgeable in infectious complications associated with chronic immunosuppression will be increasingly necessary.

Yet another example of consultative care in the ICU, particularly pertinent to the subspecialty care model, involves the treatment of patients following cardiac arrest. In recent years, the use of therapeutic hypothermia has emerged as a standard of care following successful resuscitation of out-of-hospital sudden cardiac death [42–44].

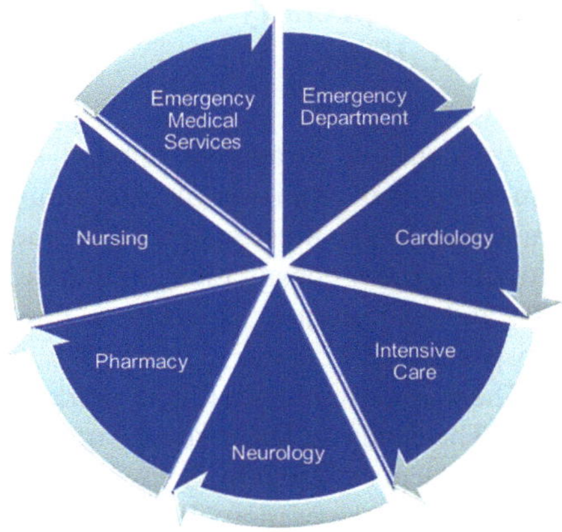

Fig. 6.2 Multidisciplinary care and consultation required for the management of the cardiac arrest patient

As a result, many of today's CICUs are now technologically well equipped to manage these complex patients. Their care, however, requires extensive multidisciplinary collaboration (Fig. 6.2). The use of hypothermia has also made neurological consultation crucial and, at the same time, accurate prognostication of recovery challenging. It seems no one criterion can effectively predict risk, and instead contemporary neurologists must now rely on integrating numerous findings and serial examinations in order to guide management decisions. The use of continuous electroencephalography (EEG), somatosensory-evoked potentials (SSEPs), and novel biomarkers have also become an important part of the neurologic consultation [45]. With more widespread adoption of therapeutic hypothermia and its broader application among diverse patient populations [46], one can expect that effective collaboration between cardiac intensivists and neurologic consultants will become increasingly more important.

The Future of Subspecialty Intensive Care

As medicine continues to diversify, patients get more complex, and technologies advance, optimal ways to involve subspecialists in the care of the critically ill will remain an important topic for discussion. In specific populations, the subspecialty ICU has been shown to improve patient outcomes. At the same time, ICU teams directed by trained intensivists have led to reductions in patient mortality, resource consumption, and lengths-of-stay.

In many cases, the evolution of subspecialty critical care and the implementation of subspecialty units have outpaced the limited evidence-base that supports their existence. Nonetheless, there is growing interest in expanding ICU settings based upon disease-specific criteria. At one time, the cardiac and neuroscience ICUs were considered newcomers to the field of critical care. Future subspecialization, however, is very likely to continue. Many expect critically ill oncology patients and those with advanced heart failure, for instance, to be the next beneficiaries of dedicated specialty units. Given the high cost and intensity of critical care delivery in general, issues pertaining to the optimal staffing, training, and multidisciplinary care within these subspecialty models must be considered. In addition, the effective involvement of specialty consultants and their timely collaboration with the critical care team should be formally addressed.

References

1. Groeger JS, Guntupalli KK, Strosberg M, et al. Descriptive analysis of critical care units in the United States: patient characteristics and intensive care unit utilization. Crit Care Med. 1993;21:279–91.
2. Knaus WA, Wagner DP, Zimmerman JE, et al. Variations in mortality and length of stay in intensive care units. Ann Intern Med. 1993;118:753–61.
3. Halpern NA, Pastores SM. Critical care medicine in the United States 2000–2005: an analysis of bed numbers, occupancy rates, payer mix and costs. Crit Care Med. 2010;38:65–71.
4. Julian DG. Treatment of cardiac arrest in acute myocardial ischaemia and infarction. Lancet. 1961;2:840–4.
5. Killip T, Kimball JT. Treatment of myocardial infarction in a coronary care unit. Two year experience with 250 patients. Am J Cardiol. 1967;20:457–64.
6. Lown B, Fakhro AM, Hood WB, et al. The coronary care unit. New perspectives and directions. JAMA. 1967;199:188–98.
7. Goldman L, Cook EF. The decline in ischemic heart disease mortality rates: an analysis of the comparative effects of medical interventions and changes in lifestyle. Ann Intern Med. 1984;101:825–36.
8. Katz JN, Shah BR, Volz EM, et al. Evolution of the coronary care unit: clinical characteristics and temporal trends in healthcare delivery and outcomes. Crit Care Med. 2010;38:375–81.
9. Wentworth DA, Atkinson RP. Implementation of an acute stroke program decreases hospitalization costs and length of stay. Stroke. 1996;27:1040–3.
10. Webb DJ, Fayad PB, Wilbur C, et al. Effects of a specialized team on stroke care: the first two years of the Yale Stroke Program. Stroke. 1998;26:1353–7.
11. Suarez JI, Zaidat OO, Suri MF, et al. Length of stay and mortality in neurocritically ill patients: impact of a specialized neurocritical care team. Crit Care Med. 2004;32:2311–7.
12. Diringer MN, Edwards DF. Admission to a neurologic/neurosurgical intensive care unit is associated with reduced mortality rate after intracerebral hemorrhage. Crit Care Med. 2001;29:635–40.
13. Mirski MA, Chang CW, Cowan R. Impact of a neuroscience intensive care unit on neurosurgical patient outcomes and cost of care: evidence-based support for an intensivist-directed specialty ICU model of care. J Neurosurg Anesthesiol. 2001;13:83–92.
14. Markandaya M, Thomas KP, Jahromi B, et al. The role of neurocritical care: a brief report on the survey results of neurosciences and critical care specialists. Neurocrit Care. 2012;16:72–81.
15. Stamou SC, Camp SL, Stiegel RM, et al. Quality improvement program decreases mortality after cardiac surgery. J Thorac Cardiovasc Surg. 2008;136:494–9.
16. Kumar K, Zarychanski R, Bell DD, et al. The impact of 24-hour in-house intensivists on a dedicated cardiac surgery intensive care unit. Ann Thorac Surg. 2009;88:1153–61.
17. Whitman GJ, Haddad M, Hirose H, et al. Thoracic surgeons providing cardiac critical care improve patient management and decrease costs. Presented at the 46th Annual Meeting of the Society of Thoracic Surgeons, Fort Lauderdale, 2010.

18. Lott JP, Iwashyna TJ, Christie JD, Asch DA, Kramer AA, Kahn JM. Critical illness outcomes in specialty versus general intensive care units. Am J Respir Crit Care Med. 2009;179:676–83.
19. Katz JN, Turer AT, Becker RC. Cardiology and the critical care crisis. A perspective. J Am Coll Cardiol. 2007;49:1279–82.
20. Brown JJ, Sullivan G. Effect on ICU mortality of a full-time critical care specialist. Chest. 1989;96:127–9.
21. Reynolds HN, Haupt MT, Thill-Baharozian MC, et al. Impact of critical care physician staffing on patients with septic shock in a university hospital medicine intensive care unit. JAMA. 1988;260:3446–50.
22. Goh AY, Lum LC, Abdel-Latif ME. Impact of 24 hour critical care physician staffing on case-mix adjusted mortality in paediatric intensive care. Lancet. 2001;357:445–6.
23. Nathens AB, Rivara FP, MacKenzie EJ, et al. The impact of an intensivist-model ICU on trauma-related mortality. Ann Surg. 2006;244:545–54.
24. Pronovost PJ, Angus DC, Dorman T, et al. Physician staffing patterns and clinical outcomes in critically ill patients. A systematic review. JAMA. 2002;288:2151–62.
25. Angus DC, Shorr AF, White A, et al. Committee on Manpower for Pulmonary and Critical Care Societies (COMPACCS). Critical care delivery in the United States: distribution of services and compliance with Leapfrog recommendations. Crit Care Med. 2006;34:1016–24.
26. Chang SY, Multz AS, Hall JB. Critical care organization. Crit Care Clin. 2005;21:43–53.
27. Mayer SA, Coplin WM, Chang C, et al. Core curriculum and competencies for advanced training in neurological intensive care: United Council for Neurologic Subspecialties guidelines. Neurocrit Care. 2006;5:159–65.
28. Neurocritical care society education and training. http://www.neurocriticalcare.org/i4a/pages/index.cfm?pageid=3345. Accessed 26 Apr 2012.
29. Morrow DA, Fang JC, Fintel DJ, et al. on behalf of the American Heart Association Council on Cardiopulmonary, Critical Care, Perioperative, and Resuscitation, Council on Clinical Cardiology, Council on Cardiovascular Nursing, and Council on Quality of Care and Outcomes Research. Evolution of critical care cardiology: transformation of the cardiovascular intensive care unit and the emerging need for new medical staffing and training models: a scientific statement from the American Heart Association. Circulation. 2012;126:1408–28.
30. European Board for the Specialty of Cardiology. Curriculum for acute cardiac care subspecialty training in Europe. www.escardio.org/communities/working-groups/acute-cardiac-care/documents/esc-curriculum-training-intensive-acc-europe.pdf. Accessed 16 Apr 2012.
31. Julian DG. The history of coronary care units. Br Heart J. 1987;57:497–502.
32. Tonnelier JM, Prat G, Le Gal G, et al. Impact of a nurses' protocol-directed weaning procedure on outcomes in patients undergoing mechanical ventilation for longer than 48 hours: a prospective cohort study with a matched historical control group. Crit Care. 2005;9:R83–9.
33. Campbell J. The effect of nurse champions on compliance with Keystone Intensive Care Unit Sepsis-screening protocol. Crit Care Nurs Q. 2008;31:251–69.
34. Gandhi PJ, Smith BS, Tataronis GR, Maas B. Impact of a pharmacist on drug costs in a coronary care unit. Am J Health Syst Pharm. 2001;58:497–503.
35. Carr DD. Building collaborative partnerships in critical care: the RN case manager/social work dyad in critical care. Prof Case Manag. 2009;14:121–32.
36. The SUPPORT Principal Investigators. A controlled trial to improve care for seriously ill hospitalized patients: the Study to Understand Prognoses and Preferences for Outcomes and Risks of Treatment (SUPPORT). JAMA. 1995;274:1592–8.
37. Bradley CT, Brasel KJ. Developing guidelines that identify patients who would benefit from palliative care services in the surgical intensive care unit. Crit Care Med. 2009;37:946–50.
38. Heyland DK, Cook DJ, Griffith L, Keenan SP, Brun-Buisson C. The attributable morbidity and mortality of ventilator-associated pneumonia in the critically ill patient. The Canadian Critical Trials Group. Am J Respir Crit Care Med. 1999;159:1249–56.

39. Cm L, Aruj P, et al. Appropriateness and delay to initiate therapy in ventilator-associated pneumonia. Eur Respir J. 2006;27:158–64.
40. Esposito S, Leone S. Antimicrobial treatment for Intensive Care Unit (ICU) infections including the role of the infectious disease specialist. Int J Antimicrob Agents. 2007;29:494–500.
41. Classen DC, Burke JP, Wenzel RP. Infectious disease consultation: impact on outcomes for hospitalized patients and results of a preliminary study. Clin Infect Dis. 1997;24:468–70.
42. Hypothermia after Cardiac Arrest Study Group. Mild therapeutic hypothermia to improve the neurologic outcome after cardiac arrest. N Engl J Med. 2002;346:549–56.
43. Bernard SA, Gray TW, Buist MD, et al. Treatment of comatose survivors of out-of-hospital cardiac arrest with induced hypothermia. N Engl J Med. 2002;346:557–63.
44. ECC Committee. Subcommittees and Task Forces of the American Heart Association. 2005 American Heart Association guidelines for cardiopulmonary resuscitation and emergency cardiovascular care. Circulation. 2005;112:1–203.
45. Blondin NA, Greer DM. Neurologic prognosis in cardiac arrest patients treated with therapeutic hypothermia. Neurologist. 2011;17:241–8.
46. Dumas F, Grimaldi D, Zuber B, et al. Is hypothermia after cardiac arrest effective in both shockable and nonshockable patients? Insights from a large registry. Circulation. 2011;123:877–86.
47. Reader R. Why the decreasing morality from coronary heart disease in Australia? Circulation. 1978;58(Suppl II):32.

Part II
Improving Intensive Care

Chapter 7
Quality Improvement in the Intensive Care Unit

Christopher Dale and J. Randall Curtis

Abstract Medical error is common and devastating, claiming the lives of an estimated 100,000 people per year in the USA. The intellectual origins of the modern intensive care unit (ICU) quality improvement (QI) movement can be traced to post-World War II Japanese industrial process management and to aviation safety. From Japanese Industrial process management, the concepts of unnecessary variation and statistical process control have been applied to the ICU to develop our current QI efforts. The Structure–Process–Outcome model of QI provides a solid theoretical approach for many efforts. From aviation safety, Human Factors Analysis, Checklists, and Crew Resource Management are tools adapted for the ICU QI team. The Institute for Healthcare Improvement has created a practical, stepwise QI process that uses a Plan-Do-Study-Act cycle to help QI teams assess and improve their ICUs. These tools provide a foundation for quality improvement efforts in the ICU.

Keywords Intensive care unit • Critical care • Quality • Quality improvement • Medical error • Variation • Checklist • Protocol

C. Dale
Value Measurement and Comparative Effectiveness, Providence Health and Services, 1801 Lind Avenue SW, Renton, WA 98057, USA
e-mail: Christopher.dale@swedish.org

J.R. Curtis (✉)
Division of Pulmonary and Critical Care, Department of Medicine, Harborview Medical Center, University of Washington, 325 Ninth Avenue, Box 359762, Seattle, WA 98104, USA
e-mail: jrc@u.washington.edu

D.C. Scales and G.D. Rubenfeld (eds.), *The Organization of Critical Care*, Respiratory Medicine 18, DOI 10.1007/978-1-4939-0811-0_7,

At the completion of this chapter the reader should be able to:

1. Understand the contributions of industrial management and aviation safety to quality improvement.
2. Describe a quality improvement framework offered by the Institute for Healthcare Improvement.
3. Be able to implement a Plan-Do-Study-Act cycle.

Every system is perfectly designed to get the results that it gets. Paul Batalden, MD [1].

In March 1984 an 18-year-old college student named Libby Zion was seen in the emergency room of a New York City hospital with a temperature of 39.7 °C and a white blood cell count of 18,000 [2]. She was diagnosed with a "viral syndrome" and admitted for IV hydration. In the early hours of the next morning, she became more agitated and received meperidine and haloperidol from her admitting intern who had been up for more than 18 h. Shortly thereafter her fever rose to 42 °C and she suffered cardiac arrest and died.

In 1994 a 39-year-old health reporter for the Boston Globe named Betsy Lehman developed breast cancer and went to the Dana Farber Cancer Institute for treatment. In December 1994, as part of her cancer treatment protocol, she received a threefold overdose of cyclophosphamide in a medication order error and died [3].

Clinicians have likely made errors as long as medicine has been practiced. The deaths of Libby Zion and Betsy Lehman put faces on the fear that many patients and clinicians have had that error is pervasive and even happens at the best hospitals. In 1999 the Institute of Medicine published a landmark report, *To Err Is Human*, which reported that just under 100,000 patients die each year because of medical error [4]. Theirs was not the first such report on the severity or extent of iatrogenic harm, but it catalyzed a patient safety movement and placed the tragic deaths of Zion, Lehman, and countless others in context [5]. Errors are not something that happens elsewhere at lesser hospitals at the hands of bad clinicians. Harm happens to my patients at my hospital and sometimes, despite how hard I work and how careful I am, on my watch. How we work to make health care better and safer is the story of quality improvement. Understanding the history of this story provides ICU clinicians with a valuable context and framework for improving quality today.

The Foundation of the Quality Improvement Movement

The modern health care quality improvement movement didn't begin in New York in 1984 or with the publication of the *To Err Is Human* report 1999. We can trace the roots of many of the principles and tools of quality improvement to two places: The post-World War II Japanese industrial management practices and the modern aviation safety movement.

Lessons from Industrial Management Practices

Just after World War II, several American thinkers, physicists and engineers by training, were interested in how companies could improve the quality of their products and the efficiency of their operations. Perhaps the most notable was W. Edwards Deming. He was a University of Wyoming and Yale-trained mathematical physicist who studied the effects of nitrogen on crops for the US Department of Agriculture and helped with statistical process control for the US Census Bureau [6]. He was interested in process control and variation and the application of statistics to process improvement. He went to Japan in 1947 to help General Douglass MacArthur rebuild Japan and his ideas that focused on the process of production and the relentless pursuit of quality found an eager audience.

One of Demming's focuses was on unnecessary variation. Variation is difference in process from moment to moment. It is inherent in every system and every process. We know from our clinical experience that heart and respiratory rates vary from minute to minute. Serum sodium levels are different from day to day. Demming and a colleague, Walter Shewhart, created Statistical Process Control wherein workers and management can monitor a process to look for variation that exceeds a desired level as an indicator of a potential quality control problem. We see this process control in many of the QI reports that are generated in today's hospitals: The plots of ventilator-associated pneumonia rates over time with upper and lower confidence error lines are a modern incarnation of Demming and Shewhart's Statistical Process Control.

To help manage quality improvement, Deming created a "system of profound knowledge" that espoused the belief that about 15–20 % of poor quality was because of workers and the remaining 80–85 % was because of bad management, improper systems and process [6]. To help improve processes, Deming and Shewart created the Plan-Do-Study-Act quality improvement cycle that, to this day, is a foundational principle of medical quality improvement and has been used by Institute for Healthcare Improvement and other hospitals and healthcare organizations nationwide. Healthcare has been somewhat slow to fully uptake the process management ideas proposed by Deming and implemented more than 60 years ago in the auto industry in Japan, but his ideas have formed the basis for many of today's quality improvement activities.

Taiichi Ohno was a 35-year-old manager of Toyota's Engine Manufacturing Department when Demming arrived in Japan in 1947. Ohno developed the Toyota Production System (TPS) that emphasizes work flow and eliminating waste or *muda*, as it is called in Japanese [7]. An integral part of the TPS is giving each worker the responsibility and ownership of the quality of the product. Each worker is encouraged to "stop the line" if he or she observes a quality defect. The logic is that if defects are detected early in the process, they are less likely to become errors and that efficiency will be enhanced. This attention to waste and defects and a focus on the production team and the role of the organization in quality echo many of Demming's thoughts.

A number of hospitals in America, including Virginia Mason in Seattle, WA and Henry Ford Hospital in Detroit, MI, use a variant of the TPS called "Lean" or various other organization-specific names [8]. At their core, these mental frameworks look at the process of production of health care and use the notion of waste (non-value added activity) to guide analysis of the process in a way that builds on the statistical analytical techniques that Deming and his contemporaries introduced to industry both in America and in Japan.

Application of Industrial Management to Health Care

Avedis Donabedian was a physician who was born in Beirut, Lebanon and immigrated to America after World War II. He obtained his Masters of Public Health from Harvard University and spent the majority of his career at University of Michigan [9]. In 1966 he authored one of the foundational papers on medical quality and created the Structure, Process and Outcome framework from which to approach healthcare quality [10]. Many healthcare organizations still use the Structure–Process–Outcome approach to quality.

Structure

The Structure component of the Donabedian triad considers fixed elements of the care environment. For example, when Peter Pronovost and his group implemented their intervention to decrease central line infection rates in Michigan hospitals, the management at each hospital had to be engaged to make sure that the central line carts were stocked with chlorhexidine cleaning solution [11]. Having central line carts stocked with chlorhexidine on each unit is a Structural element of quality.

Process

Deming, Shewhart and Ohno focused the majority of their attention on industrial processes and this is where much of quality improvement efforts to this day are focused. Using central line infection prevention as an example, the use of the chlorhexidine sterilizing washes, the use of the checklists, and the use of full barrier precautions during line placement are all process measures of quality. Process measures are often more amenable to monitoring and management than outcome measures for two reasons. First, as process measures are frequently present with each instance of the event (each time a central line is placed the clinician will or will not use full barrier precautions), the number of process events is generally much, much greater than outcome events. If that same clinician did not use full barrier precautions, it might take weeks or months to see a central line infection. Second, variations in process measures are often much more practicable to measure than outcomes. Often outcomes occur later in the course of care and the mechanisms to track and monitor them may be beyond the scope of a single ICU.

Outcome

There is no question, however, that Outcome is the component of the triad about which patients and clinicians ultimately care the most. The infection rate before Pronovost's intervention was only 2.7 infections per 1,000 catheter days. Central line-related bloodstream infections are a serious and relatively infrequent outcome. Many significant outcomes, by virtue of their relative infrequency, are not as amenable to management as process or structure measures of quality. They ought to still be measured, however, just as the function of cars coming off the Toyota production line is still measured.

Thus the quality management strategies and tactics developed by Deming, Shewhart, and Ohno are easily integrated into the Donabedian Structure–Process–Outcome paradigm. Together they form two concepts from post World War II industrial quality management that are relevant to healthcare quality improvement today: (1) Look for and manage unnecessary variation. (2) Develop, evaluate, and improve high-reliability processes as a way to create desired outcomes.

Lessons from Aviation Safety

Aviation safety is a second inspiration for modern health care quality improvement effort and recently has seeped into popular culture. Several books including Atul Gawande's *The Checklist Manifesto* and John Nash's *Why Hospitals Should Fly* have examined how the impressive improvements in aviation safety might be translated into medicine. There are three common applications of aviation safety to ICU safety and quality improvement: The Swiss cheese model of error investigation, checklists and Crew Resource Management.

Swiss Cheese Model and Human Factors Analysis

James Reason provided one of the seminal thoughts in aviation safety when he described a "Swiss Cheese" model of mishaps as a conceptual model of the reasons why errors occur [12]. Errors, he argues, are not caused by one event in isolation, rather a number of conditions must all line up (like holes in sequential pieces of Swiss cheese, hence the name) before harm befalls the patient (see Fig. 7.1). He defines the conditions as either "active failures" or "latent conditions." Active failures are the "unsafe acts committed by people who are in direct contact with the patient or the system." Latent conditions are the "invisible 'resident pathogens' in the system" that may be thought of a preconditions for unsafe acts [12].

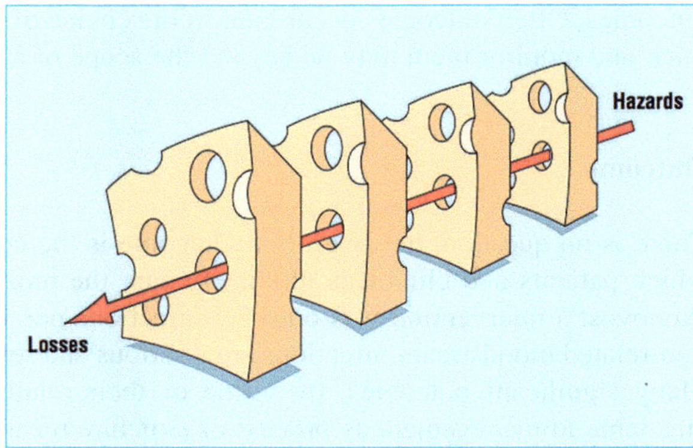

Fig. 7.1 In order for hazards to produce losses, a number of active failures and latent conditions must all line up like holes in layered pieces of Swiss cheese (from Reason [12])

The US Navy Safety Center and the Federal Aviation Administration have further refined Reason's Swiss cheese model into a robust Human Factors Analysis and Classification System (HFACS) that defines different types of latent conditions and looks for ways to mitigate them [13]. In the HFACS system, latent conditions include Organizational Influences, Supervision and Preconditions for Unsafe Acts. For example, in an ICU where the Organizational Climate values throughput and productivity (a possible Organizational latent condition) a clinician may repeatedly rush through admit orders (a possible Supervision latent condition) because he or she wants to get home for the night (a Precondition for Unsafe Acts latent condition) and one time omit orders for antibiotics in a septic patient (an Unsafe Act). Robust analysis of the reasons why the error occurred would try to discern all layers of Swiss cheese that lined up and each of the individual latent conditions that contributed to the active failure.

One of the ways that medicine lags aviation safety is that we lack a way to learn from our mistakes on a consistent or broad basis. Clinicians have long yearned to minimize harm and to improve as a central component of our mission. Morbidity and Mortality rounds provide an opportunity to examine our bad outcomes. We often informally tell stories of patient mishaps and near misses. But we lack a way to systematically improve the process of healthcare delivery across our profession. This is in distinction to aviation. For example, after a mishap, the US Navy conducts an investigation and takes the lessons learned and systematically applies them to the entire fleet. Health care lacks this coordinated improvement cycle.

There are some efforts to more towards profession-wide quality improvement. The Agency for Healthcare Research and Quality (AHRQ) hosts a monthly web M&M [14]. The Food and Drug Administration routinely publishes "Black Box" drug warnings based on feedback from clinicians and patients [15]. Some organizations like the Washington State Hospital Association have sponsored a "Safe Table" space for hospitals to share their error experiences and look to improve [16]. But we can do more as a profession to systematically learn from our outcomes. We can put in place systems to disseminate the findings of our "mishap" investigations.

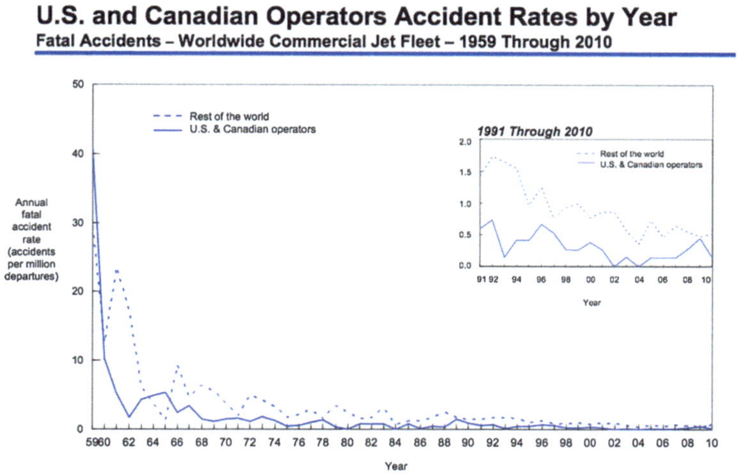

Fig. 7.2 Commercial jet mishap rate has declined significantly over the past 50 years (Courtesy the Boeing Company)

Checklists

Atul Gawande and Peter Provonovst have both popularized the concept of checklists in medicine. In 1960 the worldwide commercial jet fatal mishap rate was approximately 25 mishaps per million departures (Fig. 7.2). The early days of aviation relied heavily on pilot skill and knowledge and prized the ability of the individual to "get the job done" despite long odds and difficult situations. This resonates with the skills that are valued in clinicians today in many care situations, be it a difficult case in the OR or a tenuous patient the ICU.

As airplanes crashed out of the sky at rates that today would seem unfathomable and would make air travel untenably dangerous to the flying public, aviation leaders searched for ways to make procedures more uniform in the hopes that standard approaches could improve mishap rates. As Fig. 7.2 shows, that standardization, along with improving technology played a key role in improving aviation safety. In the period 2001–2010, the fatal mishap rate was only 1.6 % of what it was 50 years before. Standardization and checklists can play a large role in health care quality improvement efforts.

At its most simple form a checklist can be thought of as memory aid, a tool to help someone who already knows how to do her or his job to be sure that on any particular day he or she does not omit a key step. A less explicit but equally important downstream effect of checklists is that they can be designed to orient the health care activity towards the patient and the team.

Atul Gawande and The World Health Organization looked for a way to decrease operative mortality worldwide that could be implemented even in resource-poor countries. The result was the Surgical Safety Checklist, which serves both as a safety tool and as a team-orienting exercise. The checklist contains 19 elements in three sections, each for one phase of the operation [17]. For example, before the start the operation, all members of operative team introduce themselves by name and role and discuss anticipated critical events, issues that are projected to arise during the operation. This introduction not only helps form the operative team, it orients them to the task at hand and helps ensure that essential, quality-added steps are not overlooked, that patients received pre-operative antibiotics if needed, for example. It is simple and effective. In their worldwide study, Dr. Gawande and his colleagues found that implementation of the checklist was associated with a reduction in rate of death to 0.8 from 1.5 % [17].

Checklists are valuable in the ICU as well. Drawing again on the example of Peter Pronovost and his group, they showed that it is possible to use checklists as part of a statewide quality improvement initiative. The US Agency for Health Care Quality and Research (AHRQ) funded the Keystone ICU project across the state of Michigan to test the hypothesis that implementation of a bundle of ICU interventions, including a checklist to be used at the time of central line insertion, could reduce catheter-related bloodstream infections statewide. The program was quite successful and its implementation was associated with a reduction in median catheter-related bloodstream infections from 2.7 per 1,000 catheter days to 0.0 per 1,000 catheter days [11]. Similar results have been observed in a variety of other settings. Implementation of an ICU rounding checklist was associated with a 48 % reduction in ICU mortality [18]. Implementation of a Clostridium difficile prevention and treatment checklist was associated with a 40 % reduction in Clostridium difficile incidence [19]. These results show that breaking down a task into its component parts and standardizing the approach can decrease unnecessary variability and thereby improve outcomes.

Creating good checklists might be more difficult that it first appears. As Atul Gawande details in his book, *The Checklist Manifesto*, the comparison to aviation checklists can be instructive. Not all checklists perform the same function. Some checklist items call for verification that something is as it seems it is: "check: flaps down" in aviation; "patient identified with two identifiers" in healthcare. Some checklist items call for action: "make airspeed 140 knots" in aviation; "apply sterile prep to the intended central line insertion site" in medicine. Moreover, in the aviation world, checklists are dynamic instruments that are continually improved by the end user. In the case of aviation, the improvements are usually routed through a central agency. For example, the US Navy uses the NATOPS (Naval Air Training and Operating Procedures Standardization) program to aggregate input from pilots, maintainers and other interested parties and then revises the checklists so that they can then be implemented Navy-wide. This situation is different from medicine where there is not a central clearing-house with this level of authority for quality data or protocols. Often, clinicians or hospitals in need of a good checklist will look to other local hospitals, on-line or to the published literature for examples. Focusing attention at the professional level on checklist development and implementation has the potential to be a powerful lever to improve care processes and reduce unnecessary variation.

Protocols and order sets (the process by which a protocol is implemented) are cousins of checklists and serve to standardize processes. Implementation of protocols for a number of processes in the ICU has been shown to improve outcomes. For example, implementation of analgesia and sedation protocols and ventilator weaning protocols have both been shown to decrease ICU length of stay and duration of mechanical ventilation [20–22]. However, it is important to acknowledge that protocols may not improve care if the baseline quality of care is very high, as in the example of a ventilator weaning protocol implemented at Johns Hopkins University in a well-staffed, intensivist-run ICU [23]. In addition, protocol may even worsen outcomes if dangerous care is protocolized as was the case for tight glucose control in medically critically ill patients [24, 25].

Crew Resource Management

A third theme or lesson from aviation safety is a focus on the dynamic of the care team. As aviation progressed from an enterprise that valued the individual initiative and skill of the lead pilot to one that tries to optimize the performance of the cockpit team, the industry developed tools to help the teams achieve more together. Crew Resource Management is the term that is used in aviation safety to describe the process by which the collective intelligence and ability of the group can exceed that of its component individuals. An asymmetry of power and information and inefficient communication was found to be a significant contributing factor in a number of aviation disasters. The most notable example was the 1977 Tenerife disaster where two Boeing 747 s collided on a foggy runway on one of the Canary Islands, killing 583 people in the deadliest mishap in aviation history [26, 27]. Tragically crew members had data that could have prevented the mishap, but because of communication and power issues the information was not able to be used [28]. Because a high-functioning team is critical to mishap prevention, aviation safety experts began to focus more explicitly on the dynamics within the cockpit that impede the free-flow of knowledge and information.

The SCOAP checklist, for example, calls for participants in the operation to introduce themselves by their name and their role. An overly formal environment, where power relationships are highlighted in the way information is communicated can impede the flow of information and impair the functioning of the health care team. In *Outliers* Malcom Gladwell talks about the Power-Distance level of a culture. The greater the Power-Distance level, the more difficult it can be for those who are not in power to communicate important information to those who are in power, as happened in the Tenerife disaster [29]. Crew Resource Management works to decrease Power-Distance to improve information transfer.

The SBAR process for communication that has been promulgated by the Joint Commission and IHI is another example of a communication tool that strives to improve the quality of information transfer [30]. In this tool, the Situation is described, followed by the necessary Background information to place the situation in context, the reporter's Assessment of the situation is then provided along with their Recommendation. SBAR can be thought of as both a checklist for communication and a Crew Resource Management tool designed to improve teamwork and coordination. Robust randomized trial evidence of its effectiveness is lacking, but implementation of SBAR is associated with reductions in clinician order entry error and adverse drug events [30, 31].

There are three primary ways in which aviation safety thought impacts current medical quality improvement efforts: (1) Improvements to the system can improve patient outcomes. (2) Checklists can help repetitive tasks be done right and help focus high-performing teams. (3) Standard operating procedures can help clinicians do the right thing each time. (4) Teams are more effective than individuals at performing complex tasks, but require a different set of skills, many of which are not native to medicine.

Part of the reason that quality has not improved more rapidly in medicine is that the human body in illness is much more complex than any industrial process or aviation system. The counter-factual example is helpful to consider: If the tools of industrial process control or aviation safety were a panacea for the woes of the health care system, they would have already been more completely implemented and patients would be healthier. Instead, health care has lagged in quality improvement measures in large part because of the complexity of the system.

Implementing Quality Improvement in the ICU

So how then does an interested clinician go about improving the quality of care delivered by their organization?

> Give me a lever long enough and a fulcrum on which to place it, and I shall move the world.
> Archimedes

In 2005 the then former and now current governor of Oregon, John Kitzhaber, an Emergency Medicine physician, started a movement he described as The Archimedes Movement that looked to improve the state of health and healthcare for all Oregonians. The movement articulated an often-unstated principle of quality improvement: The search for the perfect lever. We all would like to improve quality but we often feel powerless or ill equipped to effect the change that we so desperately desire. Health care does not suffer from a lack of interested parties or number of (sometimes competing) quality improvement opportunities.

As Table 7.1 details, there are many interested parties. The US Federal government (CMS) is "paying for performance," reporting of certain performance measures and publically reporting hospital performance on-line. The Agency for Health Care @@Quality and Research funds research about ways to improve the quality of care. The Joint Commission, the organization that accredits most of the acute care hospitals in America, details many process improvement strategies that must be implemented for accreditation like SBAR mentioned above. Large purchasers of health care came together in the Leapfrog Group to articulate the need for improved

Table 7.1 North American quality improvement organizations

Organization name	Owners/stakeholders	Mission/vision	Example projects	How can they help me?
Institute for Healthcare Improvement (IHI) www.ihi.org	Private not-for-profit organization. Founded by Don Berwick and others in the 1980s. Funding from donations and fees from educational resources.	No needless deaths, no needless pain or suffering, no helplessness in those served or serving, no unwanted waiting, no waste, no one left out.	Open School, an online resource for people interested in QI. 100,000 and 5 million lives campaigns.	Equip professionals with tools needed to affect QI in their organization. Offers on-line learning and certificates in QI.
The Leapfrog Group www.leapfroggroup.org	Private not-for-profit organization. Founded in 2002 by a group of large employers who wanted to work together to use the way they purchased health care to have an influence on its quality and affordability. Funding from large employers (like Boeing, FedEX, General Motors) and organizations of purchasers (like Midwest Business Group on Health, Silicon Valley Employers Forum) and from health care industry "partners" (like Aetna, Lilly, Hospital Corporation of America). Also collects fees from licensing its data.	To trigger giant leaps forward in the safety, quality and affordability of health care by: Supporting informed health care decisions by those who use and pay for health care and; Promoting high-value health care through incentives and rewards.	Leapfrog Hospital Survey, an annually updated hospital survey open to any hospital in America and aimed at consumers. Survey also uses Medicare data. Leapfrog Hospital Recognition Program Health Plan Users Group. Provides a forum for purchasers and national health plan carriers to collaborate to provide employers with products that will address Leapfrog's purchasing principles.	Allows professional to see how their hospital compares to other hospitals in the selected metrics. Has called for public reporting of Intensivist staffing of ICUs.

(continued)

Table 7.1 (continued)

Organization name	Owners/stakeholders	Mission/vision	Example projects	How can they help me?
The Joint Commission (JCAHO) www.jointcommission.org	Private, not-for-profit organization. Founded in 1951 by the American College of Physicians, the American Medical Association, the American Hospital Association and the Canadian Medical Association. Funding from accreditation and on-site survey fees.	To continuously improve health care for the public, in collaboration with other stakeholders, by evaluating health care organizations and inspiring them to excel in providing safe and effective care of the highest quality and value.	Accreditation deems a hospital to be in compliance with Medicare and thus able to participate in the Medicare and Medicaid programs. Certification deems that an organization meets JCAHO's requirements in a specific area.	Operates a consumer quality check website (www.qualitycheck.org) to inform consumers about the accredited and certified hospitals and programs in their area. Has expanded topic-specific certification (Stroke certification) recently. No critical care option as of 2011.
Centers for Medicare and Medicaid Services (CMS) www.cms.gov	Agency of the US Federal Government. Part of the Department of Health and Human Services. Founded by law in 1965. Funding comes from payroll taxes and beneficiary copayments.	To ensure effective, up-to-date health care coverage and to promote quality care for beneficiaries.	Center for Medicare and Medicaid Innovation. Launched as part of the 2010 Affordable Care Act. Looks to help improve the structure of care delivery. Physician Quality Reporting System and EHR incentives provide additional money for clinicians, including Pay-for-Performance incentives.	Participate in Pay-for-Performance and other QI initiatives as they arise. HHS operates hospital compare (www.hospitalcompare.hhs.gov) which publishes process and outcome quality measures.
Agency for Healthcare Quality and Research (AHRQ) www.ahrq.gov	Agency of the US Federal government. Part of the Department of Health and Human Services. Established in 1989. Funding comes from US Federal budget.	To improve the quality, safety, efficiency and effectiveness of health care for all Americans.	Expanding Comparative Effectiveness and Health Information Technology research as part of the ACA.	Funds QI research. Helps implement Federal healthcare quality strategy.

National Quality Forum (NQF) www.qualityforum.org	Private, not-for-profit organization. Founded in 1999 by public- and private-sector leaders. Funding comes from public and private grants, including grants from the health care industry (Bristol-Myers Squibb Foundation, Cardinal Health Foundation).	To improve the quality of American healthcare by: Building consensus on national priorities and goals for performance improvement; Endorsing national consensus standards for measuring and publicly reporting on performance; Promoting the attainment of national goals through education and outreach programs	Provides input to CMS and other organizations about how to measure quality. Contracted by HHS to provide input for the National Quality Strategy.	Helps create quality standards. ICU-relevant measures include central line-related bloodstream infection prevention, incidence of venous thromboembolism, ventilator bundle.
American Association of Critical-Care Nurses (AACN) www.aacn.org	Private, not-for-profit professional organization. Founded in 1969 as the American Association of Cardiovascular Nurses. Funding comes from member dues, meetings and certifications.	Patients and their families rely on nurses at the most vulnerable times of their lives. Acute and critical care nurses rely on AACN for expert knowledge and the influence to fulfill their promise to patients and their families. AACN drives excellence because nothing less is acceptable.	Publications: *American Journal of Critical Care* Through AACN Certification Corporation offers certificates in 8 critical care disciplines. Created the Beacon Award for Excellence in Critical Care	Supports knowledge dissemination via *Practice Alerts*. Sponsors an annual conference, the National Teaching Institute and Critical Care Exposition.
Society of Critical Care Medicine (SCCM) www.sccm.org	Private, not-for-profit professional organization. Founded in 1970 by critical care professionals. Funding comes from member dues, meetings and educational activities.	To secure the highest quality care for all critically ill and injured patients.	Publications: *Critical Connections*, *Critical Care Medicine*. LearnICU (www.learnicu.org) an on-line learning environment that aggregates content, including articles, presentations and pod casts.	Offers for purchase the ICU REPORT as a QI tool to help clinicians assess their ICU. LearnICU contains learning resources for ICU care and quality improvement. Sponsors the annual Critical Care Congress.

(continued)

Table 7.1 (continued)

Organization name	Owners/stakeholders	Mission/vision	Example projects	How can they help me?
American Thoracic Society (ATS) www.thoracic.org	Private, not-for-profit professional organization. Founded in 1905 as the American Sanatorium Association. Funding comes from member dues, meetings and educational activities.	To improve health worldwide by advancing research, clinical care and public health in respiratory diseases, critical illness and sleep disorders.	Publications: *American Journal of Respiratory and Critical Care Medicine*.	Sponsors the annual ATS International Conference. Offers on-line educational resources, including videos and pod casts.
American College of Chest Physicians (ACCP) www.chestnet.org	Private, not-for-profit professional organization. Founded in 1935. Funding comes from member dues, meetings and educational activities.	To promote the prevention, diagnosis, and treatment of chest diseases through education, communication and research.	Publications: *Chest*.	Sponsors the annual Chest conference.

From the websites and publications of the organizations

process measures and used transparency as a tool by which to improve health care quality. The Institute for Health Care Improvement has supplied the health care industry with tools and resources that can help individuals and organizations lead change. This list does not even include state and local organizations or professional organizations that have an interest in quality or run a quality improvement program. The number of organizations who play some role in improving the quality of health care is dizzying.

The 2001 Crossing the Quality Chasm report from the Institute of Medicine described six aims of a safe, efficient, high-quality modern health care delivery system. Care should be: Safe, Effective, Patient-centered, Timely, Efficient and Equitable [32]. Don Berwick and the Institute for Health Care Improvement boiled this down to their Triple Aim: Improve the health of the population, Enhance the patient experience of care and Reduce (or at least control) the per capita cost of care [33].

Nuts and Bolts of Implementing Quality Improvement Steps

The IHI has developed tools that can help the busy ICU practitioner implement a quality improvement project. Table 7.1 highlights some resources that the interested practitioner can use to kindle his or her efforts. The Society of Critical Care Medicine has also published a Task Force Report outlining the practical steps for implementing a quality improvement project in the ICU [34].

The first step is to Discover a Common Purpose (Fig. 7.3). As a corollary of Crew Resource Management (CRM), we are more effective together than as individuals but only if we can work together as a team. What do the members of the ICU team think are the important quality priorities to tackle? We don't suffer for a lack of opportunity, we suffer from competing priorities. Central line infections, ventilator-associated pneumonia, and hand hygiene are all important infection control issues. But which should we choose to address first?

In selecting a project for a quality improvement effort, we would do well to recall the management saying that "you can't manage what you can't measure." In order to be readily amenable to a QI project an outcome must be measurable, frequent, and have significant variation. Death from fatal, hospital-acquired pulmonary embolism would not be a good outcome to measure for a QI project because it is relatively uncommon, although it is readily measurable and certainly represents variation from the intended result. Rather than measure that outcome, one could choose a process measure like implementation of DVT prophylaxis that occurs more frequently.

The IHI has developed a tool to help our scan of the environment to orient our attention and facilitate the development of common purpose: the ICU "Trigger Tool" [35]. It contains 23 events like transfusion, death and the initiation of dialysis that are easily identifiable in the medical record and that serve as markers of cases in which there was potential harm. Their intent is that the clinician or interested party

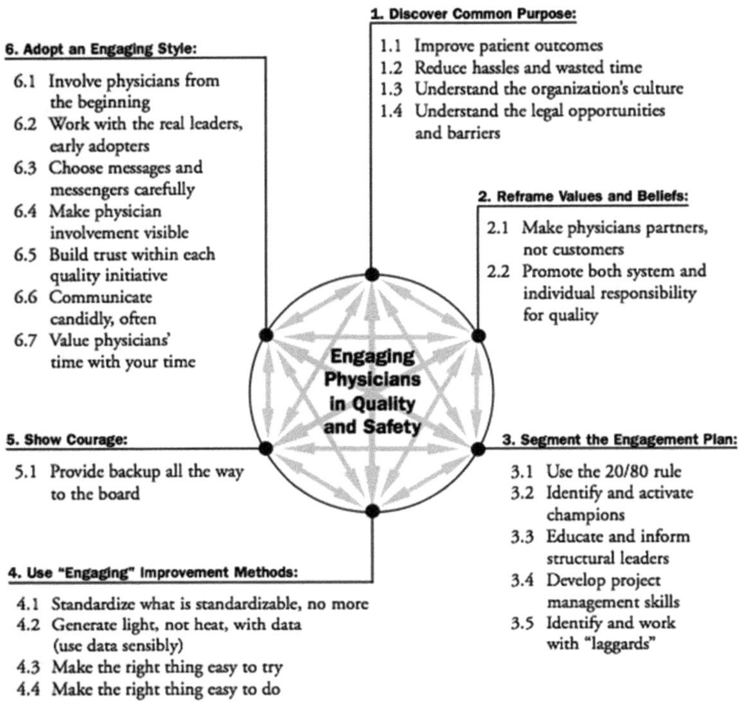

Fig. 7.3 Engaging clinicians in quality improvement

could then review the charts in which there was potential harm and then look for opportunities for quality improvement. The ICU trigger tool can also be used as a process/outcome measure for more diffuse, less focused ICU interventions.

Once an interested clinician has an idea of the best topic and has articulated a vision to help the team rally around a common purpose, the next step in the IHI's quality improvement framework is to Reframe Values and Beliefs. This begins the search for levers to move the quality of the ICU.

How can resistant clinicians be co-opted as allies? Clinician reluctance to participate in quality improvement activities often stems from a problem of competing values. Most of us share similar goals: We want patients to do well and have the best possible outcomes. For example, a clinician that is less adherent to full barrier protection might value his productivity and the use of fewer resources more than the extra time and resources that full barrier precautions take. Additionally central line infections are relatively rare outcomes and it would be plausible that the clinician had not had one of his lines infected to his knowledge. Engaging reluctant clinicians often focuses on attempts to Reframe Values and Beliefs (Step 2). We must make the patient care, business and mission-focused case for quality improvement for the proposed project to be a success and sometimes reframe the presentation of the intervention so that it can successfully compete with other priorities.

Once we have defined our common purpose and achieved tentative buy-in from the various system participants, we must examine the engagement plan, which might be described as the "art of the possible." The IHI describes this part of the process as Segmenting the Engagement Plan (Step 3). We should first look for the clinician champions, those people whose experience, temperaments, and perspectives lead them to be natural allies of the quality improvement efforts. These people can be used as levers or force-multipliers to spread the word about the quality improvement effort and to move the organization along. One valuable roll that influential clinicians can have is that they can engage the reluctant clinician and work with them from peer perspective versus a management, top-down perspective.

The method used to deploy the quality improvement project requires deliberate thought. We must consider the intervention, the way that it is rolled out and the way that data about it are collected and reported [36].

Standardize what is standardizable, no more (Step 4). It would be a significant undertaking to create a protocol that covers all the situations in which mechanical ventilation would need to be begun in the ICU. It would be less work to come up with agreement about the "standard" or default mode and settings for initial mechanical ventilation. The goal of choosing the intervention is not to come up with the perfect protocol on the first go-around. Rather the purpose is to come up with a starting point and try several different iterations until one that works the best for all involved is found.

Generate light not heat with data (Step 5). Clinicians are quite good at finding reasons why quality data don't apply to them or mean something different. "My patients are sicker." Clinicians are trained data skeptics, which often serves us well in our patient care activities. We are appropriately reluctant to accept data that seems to contradict what we think we know from other sources, a heuristic sometimes called the anchoring-bias [37]. Additionally, the message that accompanies data presentation is of paramount importance. Data that show non-ideal performance on a metric could be interpreted as "you are a bad clinician" if not presented correctly. It is more effective to present system data as system data and individual data as individual data. Risk adjusted mortality has many non-clinician contributing factors, while individual hand hygiene adherence rates are clinician-specific. It is also helpful to compare clinicians to the ideal standard or goal and not to each other or an external benchmark.

Make the right thing easy to try and to do (Step 6). A new order set reconciliation process that takes 200 % more time will fight against the competing value of efficiency and the opportunity cost of the additional minutes that it will take. If that same activity is easier it becomes, in the phrasing of health economics, the dominant solution that is both cheaper (in terms of time) and better (in terms of outcome). It is not logical that we will always get to the better solution on the first try and clinicians are a naturally risk-adverse group. It is helpful to enter the process with the mindset of trying a number of small steps or ideas. This will soften some resistance to trying new things and may make clinicians less wedded to their own idea. The goal is to create a system that continually strives to improve itself.

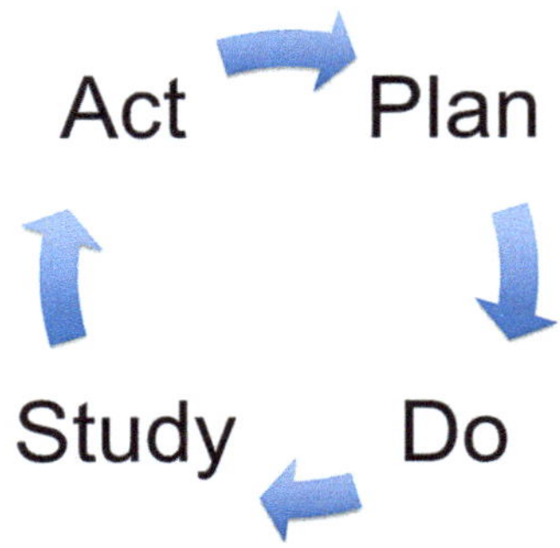

Fig. 7.4 The Plan-Do-Study-Act cycle

The final step in the IHI plan is a strategy to be employed throughout the quality improvement process: Show Courage. The proposed quality improvement project has to fit within the organization's strategic plan. For larger, more resource intense projects that means having support and back-up all the way to the organization's board of directors. In smaller projects that operationally means that the leaders of the involved segment of the organization have buy-in and value the underlying philosophy or belief of the quality improvement project. The final step in the IHI process is to Adopt an Engaging Style. This could be rephrased as "look for levers." Impacted parties, including the real opinion leaders in the group, should be involved from the beginning. Communication should be frequent, open, and honest. These seven steps from the IHI detail a conceptual framework from which to approach a quality improvement project, but they don't describe the nuts and bolts of how to get the project done.

If we return to Industrial Quality Management in the 1920s, we find the single most helpful and powerful quality improvement tool, the Plan-Do-Study-Act (PDSA) cycle (Fig. 7.4). Developed by Walter Shewart in the 1920s, this tool can focus and direct quality improvement efforts [7]. Indeed, the PDSA cycle is the engine that powers Toyota's process improvement method and the IHI's seven step tool.

Plan

The first element in the PDSA cycle is the plan. What is it that we are trying to accomplish? How will we do it? The IHI model for engaging clinicians in quality improvement focuses on this key step in the PDSA cycle. The right people in the organization need to be ready to affect change. The change needs to be rolled out in the right way. We need to be able to measure the process or outcome that we're changing as well as be able to measure any relevant amount of change. We also need baseline data to suggest that we have a problem we think we can fix. All of these elements are in the planning phase of the PDSA cycle.

Do

After we have our Plan in place, we need to Do it. There will be hiccups and unintended and unanticipated consequences. This is an iterative process. The goal is not to be perfect the first time. The goal is to keep working together as a team towards the common objective. As we "Do" it, we must make sure that we are measuring what we are trying to manage. Congratulate people for going through the process. Reward small steps. Build momentum.

Study

How do the consequences of our project compare to our intended effects? The results of the project should be summarized and the lessons learned shared. Harkening back to the IHI model, we should strive to communicate candidly and often. For this step, it can be helpful to have experienced database manager and statistical analysts who are familiar with the presentation of quality improvement data. We should compare our process and outcome data with our desired goal.

Act

How can we modify our plan to improve it? Are we measuring the right processes and outcomes? Do we have the right stakeholders engaged? What can be done to improve our intervention? We then go back to the drawing board and Plan on ways to improve the intervention and the cycle begins again.

This PDSA activity obviously consumes a significant amount of staff time, resources, and mental energy. This is a difficult thing. Our QI project should be chosen based on clinical need and the availability and practicability of the various quality improvement levers from which we can choose. Quality improvement is truly the art of the possible. We should engage those around us and look for levers to improve quality.

Where Do We Go from Here?

Damon Scales and his team have shown in Ontario and Peter Pronovost and his team have shown in Michigan that large-scale and successful quality improvement efforts are possible [11, 38]. We all have seen QI projects both flourish and flounder in our ICUs. Despite the tragedies of Libby Zion and Betsy Lehman, medication errors still happen today. Some have estimated that the number of deaths from medical harm has not decreased significantly since publication of the IOM *To Err Is Human* report in 1999 [39]. Despite all the good efforts to improve the quality of care delivered in our ICUs, they remain lifesaving and dangerous places. But this is our starting point. We have a great opportunity to work together as a multidisciplinary team to measure and improve the quality of our care processes and patient outcomes.

> Never doubt that a small group of thoughtful, committed citizens can change the world. Indeed, it is the only thing that ever has. Margarget Mead

References

1. Batalden P, Davidoff F. Teaching quality improvement: the devil is in the details. JAMA. 2007;298(9):1059–61.
2. Asch DA, Parker RM. The Libby Zion case. One step forward or two steps backward? N Engl J Med. 1988;318(12):771–5.
3. Conway J, Nathan D, Benz E. Key learning from the Dana–Farber Cancer Institute's 10-year patient safety journey. Alexandria: American Society of Clinical Oncology; 2006 (2006 Educational Book).
4. Institute of Medicine. To err is human: building a safer health system. 1st ed. Washington, DC: National Academies Press; 2000.
5. Brennan TA, Gawande A, Thomas E, Studdert D. Accidental deaths, saved lives, and improved quality. N Engl J Med. 2005;353(13):1405–9.
6. Best M, Neuhauser D. W Edwards Deming: father of quality management, patient and composer. Qual Saf Health Care. 2005;14(4):310–2.
7. Ransom ER, Joshi MS, Nash DB, Ransom SB. The healthcare quality book: vision, strategy, and tools. 2nd ed. Chicago: Health Administration Press; 2008.
8. Zarbo RJ, D'Angelo R. Transforming to a quality culture: The Henry Ford production system. Pathol Patterns Rev. 2006;126 Suppl 1:21–9.
9. Sunol R. Avedis Donabedian. International J Qual Health Care. 2000;12(6):451–4.
10. Donabedian A. Evaluating the quality of medical care. Milbank Memorial Fund Q. 1966;44:166–203.
11. Pronovost P, Needham D, Berenholtz S, Sinopoli D, Chu H, Cosgrove S, et al. An intervention to decrease catheter-related bloodstream infections in the ICU. N Engl J Med. 2006;355 (26):2725–32.
12. Reason J. Human error: models and management. BMJ. 2000;320(7237):768–70.
13. Wiegmann D, Shappell S. Human error analysis of commercial aviation accidents: application of the Human Factors Analysis and Classification System (HFACS). Aviat Space Environ Med. 2001;72(11):1006–16.
14. AHRQ WebM&M: Morbidity & mortality rounds on the web. http://www.webmm.ahrq.gov/perspective.aspx?perspectiveID=3. Cited 15 November 2011.
15. O'Connor NR. FDA boxed warnings: how to prescribe drugs safely. Am Fam Physician. 2010;81(3):298–303.
16. Washington State Hospital Association: Quality & safety. http://www.wsha.org/qualitySafety.cfm. Cited 22 November 2011.
17. Haynes AB, Weiser TG, Berry WR, Lipsitz SR, Breizat A-HS, Dellinger EP, et al. A surgical safety checklist to reduce morbidity and mortality in a global population. N Engl J Med. 2009;360(5):491–9.

18. Weiss CH, Moazed F, McEvoy CA, Singer BD, Szleifer I, Amaral LAN, et al. Prompting physicians to address a daily checklist and process of care and clinical outcomes: a single-site study. Am J Respir Crit Care Med. 2011;184(6):680–6.
19. Abbett SK, Yokoe DS, Lipsitz SR, Bader AM, Berry WR, Tamplin EM, Gawande AA. Proposed checklist of hospital interventions to decrease the incidence of healthcare-associated Clostridium difficile infection. Infect Control Hosp Epidemiol. 2009;30:1062–9. http://dx.doi.org/10.1086/644757.
20. Ely EW, Baker AM, Dunagan DP, Burke HL, Smith AC, Kelly PT, et al. Effect on the duration of mechanical ventilation of identifying patients capable of breathing spontaneously. N Engl J Med. 1996;335(25):1864–9.
21. Kress JP, Pohlman AS, O'Connor MF, Hall JB. Daily interruption of sedative infusions in critically ill patients undergoing mechanical ventilation. N Engl J Med. 2000;342(20):1471–7.
22. Girard TD, Kress JP, Fuchs BD, Thomason JWW, Schweickert WD, Pun BT, et al. Efficacy and safety of a paired sedation and ventilator weaning protocol for mechanically ventilated patients in intensive care (Awakening and Breathing Controlled trial): a randomised controlled trial. Lancet. 2008;371(9607):126–34.
23. Krishnan JA, Moore D, Robeson C, Rand CS, Fessler HE. A prospective, controlled trial of a protocol-based strategy to discontinue mechanical ventilation. Am J Respir Crit Care Med. 2004;169(6):673–8.
24. NICE-SUGAR Study Investigators, Finfer S, Chittock DR, Su SY-S, Blair D, Foster D, et al. Intensive versus conventional glucose control in critically ill patients. N Engl J Med. 2009;360(13):1283–97.
25. Finney SJ, Zekveld C, Elia A, Evans TW. Glucose control and mortality in critically ill patients. JAMA. 2003;290(15):2041–7.
26. Gawande A. The checklist manifesto: how to get things right. 1st ed. New York: Picador; 2011.
27. Nance JJ. Why hospitals should fly: the ultimate flight plan to patient safety and quality care. 1st ed. Bozeman: Second River Healthcare Press; 2008.
28. Sax HC, Browne P, Mayewski RJ, Panzer RJ, Hittner KC, Burke RL, et al. Can aviation-based team training elicit sustainable behavioral change? Arch Surg. 2009;144(12):1133.
29. Gladwell M. Outliers: the story of success. New York: Back Bay Books; 2011.
30. Haig KM, Sutton S, Whittington J. SBAR: a shared mental model for improving communication between clinicians. Jt Comm J Qual Patient Saf. 2006;32(3):167–75.
31. Telem DA, Buch KE, Ellis S, Coakley B, Divino CM. Integration of a formalized handoff system into the surgical curriculum: resident perspectives and early results. Arch Surg. 2011;146(1):89–93.
32. IOM. Crossing the quality chasm: a new health system for the 21st century. Washington, DC: National Academy Press; 2001. p. 1–8.
33. Berwick DM, Nolan TW, Whittington J. The triple aim: care, health, and cost. Health Aff. 2008;27(3):759–69.
34. Curtis JR, Cook DJ, Wall RJ, Angus DC, Bion J, Kacmarek R, et al. Intensive care unit quality improvement: a "how-to" guide for the interdisciplinary team. Crit Care Med. 2006;34 (1):211–8.
35. Resar RK, Rozich JD, Simmonds T, Haraden CR. A trigger tool to identify adverse events in the intensive care unit. Jt Comm J Qual Patient Saf. 2006;32(10):585–90.
36. Reinertsen J, Gosfield A, Rupp W, Whittington J. Engaging physicians in a shared quality agenda. Cambridge: IHI Innovation Series white paper; 2007. http://www.ihi.org
37. Tversky A, Kahneman D. Judgment under uncertainty: heuristics and biases. Science. 1974;185(4157):1124–31.
38. Scales DC, Dainty K, Hales B, Pinto R, Fowler RA, Adhikari NKJ, et al. A multifaceted intervention for quality improvement in a network of intensive care units: a cluster randomized trial. JAMA. 2011;305(4):363–72.
39. Goodman JC, Villarreal P, Jones B. The social cost of adverse medical events, and what we can do about it. Health Aff. 2011;30(4):590–5.

Chapter 8
Facilitating Interactions Between Healthcare Providers in the ICU

Andre Carlos Kajdacsy-Balla Amaral

Abstract Healthcare organizations are dynamic and complex systems that require multiple subjects to achieve its goals. Therefore it is no surprise that communication is a fundamental process in these systems, and that failures in communication are associated with worse outcomes. However, the term communication without a formal definition is nothing more than an elusive concept. In this chapter we borrow from an established mathematical framework of communication and use it as the basis to identify sources of errors in communication, discuss the main moments of communication in the ICU, and contextualize how communication tools, such as interdisciplinary rounds, standardization, pre-printed orders (PPOs), algorithms and language style, can help improve communication and increase the efficiency of healthcare and patient safety.

Keywords Communication • Mathematical theory • Patient safety • Efficiency • Interdisciplinary rounds • Protocols • Language

The Importance of Communication

Communication lies in the center of all socio-cultural interactions [1]. Human actions are a product of social interactions and are preceded by some sort of communication. Therefore, it follows that communication is a necessary component of systems composed of more than one subject, to initiate and guide actions towards achieving a goal.

A.C. Kajdacsy-Balla Amaral (✉)
Department of Critical Care Medicine, Sunnybrook Health Sciences Centre, Office D1 08, 2075 Bayview Avenue, Toronto, ON, Canada

Interdepartmental Division of Critical Care Medicine, University of Toronto, Toronto, ON, Canada
e-mail: AndreCarlos.Amaral@sunnybrook.ca

D.C. Scales and G.D. Rubenfeld (eds.), *The Organization of Critical Care*, Respiratory Medicine 18, DOI 10.1007/978-1-4939-0811-0_8,

Healthcare organizations are dynamic and complex systems that require multiple subjects to achieve its goals. Therefore it is no surprise that communication is frequently described as a fundamental process in these systems. However, the term communication without a formal definition is nothing more than an elusive concept. To further improve our understanding on communication processes a clearly defined model is necessary. The most frequently cited mathematical model of communication is based on the seminal work of Shannon [2], which describes communication as the flow of information between two points. However this definition is insufficient to support models of communication in complex organizations, as it doesn't take into account two other fundamental aspects of communication: the social determinants of communication and the cognitive processes that happen when a subject receives some sort of stimulus. In this chapter we will borrow from an established mathematical framework of communication [3] that will serve as the basis to identify sources of errors in communication, discuss the main moments of communication in the ICU, and contextualize how communication tools can improve patient care.

A Theory of Communication

A broader definition states that communicative processes occur in complex dynamical systems and are modulated by cognitive dynamics and social context.

For the sake of communication in healthcare, the complex dynamical systems are the people involved in communicative processes. When a person is exposed to an external stimulus, defined as any type of visual, auditory, olfactory, or auditory signal, he or she will infer a certain meaning and create a certain degree of information associated with the stimulus. Communication is thus the exchange of *information* and *meaning* between at least one pair of subjects, which is modulated by social aspects of this interaction and ultimately leads to an action agreed by the two subjects [3].

Subjects involved in the process of communication have different cognitive processes and generate different degrees of information and meanings after the initial stimulus. Furthermore, the *social aspects* of the interaction—such as hierarchical position, professional background, age, gender—will influence the amount, type and quality of information and meaning. For communication to occur properly, it is necessary that the subjects achieve a shared meaning about the situation. This definition will prove very useful in understanding sources of errors, in making diagnostic considerations on why communication is failing and in identifying solutions.

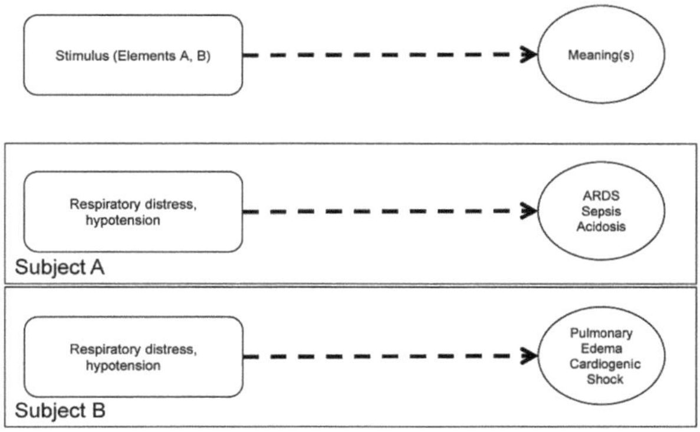

Fig. 8.1 The formation of meaning after an stimulus

Meaning of a Stimulus

Meaning is the generation of a specific mental image in relation to a specific external stimulus, composed of a certain number of elements (Fig. 8.1). Subjects generate several mental images in response to a certain stimulus and unconsciously attribute probabilities to each of them, which are dependent on previous experiences. For example, an intensivist who sees a patient in respiratory distress may think "intubation," "acute respiratory distress syndrome," "sepsis." The same stimulus may lead to different meanings depending on the background of the person receiving the information. A cardiologist seeing the same patient may immediately think "pulmonary edema," "noninvasive ventilation," "myocardial infarction." A simpler example is to consider the word "food" in a language and present it to a native speaker and to someone who has no knowledge of that language. Although the stimulus is the same, the meanings will be completely different. The native speaker will understand the immediate meaning and may generate other mediate meanings such as "I'm hungry," "what will I have for dinner," etc..., while the other person will generate meanings that may relate to how the word sounds in their own language. In healthcare a large part of training is dedicated to teaching the meaning of certain stimulus to facilitate shared understanding by all subjects; but there are elements that may still generate different meanings, especially between professions (e.g., physicians and nurses) and between disciplines (e.g., surgeons and internists). One of the goals of improving communication is to find solutions that facilitate sharing the meaning of terms by clinicians.

Information Contained in a Stimulus

The degree of information contained in a stimulus is proportional to its negative probability [2]. This is to say that the more unexpected the stimulus, the more

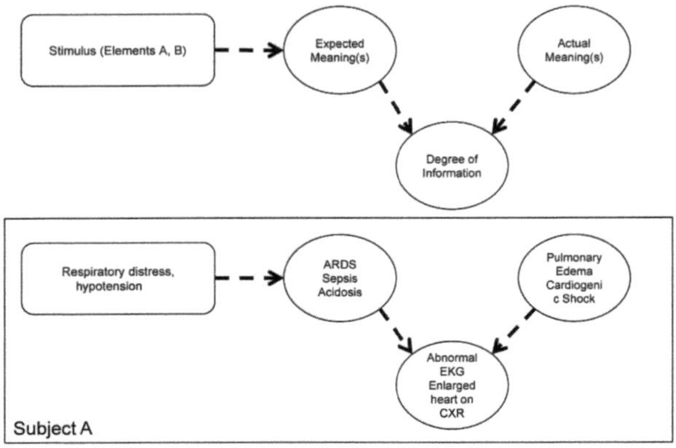

Fig. 8.2 Degree of information contained in a stimulus

information it contains for that subject (Fig. 8.2). This is akin to hearing a joke, where one creates a certain expectation (or meaning) based on the story (stimulus), but is usually surprised by events that unfold. The difference in the final events and the expectation created by the person is the degree of information contained in the joke (the better the joke, the higher the degree of information, or surprises, it contains). For a pair of subjects involved in communication the degree of information received by each can vary by several degrees, depending on each subject's previous knowledge on the subject. For an experienced intensivist the stimulus "septic shock" triggers an association with multiple organ failure. A trainee may not have developed the same association to the word "septic shock" and may be surprised by seeing the patient developing thrombocytopenia, acute renal failure, and acidosis. Thus, the degree of information contained in septic shock with multiple organ failure is higher for the trainee than for the experienced intensivist. Of course, the higher the degree of information available (or the more "surprises" are observed in the new information), the more meanings a person creates to understand the situation, and the longer it will take for the two communicators to achieve a shared understanding. Therefore, a case discussion between two experienced intensivists is likely to take less time than a case discussion between an intensivist and a trainee.

Sharing Meaning and Information

The cognitive processes of creating meaning and generating a certain degree of information occur within a subject. Communication occurs when these meanings and information are shared with another subject, who will then assimilate this new stimulus to create new meanings and/or provide information on elements that were as yet not discussed. The exchange of meanings and information will ultimately

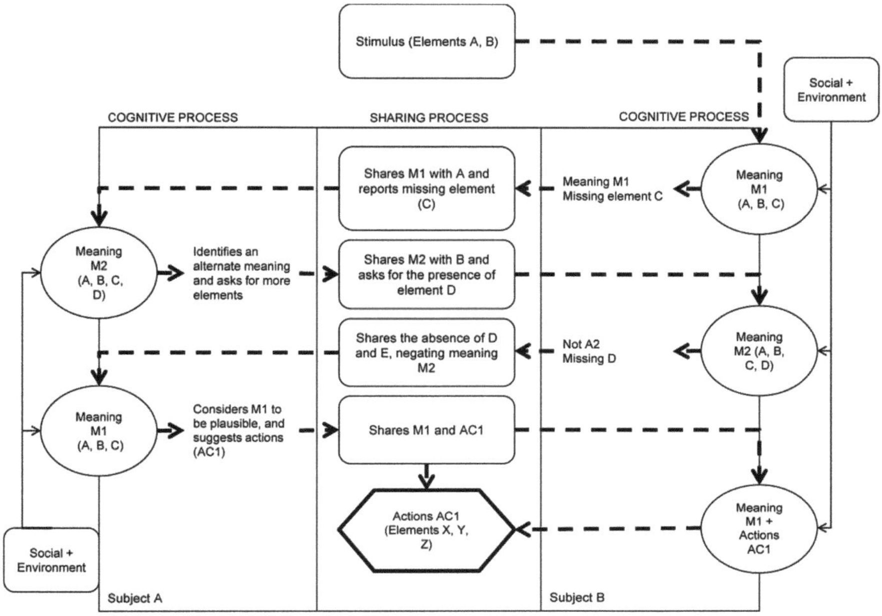

Fig. 8.3 Framework for a communicative process

lead to a proposition for actions, agreed between the two subjects (Figs. 8.3 and 8.4). If the process of communication always occurred in such a rational and elegant way, it would be simple to have great communication, because it only depends on the cognitive processes of each subject. Therefore perfect cognition should lead to perfect communication. However, social and environmental aspects of the interaction influence both cognitive and sharing processes.

Environmental Influences on Communicative Processes

The discussion above assumes that subjects are always working at an ideal state to work on cognitive processes. However, environmental factors may influence cognitive processes and decrease the number of different meanings generated after a stimulus, as well as limit the comparison to other meanings (or analogies) based on the previous experiences of the subject. In this sense, the cognitive functions of the subject are the same, but they are decreased by a factor "X," that is present in the environment. We define these environmental factors as external conditions that may decrease the ideal cognitive function of a subject, limiting the identification of meanings, the association of the perceived meaning with previous experiences and their ability to share concepts (Fig. 8.5).

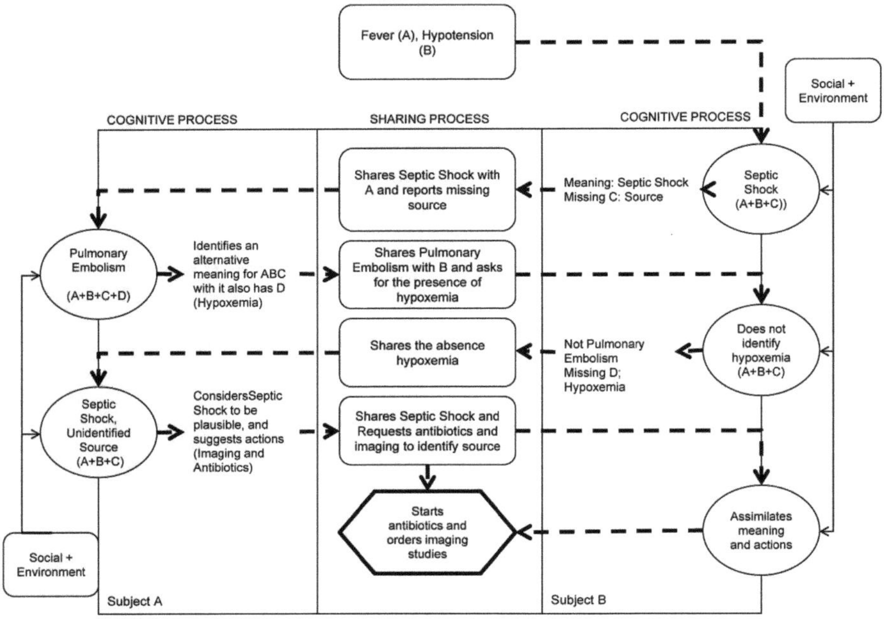

Fig. 8.4 Example of a framework for a communicative process

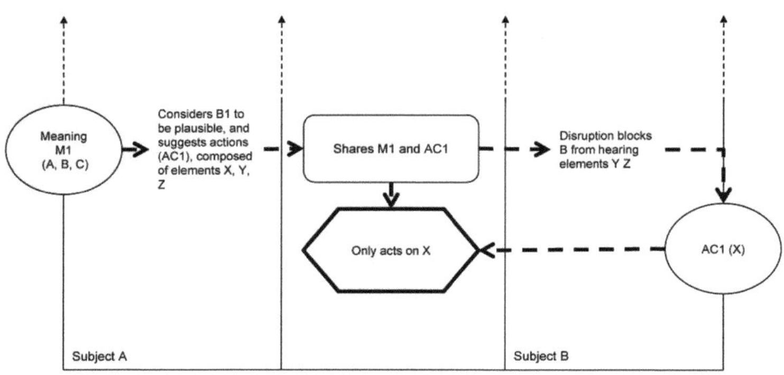

Fig. 8.5 An environmental factor (disruption of rounds) blocking the sharing process from A to B

Typical environmental factors that can influence communication processes are (1) strenuous conditions (such as being awake at night or having an excessive number of patients); (2) emotional distress; and (3) time constraints. For example, if an intern spends the night awake on call, it is more likely that some information may not be shared, such as pointing out that a patient became hypotensive over night and required the initiation of vasopressors. Likewise, if the nurse caring for this patient is having family problems, it is more likely that the meaning "septic shock" will not be generated as a limitation of the current cognitive processes.

Thus, if this patient has septic shock, it is possible that antibiotics will be delayed until rounds occur. If a decision needs to be made within a certain time frame, such as when making decisions during acute resuscitation or a medical crisis, the amount of time to generate several different meanings, compare them to previous experiences, share between the members of the groups, and decide on the best way to act is limited, therefore the communicative process will be fairly limited and designed to optimize actions that are relevant to the most common meanings.

Social Influences on Communicative Processes

We will briefly explore a theory of social differentiation [4], which will lead to the concepts of social dimensions. We will use these dimensions to add social influences as another parameter in our framework of communicative processes. All societies evolve through three stages: (1) *segmentation*, characteristic of early tribe societies, where the differentiation between subjects is determined by social segments, mainly defined by kinship relations, such as the formation of clans; (2) *stratification*, where a new structure evolved to include the distinction between "higher" and "lower" persons, characteristic of the middle-ages, with the well-known development of social inequalities. In stratified societies segmentation ("clans") is still relevant *within* each stratum; (3) *functionalism*, where members are differentiated by their societal function (e.g., scientists, politicians, economists, teachers…), each of them being functionally autonomous. Society members are usually active in a single functional segment, although they participate in the other segments as well. For example, a politician benefits from the educational segment when his or her children attend school. Within each segment, the goal is to maximize growth, be it economic, scientific, educational, etc.… Again, within a functional structure the preceding rules of social differentiation are still valid. For example, there may be different ranks of professors in a university and within each rank there may be "clans" organized by affinity.

As the three stages of differentiation co-exist, we can think of each of them in terms of *social dimensions* [3]. The first social dimension is how "alike" two individuals are, and this is of course a very fluid concept, and may include concepts such as citizenship, where someone lives, stage in life and background. We define the *affinity distance* between subjects as how similar they see the other subject to themselves. Greater affinity distances impair communication. A second social dimension is rank. Individuals assign each other ranks in specific social situations and may see themselves as "higher," "lower," or in the "same" rank as the other subject. For example, a soldier will recognize the higher rank of a lieutenant while in the army, but may (or may not!) assign the same rank when they meet in a non-military party. Greater rank distances impair communication. A third social dimension is the amount of knowledge on a specific function that a subject has. More knowledgeable subjects will assume a more active role in communications, while less knowledgeable subjects will assume a more passive role. Greater

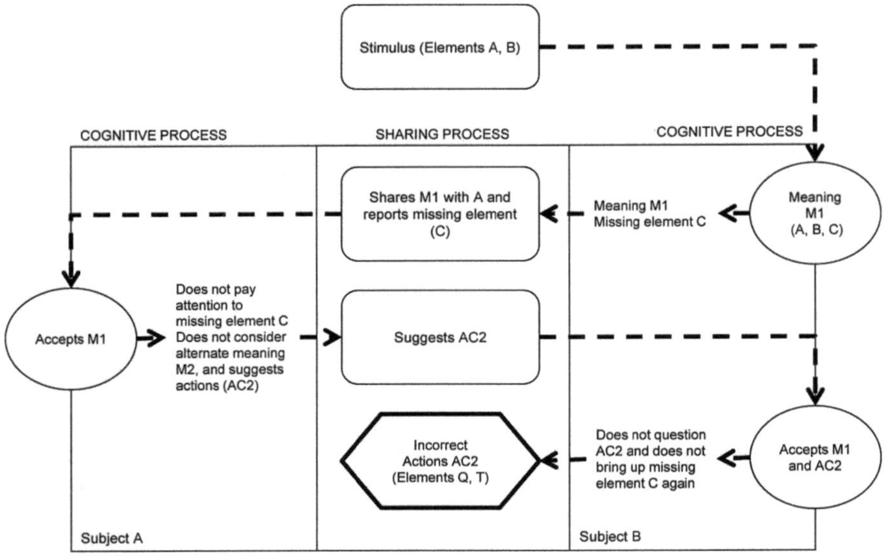

Fig. 8.6 Communicative process when social distance is high

knowledge distances impair communication. Mathematically, the previous three terms can be combined to generate a summary *social distance*. Greater social distances impair communication. For example, the communication between an elderly professor of critical care medicine and a young intern rotating through critical care who has no interest in critical care has an elevated social distance, as there are great distances in affinity, rank, and knowledge. It is likely that the intern will simply do as told, not engaging in discussions regarding diagnosis or plans of care by the professor (Fig. 8.6). This situation may change if the subjects recognize the social distances and try to overcome these barriers to communication. It is easy to think about numerous examples that are influenced by social distances in critical care (conflicts among different specialties, related to *knowledge distance*; inattention to important clinical information given by a junior resident by staff, related to *rank distance*; and poor handoffs between residents, related to *affinity distance*).

The Effects of Memory on Communication

Although not a formal part of the theory of communication, the amount of memory processing capacity of human beings has an important influence on communication.

In the special case of complex communications, where a large amount of new information is available (e.g., case discussions) or a large number of possible meanings exist (e.g., complex case with a large list of differential diagnosis), a subject's memory span may limit the processing of stimuli and meanings. Human memory span has a limit of dealing with 7 (±2) items in a single dimension at a time [5], which may block handling new information and creating a large number of meanings at the same time when this value is exceeded. There are two important elements to deal with this limitation in healthcare, the first is to increase the number of cognitive units, or subjects, dealing with the same problem, which may expand the processing capacity of the group, such as during interdisciplinary rounds. The second element is related to expertise. Since the degree of information contained in a stimulus is the difference between the observed and the expected concepts, people who have a larger number of pre-established concepts will generate a smaller degree of information when faced with a new stimulus, therefore requiring the memorization of a smaller number of elements to generate meanings and decide on actions. This is the role of experienced clinicians during case discussions and rounds.

Moments of Communication in Healthcare

Healthcare is a teamwork profession because we cannot achieve adequate results by the work of a single individual [6]. Teamwork is essentially communication and co-ordination of information and actions between subjects working towards a common goal, therefore communication underpins the results of teamwork and directly influences the quality of care. In healthcare there are different moments of communication, such as rounds and case discussions, orders or transitions of care; and different types of communication, such as verbal or written, on or off-site and synchronous or asynchronous.

Each form of communication has its pros and cons and may be better suited to specific tasks. *Verbal* communication is richer than *written*, can generate a very complex discussion, allows the subjects to clarify meanings and concepts, but also requires synchronicity (subjects must be available at the same time), may take a longer time than written communication, and also requires the limitation of environmental factors to a minimum. Written communication makes clarification more difficult, is prone to misunderstandings, but can help overcome memory limitations, may be asynchronous, which permits people to work on their own time, and may use aids such as note templates and pre-printed orders (PPOs), which enhance efficiency. *On- or off-site* communication refers to communication done with the presence of the subjects in the same space or in different spaces via phone, Internet, text messaging, amongst others. Off-site is more inclusive, as it does not depend on sharing the same physical space, but the loss of visual contact may impede the communication of nonverbal signs that make an important part of face-to-face communication. *Synchronicity* refers to sharing information at the same time. Some communications, especially those that are not time sensitive, may not require the subjects to share information at the same time. One subject may write an email that the other will only read and reply later on.

We will review each moment of communication focusing on participants, types of communication, social distances, and environmental factors.

Multidisciplinary Rounds and Case Discussions

Multidisciplinary rounds are one of the most important moments for communication, as they are the main moment to discuss diagnoses, uncertainties and make decisions on a plan of care for each patient, while taking into consideration the perceptions of every member of the team. Rounds are composed of several different members of the healthcare team, such as physicians, nurses, respiratory therapists, dietitians, pharmacists, physical therapists, occupational therapists, families, social workers, chaplaincy, and others, in variable formats and in variable ranks within each group (for example, attending physician, fellow and resident). The opportunity to gather such a heterogeneous group means that several distinct cognitive processes are available, which enlarges the cognitive pool, enriching the discussion and the generation of different and relevant meanings for a given patient. Communication is usually conducted verbally, synchronous and on-site, with the possibility of using written tools as well, such as daily goals [7]. The introduction of multidisciplinary rounds is associated with better outcomes for patients [8] and is certainly an important tool to improve communication. However it is a tool that is difficult to generalize, as social distances are usually high and an adequate flow of communication may depend on the abilities of the person leading discussions to decrease potential barriers. Rounds are also affected by environmental factors as it needs to be finished within a certain time, participants may get tired and disruptions are common due to the acute demands of other patients.

Case discussions are communications about specific patients outside the formal, scheduled rounds. They may involve updates on a patient during or after rounds, the admission of a new patient to the service or discussions with consulting services. Updates on a patient and new admissions share many similarities with rounds, except for the presence of a smaller group and the possibility of off-site communication (for example, when a nurse calls the resident to give an update on the patient). Although one may think that case discussions with consultants would also be similar, there is one important difference. Communications between two medical teams have the threat of conflict due to a large symmetric knowledge distance. Each team possesses greater knowledge in their field and may fail to recognize the other team's expertise in their specific field. This situation may create large social distances, making communication very difficult. Smaller distances in the other areas, such as affinity and function, can attenuate this effect.

Case discussions are also highly influenced by environmental factors. For example, take the situation where a resident is discussing a new admission with the staff. If the patient is stable, there is time to consider several differential diagnoses and design a plan of care that may involve treatment for the most likely diagnosis, as well as investigations and consultations to clarify uncertain elements. If the same patient is hypotensive and in respiratory failure, many important actions need to carried out immediately, thus limiting the amount of discussion.

Transitions of Care

Different teams see patients over the course of their hospital stay. As patient care responsibility is transitioned to different services in the hospital ("between teams handoff") and to different professionals during successive work shifts ("within team handoff"), the communication of information pertinent to patient care is fundamental for continuity of care. This process is known as "handoff" and closely related names, such as "sign-out," "sign-over," or "handover" [9]. The primary focus of a handoff is to provide information about patients that will allow for increased effectiveness and safety of actions from the receiving party [10]. The medical literature is abundant with examples on the linkage between handoffs and quality of care. There is indirect and direct empiric evidence linking handoff to several unwanted outcomes, such as adverse events, surgical errors, malpractice claims, increased costs, and decreased efficiency [11–17]. Several observations, demonstrating that handoffs are poorly conducted, provide the rationale for these outcomes. For example, trainees reported "surprises" after a handoff in 14 % of 426 days [18]. In the pediatric setting, trainees identified that they lacked clinical information to manage 80 % of events that occurred at night, and observed that 75 % of these could have been anticipated and discussed during handoffs [19].

There is a large variation in the practice of handoffs [20]. They may occur verbally, in written format or using a combination of both. They are mostly synchronous, but may occur asynchronously, when a resident leaves a written sign-out for another one. They may occur on- or off-site. As with the previous example of rounds, handoffs are especially prone to social and environmental factors. For example, there is a large variation in the time dedicated to handoffs, ranging from 5 min to 1 h [21, 22]. Time is an important factor in the quality of handoffs and explains why trainees identified over-the-phone handoffs (which are time-constrained) to be less appropriate than face-to-face communication [11], even though phone handoffs still present with the opportunity for clarification. The location where handoffs are conducted also changes the dynamics of the communication: moving away from the bedside decreases the number of interruptions and background noise [23], whereas proximity to the bedside allows for (1) visual observation of the patient, which provides cues for subjects to engage in the conversation [24], and (2) direct access to information resources, such as medical records and other team members who will frequently join the discussion to complement the information [25, 26].

Orders

Orders are a special type of communication. They are the last step of converting communication into action. Orders are usually documented in a written format, although some may exist temporarily in verbal form only, if there are time constraints that limit documentation. Orders are synchronous or asynchronous, depending on the urgency, and can be taken on or off-site (such as telephone orders). The ideal order should be written, synchronous and on-site, as the other forms of communication are more prone to lack of clarity. Although this is one of the simpler types of communication, it is nonetheless still subject to social and environmental interactions. Social distances may inhibit the person who has to implement an order to ask for clarification on the order or to challenge the order if it is felt to be incorrect. Environmental factors may impede the enactor of an order from hearing all the elements, due to disruptions or time constraints. Furthermore, the person formulating the plan of action may be fatigued and unable to include all the necessary elements.

Tools and Strategies to Improve Communication in the ICU

Rounds

As we have previously discussed, multidisciplinary rounds are an effective way to gather different perspectives in the same time and space to discuss a patient. This initiative is in itself a tool to improve communication, and mortality in units that have multidisciplinary rounds are 22 % lower [8]. These results were robust in subgroup analyses of sicker patients, ventilated patients and patients with sepsis, and was independent of the effect of intensivist staffing.

Communication Tools

Several types of communication tools exist, mainly focused on transitions of care. They may vary from very simple, such as taking notes during the conversation, to more complex, such as fully electronic handoff systems. Using some form of written aid seems to be the most important step. In a simulation study of information discontinuity, where residents were asked to transfer information up to five times (akin to the playing "broken telephone"), the isolated use of verbal communication led to a loss of 70 % of information in the first communication, up to almost 100 % by the fifth communication. In contrast, the use of a pre-printed format or simply allowing note taking led to loss of less than 10 % of information in the first communication to a maximum of 20 % after the fifth communication [27].

Standardization and templates

Quality improvement organizations encourage the use of certain communication tools [28], such as SBAR [29] (situation, background, assessment, recommendations) and others. However very little empirical evidence supports improvement in the quality of communication with these tools [30], which is not unexpected, as they do not cover the relevant social and environmental factors modulating communication. Furthermore, experienced clinicians do not use such a fixed format of communication [31], which suggests that these formats do not follow a natural linguistic process. Also, subjectively, residents perceive that close adherence to pre-designed data forms was conducive to more errors [18].

Electronic Systems

The use of electronic generated handoff systems reduces the length of handoffs [32] and provides a more accurate and consistent content [33]. Despite generating legitimate fears of introducing new problems (such as the persistence of incorrect information), the introduction of a computerized system was associated with a decrease in adverse events in at least one report [34]. However, problems may still exist with the use of electronic systems, such as the persistence of incorrect or outdated information in the record [35].

Protocols

We define protocols as a set of instructions on how to provide care specific to a clinical condition. This can involve the use of PPOs and can be combined with flow-diagrams when the process involves multiple steps that depend on the individual response of patients. Protocols have four specific attributes that facilitate communication and adoption of evidence-based interventions: (1) Protocols summarize actions: protocols provide a practical summary of the evidence-based intervention. Clinicians are then exposed to this summary, which makes meanings and actions relevant to a certain diagnosis immediately discuss these items. (2) Protocols act as memory aids: when protocols take the form of PPOs, they also behave as checklists, providing a memory aid [36]. This may be a particularly useful aspect of protocols when dealing with complex interventions, where actions may be only partially completed due to failure in recollection. Thus, protocols help deal with the limitation of our cognitive processes in memorizing items. The protocol actually frees cognitive processing functions to other purposes. (3) Protocols rely on the use of the same terms, repeatedly. The repetition of terms help subjects get used to a common meaning for them, which simplifies communication and avoids dubious alternate meanings. (4) Standardization of processes and terms decrease social distances, allowing better communication. For example, if a higher ranked person asks for an action that is not in the protocol, it is easier for the other subject to question that decision as it is a deviation from the protocol. The higher ranked person is now in a position where he or she needs to provide a good argument on why the deviation from the protocol is the correct action.

These potential benefits of protocols on communicative processes, however, hinge on how the protocols are designed. A poorly designed protocol could make adopting the intervention seem to be more complicated and time consuming than it actually is. Also, a poorly designed protocol can fail to serve as an effective memory aid. In fact, a pre-printed order with a poorly designed checklist has led to an adverse event [37]. Moreover, a review of medication errors reported to the United States Pharmacopeia (USP) from 1998 to 2003 found 4,437 case reports that identified PPOs as a cause of error [38]·

Language, Style, and Form

Several aspects of how the message is shared between subjects impact on the accuracy of information. We will review a limited set of these aspects where there is evidence to support recommendations for communication.

The airline industry is rich in examples of the importance of style of communication. The most relevant to healthcare is the study of "politeness theory" [39] which shows that polite orders or suggestions and topic changes were rejected more often than direct ones by pilots, and many have led to accidents. These rejections indicate that the recipient did not take the meaning and information contained in the shared messages into account. It is likely that polite messages also suggest a *rank distance* between subjects, which allows the recipient to ignore messages. There are similar examples in healthcare, especially in time sensitive situations, such as acute resuscitation and operation room emergencies. Teams that used more polite suggestions, as opposed to assertive communication, were more likely to perform poorly in simulated trauma bay scenarios [40].

One of the ways of coping with time constraints is to communicate several items simultaneously. As we observed before, there is a certain limitation to our memory span and this technique may lead to more errors. In aviation, when controllers use long command strings containing several separate actions pilots make more mistakes because of the message length [41].

Another technique of language to improve communication is the standardization of read-back orders, so frequently done in aviation. Read-back orders help close the final loop, where the final information, meaning and/or actions shared from subject A to subject B are then repeated back to A, who confirms the correctness of the message. As we have demonstrated above in the theory of communication, this simple strategy can be very helpful in avoiding errors in the final stage of communication, when the decisions and actions are ready and need to be implemented.

As we discussed above, it is possible that subjects may not question or ask for clarification on orders or diagnosis in situations where a great rank distance exists [42]. One of the solutions for this is to "increase the ranks" of everyone. The person who has a perceived higher rank (for example, the staff physician leading rounds) can ask everyone in the team if the plan seems satisfactory and if there are any other problems that we need to deal with. This active empowerment of the other members of the team can theoretically improve communications and avoid errors.

Conclusion

We presented a theory of communication and defined communicative processes as the sharing of meaning and information between at least two subjects, which is modulated by social and environmental factors. We delineated several aspects of this theory that are related to failures in communication, especially in the social and environmental modulation of communication, and discussed how certain strategies can improve or hinder communication, such as multidisciplinary rounds, protocols, handoff tools, and language.

References

1. Eco U. A theory of semiotics. Bloomington: Indiana University Press; 1978.
2. Shannon CE. A mathematical theory of communication. Bell Syst Tech J. 1948;27:379–423.
3. Kluver J, Kluver C. On communication: an interdisciplinary and mathematical approach. Dordrecht: Springer; 2007.
4. Buckley W. Social stratification and the functional theory of social differentiation. Am Sociol Rev. 1958;23:369–75.
5. Miller GA. The magical number seven plus or minus two: some limits on our capacity for processing information. Psychol Rev. 1956;63:81–97.
6. Paris CR, Salas E, Cannon-Bowers JA. Teamwork in multi-person systems: a review and analysis. Ergonomics. 2000;43:1052–75.
7. Pronovost P, Berenholtz S, Dorman T, Lipsett PA, Simmonds T, Haraden C. Improving communication in the ICU using daily goals. J Crit Care. 2003;18:71–5.
8. Kim MM, Barnato AE, Angus DC, Fleisher LF, Kahn JM. The effect of multidisciplinary care teams on intensive care unit mortality. Arch Intern Med. 2010;170:369–76.
9. Cohen MD, Hilligoss B, Kajdacsy-Balla Amaral AC. A handoff is not a telegram: an understanding of the patient is co-constructed. Crit Care. 2012;16:303.
10. Cohen MD, Hilligoss PB. The published literature on handoffs in hospitals: deficiencies identified in an extensive review. Qual Saf Health Care. 2010;19:493–7.
11. Arora V, Johnson J, Lovinger D, Humphrey HJ, Meltzer DO. Communication failures in patient sign-out and suggestions for improvement: a critical incident analysis. Qual Saf Health Care. 2005;14:401–7.
12. Petersen LA, Brennan TA, O'Neil AC, Cook EF, Lee TH. Does housestaff discontinuity of care increase the risk for preventable adverse events? Ann Intern Med. 1994;121:866–72.
13. Fins JJ. Professional responsibility: a perspective on the Bell Commission reforms. Bull N Y Acad Med. 1991;67:359–64.

14. Laine C, Goldman L, Soukup JR, Hayes JG. The impact of a regulation restricting medical house staff working hours on the quality of patient care. JAMA. 1993;269:374–8.
15. Gawande AA, Zinner MJ, Studdert DM, Brennan TA. Analysis of errors reported by surgeons at three teaching hospitals. Surgery. 2003;133:614–21.
16. Gandhi TK, Kachalia A, Thomas EJ, et al. Missed and delayed diagnoses in the ambulatory setting: a study of closed malpractice claims. Ann Intern Med. 2006;145:488–96.
17. Kachalia A, Gandhi TK, Puopolo AL, et al. Missed and delayed diagnoses in the emergency department: a study of closed malpractice claims from 4 liability insurers. Ann Emerg Med. 2007;49:196–205.
18. Philibert I. Use of strategies from high-reliability organisations to the patient hand-off by resident physicians: practical implications. Qual Saf Health Care. 2009;18:261–6.
19. Borowitz SM, Waggoner-Fountain LA, Bass EJ, Sledd RM. Adequacy of information transferred at resident sign-out (inhospital handover of care): a prospective survey. Qual Saf Health Care. 2008;17:6–10.
20. Catchpole K, Sellers R, Goldman A, McCulloch P, Hignett S. Patient handovers within the hospital: translating knowledge from motor racing to healthcare. Qual Saf Health Care. 2010;19:318–22.
21. Lamond D. The information content of the nurse change of shift report: a comparative study. J Adv Nurs. 2000;31:794–804.
22. Fassett MJ, Hannan TJ, Robertson IK, Bollipo SJ, Fassett RG. A national survey of medical morning handover report in Australian hospitals. Med J Aust. 2007;187:164–5.
23. Solet DJ, Norvell JM, Rutan GH, Frankel RM. Lost in translation: challenges and opportunities in physician-to-physician communication during patient handoffs. Acad Med. 2005;80:1094–9.
24. Chaboyer W, McMurray A, Wallis M. Bedside nursing handover: a case study. Int J Nurs Pract. 2010;16:27–34.
25. Odell A. Communication theory and the shift handover report. Br J Nurs. 1996;5:1323–6.
26. Miller A, Scheinkestel C, Limpus A, Joseph M, Karnik A, Venkatesh B. Uni- and interdisciplinary effects on round and handover content in intensive care units. Hum Factors. 2009;51:339–53.
27. Bhabra G, Mackeith S, Monteiro P, Pothier DD. An experimental comparison of handover methods. Ann R Coll Surg Engl. 2007;89:298–300.
28. Accreditation C. Required organizational practices. Ottawa: Accreditation Canada; 2009.
29. Haig KM, Sutton S, Whittington J. SBAR: a shared mental model for improving communication between clinicians. Jt Comm J Qual Patient Saf. 2006;32:167–75.
30. Riesenberg LA, Leitzsch J, Little BW. Systematic review of handoff mnemonics literature. Am J Med Qual. 2009;24:196–204.
31. Ilan R, LeBaron CD, Christianson MK, Heyland DK, Day A, Cohen MD. Handover patterns: an observational study of critical care physicians. BMC Health Serv Res. 2012;12:11.
32. Van Eaton EG, Horvath KD, Lober WB, Rossini AJ, Pellegrini CA. A randomized, controlled trial evaluating the impact of a computerized rounding and sign-out system on continuity of care and resident work hours. J Am Coll Surg. 2005;200:538–45.
33. Anderson J, Shroff D, Curtis A, et al. The Veterans Affairs shift change physician-to-physician handoff project. Jt Comm J Qual Patient Saf. 2010;36:62–71.
34. Petersen LA, Orav EJ, Teich JM, O'Neil AC, Brennan TA. Using a computerized sign-out program to improve continuity of inpatient care and prevent adverse events. Jt Comm J Qual Improv. 1998;24:77–87.
35. Ash JS, Sittig DF, Campbell EM, Guappone KP, Dykstra RH. Some unintended consequences of clinical decision support systems. AMIA Annu Symp Proc. 2007:26–30.
36. Cheney C, Ramsdell JW. Effect of medical records' checklists on implementation of periodic health measures. Am J Med. 1987;83:129–36.
37. Institute for Safe Medication Practices. ISMPs guidelines for standard order sets; 2011.
38. Hicks RW, Nelson J, Santell JP. Medication errors associated with preprinted orders. USP Drug Saf Rev Syst. 2004;148:pHSE28.

39. Brown P. Politeness: some universals in language usage. Cambridge: Cambridge University Press; 1987.
40. Westli HK, Johnsen BH, Eid J, Rasten I, Brattebo G. Teamwork skills, shared mental models, and performance in simulated trauma teams: an independent group design. Scand J Trauma Resusc Emerg Med. 2010;18:47.
41. Barshi I. The effects of mental representation on performance in a navigation task. ProQuest Dissertations and Theses, University of Colorado at Boulder, 1998, p. 93.
42. Snook SA. Friendly fire: the accidental shootdown of U.S. Black Hawks over Northern Iraq. New Jersey: Princeton University Press; 2000.

Chapter 9
Teamwork and Leadership in the Critical Care Unit

Tom W. Reader and Brian H. Cuthbertson

Abstract Effective multidisciplinary teamwork and team leadership have been shown as essential for the safe management of patients in intensive care medicine (ICM). Solutions to improve teamwork and leadership have been developed, but with mixed success. It is observed that to improve teamwork in ICM, interventions must reflect (1) the demands and constraints of ICM, and how they influence team behaviour and (2) the specific teamwork skills and behaviours that are associated with safe patient care. Research in ICM shows that effective team leadership is the key determinant of team functioning, and that interventions should focus on enhancing leadership. Yet, simply applying leadership solutions developed in other domains (e.g. aviation) is not appropriate. Specifically, the flow and nature of work, and the changeable and complex construction of teams, means that tools for improving and assessing leadership need to be designed to reflect the very specific constraints of ICM.

Keywords Teamwork • Leadership • Training • Error • Communication

Introduction

Applied psychology research investigates the relationship between teamwork and organisational outcomes [1]. This work shows that group norms and behaviours have a profound effect upon the success of teams in numerous complex work

T.W. Reader (✉)
Department of Social Psychology, London School of Economics, Houghton Street, London WC2A 2AE, UK
e-mail: t.w.reader@lse.ac.uk

B.H. Cuthbertson
Department of Critical Care Medicine, Sunnybrook Health Sciences Centre, 2075 Bayview Avenue, Toronto, ON, Canada M4N 3M5
e-mail: brian.cuthbertson@sunnybrook.ca

D.C. Scales and G.D. Rubenfeld (eds.), *The Organization of Critical Care*, Respiratory Medicine 18, DOI 10.1007/978-1-4939-0811-0_9,

settings, including aviation, energy, oil and gas, management, and the military [2–4]. Broadly, teamwork refers to the way in which team members work together to produce “synchronised” output [5]. In a practical sense, this describes the communication, coordination, decision-making, and leadership processes that occur as a team attempts to complete a shared task. Group processes are influenced by the nature of a task (e.g. an emergency), the norms of a group (e.g. for managing error), and institutional constraints (e.g. rewards, penalties, culture). Over the past 10 years, the importance of teamwork for ensuring high-quality patient care in healthcare environments has been repeatedly demonstrated [6]. Specifically, medical error research has shown adverse events to frequently emerge from problems in how groups of multidisciplinary healthcare workers function together [7]. Furthermore, effective teamwork is shown as important not only for avoiding medical error but also for managing situations that are risky, stressful, and susceptible to error [8]. This is particularly true in the domain of critical care medicine, within which multidisciplinary teams of nurses and doctors provide care to critically ill patients.

Teamwork and leadership are both considered “non-technical skills”. These relate to the social and cognitive skills (e.g. communication, decision-making, situation awareness) that underpin behaviour in work environments. Problems in non-technical skills have been associated with approximately half of critical incidents in critical care [9]. Frequently, problems in teamwork, situation awareness, and decision-making underlie threats to patient safety. The ability to manage risk, complex technologies, changeable workloads, and uncertainty is essential [10], and fatigue and stress are key performance-shaping factors [11]. Of the various non-technical skills important for safe patient care in the ICU, teamwork and leadership are frequently highlighted as the most significant. This is because the association between teamwork and positive patient outcomes in ICU has been demonstrated repeatedly [12–14]. Although a multitude of examples exist, commonly cited factors leading to errors include problems in team structures, leadership verbal or written communication during routine care and handovers, and communication during crisis situations [15]. Conversely, good teamwork is also associated with good patient outcomes. For example, the degree to which nurses and doctors collaborate is associated with reduced patient mortality rates and lower average patient lengths of stay [16, 17].

The recognition that effective teamwork can underlie good patient care has led to a drive to introduce solutions for improving teamwork within multidisciplinary ICU settings. Solutions focus on developing tools or organisational culture to enhance team functioning [18, 19], and also improving attitudes towards teamwork [20]. Efforts to improve teamwork in healthcare often utilise team training solutions designed in the aviation industry to improve pilot communication and leadership skills. Whilst these solutions may be relevant for ICU, it is necessary that interventions to improve teamwork reflect (1) the demands and constraints of intensive care medicine (ICM) and how they influence team behaviour, and (2) the teamwork skills and behaviours that are associated with safe patient care. In particular, the team leadership skills of senior doctors (ICU specialists) are recognised as critical for engendering effective teamwork multidisciplinary teamwork in the ICU.

Team Leadership

Intensive care research increasingly points towards the importance of the leadership of ICU specialists for shaping how team members coordinate and combine to provide patient care [21]. Team leadership refers to how a team leader ensures the needs and goals of a team are met [22]. In the psychological literature, a team leader can be described as the team member responsible (formally or informally) for guiding a team to complete a task or work cycle [22]. In ICU, teams are normally led by ICU specialists; however, a number of other team members will have leadership roles [23, 24]. For example, senior trainee physicians lead teams at night or during emergency events (e.g. resuscitations), and senior nurses lead groups of nursing staff (and also, informally, junior trainee physicians). Nonetheless, ICU specialists largely retain executive authority for patients and are ultimately responsible for patient care. Their expertise is used to train junior physicians, to develop patient treatment strategies, and to structure and direct the ICU team. Their leadership abilities are crucial for ensuring that multidisciplinary teams provide effective patient care [17, 25–27].

ICU research shows specialist' team leadership can influence team functioning and patient outcomes through a range of mechanisms. Within both simulated and real-life studies, team performance is shaped by leadership behaviours such as encouraging junior team member inputs, stating and evaluating plans, gathering feedback on plans, effective task delegation, and clear prioritisation of patient care tasks [28–30]. The ability of specialists to communicate with the ICU team, to manage limited resources, to create and demonstrate standards, and to provide support for team development is found to be associated with outcome measures such as task completion within NICUs [31]. Leader inclusiveness (e.g. listening and encouraging junior team members to state and discuss their ideas) is found to result in team members becoming more involved in activities such as quality improvement initiatives [32].

The above studies indicate how the team leadership behaviours of specialists can have a profound influence upon the team communication behaviours of junior physicians and nursing staff. *Team communication* refers to team members transferring information, ideas, and opinions [33]. A range of behaviours are seen as constituting "good communication" in the ICU [27]. For example, the accurate transfer of information during events such as handovers and admitting new patients, sharing patient treatment plans, and junior team members engaging in speaking up behaviours if they identify an error or have a knowledge gap. More specific behaviours, such as directed communication during crisis events, directed verbal and non-verbal communication, and closed loop communication (where team members acknowledge communications) are also important. Critically, the quality of communication within an ICU team is shaped by norms and expectations established by the leadership. Poor communication is often caused by beliefs that junior staff that they will be penalised for erroneously reporting problems in patient care (or errors that they have observed), or a lack of shared understanding for standards of communication [34]. Teams can develop quite divergent understandings of how they should communicate together. Specialists can believe communication in a team is open, but junior team members do not perceive this [35].

Research investigating team situation awareness in the ICU has demonstrated how leadership and communication can shape the cognitions of team members during tasks such as the ICU rounds [36]. *Situation awareness* (SA) refers to an individual's perception of the information within their task environment, comprehension of what the information means, and anticipation of how a situation will evolve over time [37]. *Team situation awareness* refers to how teams form a shared and accurate understanding of their work environment. Within the ICU, the development of shared and accurate SA between team members (e.g. for daily goals) is important for patient safety [38, 39].

Indeed, events such as daily rounds should be orientated towards developing shared SA [40]. Forming a shared awareness of aspects of a patient's condition and future trajectory influences team activities such as patient monitoring, task prioritisation, and in the anticipation of adverse events. Critical to this is (1) giving opportunities for junior team members to contribute information to patient planning, (2) working with team members to understand patient treatment goals and interpret information, and (3) allowing ICU specialists to identify and remedy gaps in the knowledge and understanding of team members. Crucially, the involvement of junior team members in decision making during the morning round is shaped by their beliefs of how senior team members expect junior team members to behave. For example, nursing staff can feel there is a lack of opportunity/need to contribute to decision-making, and trainee physicians that asking an inappropriate question or not understanding an aspect of a patient's condition will compromise senior doctor beliefs about their competence. Such beliefs make it less likely that teams will form shared and accurate SA during the round, and specialist leadership (e.g. asking junior staff to present patients, to lead decision making) is critical for shaping junior team member attitudes and behaviours.

Challenges in the Leadership of ICU Teams

In understanding the relationship between team leadership and teamwork in the ICU, it is necessary to consider how the ICU environment itself shapes behaviour and constraints activity. Human factors research shows that each working environment has its own unique non-technical challenges and requirements [41]. To ensure interventions for improving teamwork are effective, it is important to diagnose and specify the teamwork and leadership skills important for a given situation. Although the principle skills underlying effective teamwork may be generic (e.g. communication and leadership), how they manifest themselves in different situations is critical for safety. Thus, the behaviours that demonstrate proficiency for teamwork in a particular setting will be reflective of the demands within that domain [33]. Reader and Cuthbertson [42] have detailed how the challenges to improving teamwork in the ICU (e.g. in understanding factors that affect teamwork, and in developing and implementing training) differ from those in the aviation, where pilots regularly experience team training (this is increasingly the case for surgical teams). Prior to develop solutions for improving leadership or teamwork in the ICU, these challenges must be considered.

First, the types of risks and problems faced by ICU teams differ to those in domains such as aviation and surgery. Within these settings, there are similarities in procedures (e.g. pre-operative checks, post-operative checks, induction, commencement of surgery, extubation, and awakening), and teams generally focus on a clear objective end-point (e.g. landing, successful completion of an operation) within a fixed geographic area (i.e. the cockpit or operating room). Improving teamwork often focuses on managing emergency events where the stable functioning a system (whether a technological system or a patient) is threatened. In ICU, teams must form treatment plans for patients who are sometimes incompletely understood, unstable, and have multiple problems. Team members are often not apprised of patient histories, and patient populations have diverse risk factors, pathologies, and demographic characteristics. ICU teams frequently encounter emergencies situations, and must tolerate quite high levels of risk (e.g. using treatments where the outcomes are uncertain). They must also develop an understanding of complex interactions between medical treatments and patient physiology that changes with time. Thus, leadership occurs in a very uncertain environment, where risks are constantly changing and difficult to appraise.

Second, the flow of work in intensive care medicine also complex, and this poses significant challenges to teamwork and leadership. Within a single ICU, teams will perform a diverse range of hands-on, problem-solving, and monitoring tasks [43]. The number of patients being treated, and length of patient care, fluctuates and depends on patient factors (e.g. stage of treatment, severity of illness) and also system factors. The team skills and behaviours important for managing patients and situations vary, and strategies used by teams will differ according to a range of constraining factors (e.g. available team members, resources, external support within a hospital). Furthermore, there is no "safe landing" for a patient. Their care does not cease on discharge from ICU, and patients may return or require further monitoring and follow-up. Also in comparison with domains such as aviation, errors and failures in safety are more difficult to detect (e.g. due to less sophisticated monitoring systems), and errors are only likely to influence a single patient, their family, and their healthcare providers [6]. The leader must try to lead through a variety of situations, each with their own demands and needs (e.g. long-term planning vs. emergency management).

Third, to understand the team performance requirements in intensive care medicine, it is also important to examine the composition and structure of ICU teams. Critical care teams often consist of large number of medical and nursing team members who must cooperate together to provide safe patient care. Care can occur over a period of weeks, with care being provided by different teams, and teams communicate through handovers of care that tend to be non-standardised [44]. ICUs can also have several specialists leading the unit, and a key challenge for ICU teams in combining the expertise of varying ICU specialists with the skills of junior trainees. Trainees often perform much of the "hands-on" clinical work so teams must develop high levels of coordination and supervision to ensure that trainees skills can develop whilst patient safety is maintained. Advance trainees must often manage the ICU and make decisions on their own, and their relationship with nursing staff is critical and sometimes challenging. Whilst senior intensivists are available to provide support, the level of this supervision and support can vary appropriately depending on the leadership style of ICU specialists as well as the seniority of the trainee. For example, senior leadership support for trainees can differ due to variations in how specialists conceptualise effective teamwork (e.g. beliefs on how team members should work together, attitudes towards supervision and support), and beliefs on how and when standards and procedures should be applied (e.g. allowing risk-taking activities, variation between consultants in beliefs on treatment strategies) [45]. Furthermore, ICU specialists can differ in their attitudes towards concepts such as human factors, with some being reluctant to acknowledge the detrimental impact of factors such as stress and fatigue upon safety and performance [46].

Thus, team leadership in the ICU is a shared phenomenon that occurs between and across specialists. This is particularly important when considering the leadership and direction of care during an individual patient's treatment, with potential multiple leaders influencing the process, direction and activities of the team.

Effective Team Leadership in the ICU

Our own research has detailed the skills and behaviours that constitute effective team leadership in the ICU [45]. This is underpinned by both psychological frameworks for interpreting leadership within complex work settings, and also the complexities that must be managed by specialists in intensive care. Typically, ICU specialists describe effective team leadership as a highly adaptive process, whereby leadership activities (e.g. styles, behaviours) are shaped according to the task (e.g. rounds vs. emergencies) and the team (e.g. inexperienced vs. experienced). The ability of specialists to adjust their behaviour to these dimensions is seen as key for ensuring teams can function to the best of their ability, and also for aiding the training of trainees. Furthermore, and perhaps more challenging, developing a sense of continuity in leadership is also important.

In terms of adaptive leadership, specialists generally distinguish between three activities (rounds, treatment, emergencies). During rounds, good leadership refers to guiding the ICU team to develop an understanding of the patient's conditions, and facilitating the team to develop a shared patient treatment plan. This more consensual process is important for eliciting information key to patient decision-making, for developing shared knowledge structures (e.g. daily goals), and for ensuring tasks are designed to meet the skills and training needs of team members. As work is performed in the ICU (during the post-round period), specialists step back from their leadership role, and move into a supporting role. Here, leadership constitutes identifying problems and assessing team members in providing patient care. This involves retaining a bird's-eye view of the unit, identifying problems before they emerge or take root, and where necessary giving guidance. However, the extent to which specialists provide hands-on leadership depends on their training objectives for trainees, the other challenges being faced within the ICU, and the threat to patient safety. Finally, a far more proactive form of leadership occurs during emergency phases of work. This can involve a more directive approach to task delegation, and information sharing, and depending on the context, a reduced involvement of team members in patient decision-making or in the development of short-term solutions. Thus, there is not a single type or style of leadership that is effective for managing teams in ICU. Rather, leadership behaviours need to reflect the changeable nature of work and teams.

Finally, alongside the leadership of day-to-day work, the development of unit culture is also important. Psychology research investigating leadership in organisational settings shows the importance of actions such as developing a vision, shared norms, and demonstrating standards of excellence. These are also important for the ICU environment, and a key function of ICU specialists is to develop a stable and safe environment where team members (who constantly change and rotate) can develop their skills and knowledge. Within an ICU there may be several specialists, and developing and communicating a shared perspective of patient care and teamwork is challenging (e.g. on treatments strategies, expectations for junior team member contributions during decision-making). Where this does not occur, junior team members receive mixed messages on the behaviours that are expected of them, and the standards to which they should aspire. This can create a culture where junior team members (and in particular junior trainee trainees) adapt their behaviour to meet the perceived (and sometimes contradicting) demands of individual team leaders. In turn, it can cause behavioural inconsistency, and increase the likelihood of error through team members trying to adapt their behaviour to satisfy a team leader rather than the clinical situation.

Conclusions

Understanding the skills and behaviours that underpin effective teamwork and team leadership in critical care medicine is crucial for ensuring the safe treatment of patients. Although there is considerable research on what makes an effective leader in domains such as anaesthesia and surgery (and how to measure leadership), critical care medicine poses a number of different challenges. Specifically, the flow and nature of work, and the changeable and complex construction of teams, means that tools for observing leadership behaviour and theories need to be designed to reflect the very specific constraints of critical care medicine. Research has begun to investigate how team leaders in ICU shape aspects of team functioning amongst trainee doctors and nurses (e.g. communication, situation awareness), and this would seem a very fruitful avenue for future investigation.

References

1. Salas E, Bowers C, Edens E. Improving teamwork in organizations: applications of resource management training. Mawah: LEA; 2001.
2. O'Connor P, Campbell J, Newon J, Melton J, Salas E, Wilson K. Crew resource management training effectiveness: a meta-analysis and some critical needs. Int J Aviat Psychol. 2008;18:353–68.
3. Bell ST. Deep-level composition variables as predictors of team performance: a meta-analysis. J Appl Psychol. 2007;92:595–615.
4. Burke CS, Stagl K, Salas E, Pierce L, Kendall D. Understanding team adaptation: a conceptual analysis and model. J Appl Psychol. 2006;91:1189–207.
5. Paris C, Salas E, Cannon-Bowers J. Teamwork in multi-person systems: a review and analysis. Ergonomics. 2000;43:1052–75.
6. Vincent C. Patient safety. London: Elsevier; 2006.
7. Gawande AA, Studdert D, Zinner M, Brennan TA. Analysis of errors reported by surgeons at three teaching hospitals. Surgery. 2003;133:614–21.
8. Flin R, Maran N. Identifying and training non-technical skills for teams in acute medicine. Qual Saf Health Care. 2004;13(Suppl 1):80–4.
9. Reader T, Flin R, Lauche K, Cuthbertson B. Non-technical skills in the intensive care unit. Br J Anaesth. 2006;96:551–9.
10. Bion J, Heffner JE. Challenges in the care of the acutely ill. Lancet. 2004;363:970–7.
11. Reader T, Cuthbertson B, Decruyenaere J. Burnout in the ICU: potential consequences for staff and patient well-being. Intensive Care Med. 2008;34:4–6.
12. Donchin Y, Gopher D, Olin M, et al. A look into the nature and causes of human errors in the intensive care unit. Crit Care Med. 1995;23:294–300.
13. Walker S, Brett S. Oiling the wheels of intensive care to reduce "machine friction": the best way to improve outcomes? Crit Care Med. 2010;38(10 Suppl):S642–8.
14. Valentin A, Bion J. How safe is my intensive care unit? An overview of error causation and prevention. Curr Opin Crit Care. 2007;13:697–702.
15. Pronovost PJ, Thompson D, Holzmueller C, et al. Toward learning from patient safety reporting systems. J Crit Care. 2006;21:305–15.
16. Baggs JG, Schmitt MH, Mushlin AI, Mitchell PH, Eldrege DH, Oakes D. Association between nurse-physician collaboration and patient outcomes in three intensive care units. Crit Care Med. 1999;27:1991–8.
17. Shortell SM, Zimmerman JE, Rousseau DM, et al. The performance of intensive care units: does good management make a difference? Med Care. 1994;32:508–25.
18. Pronovost PJ, Berenholtz SM, Ngo K, et al. Developing and pilot testing quality indicators in the intensive care unit. J Crit Care. 2003;18:145–55.
19. Huang D, Clermont G, Sexton J, et al. Perceptions of safety culture across the intensive care units of a single institution. Crit Care Med. 2007;35:165–76.
20. Salas E, Wilson-Donnelly K, Sims D, Burke CS, Priest H. Teamwork training for patient safety: best practices and guiding principles. In: Carayon P, editor. Handbook of human factors and ergonomics in health care and patient safety. Mahwah: LEA; 2007. p. 803–22.
21. Thomas EJ, Sexton J, Helmreich RL. Discrepant attitudes about teamwork among critical care nurses and physicians. Crit Care Med. 2003;31:956–9.

22. Morgeson F, DeRue D, Karam E. Leadership in teams: a functional approach to understanding leadership structures and processes. J Manag. 2010;36:5–39.
23. Bion J, Fox-Kirk W. Eighteenth century mindsets, twenty-first century challenges: the physician as team player. Crit Care Med. 2009;37:1288–9.
24. Reader T, Flin R, Cuthbertson B. Factors affecting team communication in the intensive care unit. In: Nemeth C, editor. Improving healthcare team communication: building on lessons from aviation and aerospace. Aldershot: Ashgate; 2008. p. 117–34.
25. Malhotra S, Jordan D, Shortliffe EH, Patel V. Workflow modeling in critical care: piecing together your own puzzle. J Biomed Inform. 2007;40:81–92.
26. Manser T. Teamwork and patient safety in dynamic domains of healthcare: a review of the literature. Acta Anaesthesiol Scand. 2009;53:143–51.
27. Reader T, Flin R, Mearns K, Cuthbertson B. Developing a team performance framework for the intensive care unit. Crit Care Med. 2009;35:1787–93.
28. Kim J, Neilipovitz D, Cardinal P, Chiu M, Clinch J. A pilot study using high-fidelity simulation to formally evaluate performance in the resuscitation of critically ill patients: The University of Ottawa Critical Care Medicine, High-Fidelity Simulation, and Crisis Resource Management I Study. Crit Care Med. 2006;34:2167–74.
29. Ottestad E, Boulet J, Lighthall G. Evaluating the management of septic shock using patient simulation. Crit Care Med. 2007;35:769–75.
30. Thomas EJ, Sexton J, Lasky R, Helmreich RL, Crandell D, Tyson J. Teamwork and quality during neonatal care in the delivery room. J Perinatol. 2006;26:163–9.
31. Stockwell D, Slonim A, Pollack M. Physician team management affects goal achievement in the intensive care unit. Pediatr Crit Care Med. 2007;8:840–5.
32. Nembhard I, Edmondson AC. Making it safe: the effects of leader inclusiveness and professional status on psychological safety and improvement efforts in health care teams. J Organ Behav. 2006;27:941–66.
33. Flin R, O'Connor P, Crichton M. Safety at the sharp end. A guide to non-technical skills. Aldershot: Ashgate; 2008.
34. Reader T, Flin R, Cuthbertson B. Communication skills and error in the intensive care unit. Curr Opin Crit Care. 2007;13:732–6.
35. Reader T, Flin R, Mearns K, Cuthbertson B. Interdisciplinary communication in the intensive care unit. Br J Anaesth. 2007;98:347–52.
36. Reader T, Flin R, Mearns K, Cuthbertson B. Team situation awareness and the anticipation of patient progress during ICU rounds. BMJ Qual Saf. 2011;20:1035–42.
37. Endsley M. Towards a theory of situation awareness in dynamic systems. Hum Factors. 1995;37:32–64.
38. Wright M, Endsley M. Building situation awareness in healthcare teams. In: Nemeth C, editor. Improving healthcare team communication. Aldershot: Ashgate; 2008. p. 97–114.
39. Patel V, Zhang J, Yoskowitz N, Green RA, Osman RS. Translational cognition for decision support in critical care environments: a review. J Biomed Inform. 2008;41:413–31.
40. Gurses A, Xiao Y. A systematic review of the literature on multidisciplinary rounds to design information technology. J Am Med Inform Assoc. 2006;13:267–76.
41. Stanton N, Salmon P, Walker G, Baber C, Jenkins D. Human factors methods: a practical guide for engineering and design. Aldershot: Ashgate; 2005.
42. Reader T, Cuthbertson B. Teamwork and team training in the ICU: where do the similarities with aviation end? Crit Care. 2011;15:313–9.
43. Fackler J, Watts C, McHugh A, Miller T, Crandall B, Pronovost P. Critical care physician cognitive task analysis: an exploratory study. Crit Care. 2009;13:R33.
44. Raduma-Tomàs M, Flin R, Yule S, Williams D. Doctor's handovers in hospitals: a literature review. BMJ Qual Saf. 2011;20:128–33.
45. Reader T, Flin R, Cuthbertson B. Team leadership in the intensive care unit. The perspective of specialists. Crit Care Med. 2011;39:1683–91.
46. Sexton J, Thomas EJ, Helmreich RL. Error, stress and teamwork in medicine and aviation: cross sectional surveys. Br Med J. 2000;320:745–9.

Chapter 10
Caring for ICU Providers

Ruth M. Kleinpell, Omar B. Lateef, Gourang P. Patel, and Rachel Start

Abstract The intensive care unit (ICU) environment can pose adverse risks to ICU care providers including psychological and physical stressors. Managing care for critically ill patients with life-threatening conditions can result in conflicts related to end-of-life decisions, ICU burnout, and moral distress. Other factors such as exposure to patient suffering and family distress, prolonged work hours, or inadequate resources or staffing can result in stress for ICU healthcare professionals. Addressing burdens placed upon ICU providers and promoting a healthy work environment are important in ensuring respectful relationships, interdisciplinary teamwork, and active engagement as well as promoting job satisfaction and ensuring retention.

Keywords ICU providers • ICU caregivers • Healthy work environment • ICU work environment • ICU staff burnout • ICU staff moral distress

R.M. Kleinpell (✉)
Center for Clinical Research and Scholarship, Rush University Medical Center, Chicago, IL, USA

Rush University College of Nursing, Chicago, IL, USA

Mercy Hospital and Medical Center, Chicago, IL, USA
e-mail: Ruth_M_Kleinpell@rush.edu

O.B. Lateef (✉) • G.P. Patel (✉)
Rush University Medical Center, Chicago, IL, USA
e-mail: Omar_B_Lateef@rush.edu; Gourang_P_Patel@rush.edu

R. Start
Magnet Program Director, Rush Oak Park Hospital
e-mail: Rachel_e_Start@rush.edu

D.C. Scales and G.D. Rubenfeld (eds.), *The Organization of Critical Care*,
Respiratory Medicine 18, DOI 10.1007/978-1-4939-0811-0_10,

Overview

By virtue of high patient acuity, uncertainty about the outcome of critical illness, and the stressful environment of the intensive care unit (ICU), ICU care providers are at risk for a number of adverse work associated psychological and physical stressors. It has been identified that ICUs are probably the most stressful places in hospitals [1]. Conflicts related to end-of-life decisions, ICU burnout, and moral distress is among some of the psychological stressors. Physical stressors can result from prolonged work hours, inadequate staffing ratios, and job-related hazards such as patient lifting and personal injury. There are many factors that serve to increase the stress of caring for critically ill patients including communication problems with patients and their family members, as well as other healthcare professionals, inadequate resources or staffing, role conflict, exposure to family distress, and exposure to patient suffering [2]. It becomes evident that promoting a healthy work environment for ICU care providers is important to mitigate the risk of adverse stressors. Addressing burdens placed upon ICU caregivers and improving the ICU work environment is paramount in improving the work life of ICU clinicians, promoting job satisfaction, and ensuring retention. This chapter reviews concepts related to caring for the ICU clinicians including strategies for promoting a healthy work environment, reducing moral distress and burnout, and supporting ICU providers.

Promoting a Healthy Work Environment in the ICU

It is well acknowledged that the ICU is a stressful work environment involving acute life-threatening illness, complex therapies, and frequent deaths [3]. The challenge of caregiving for the critically ill is compounded by the uncertainty that characterizes critical care including uncertainty about prognosis, uncertainty about ultimate quality of life, uncertainty about medical decision making, and the uncertainty about the time course of disease [2]. The Conflicus study which examined the prevalence and factors related to ICU conflicts from 7,498 ICU staff members from 323 ICUs in 24 countries found that 71.6 % experienced conflicts in the ICU ranging from communication gaps, workload stressors, and job strain [1]. A number of factors were associated with perceive conflicts including staff working more than 40 h/week, caring for dying patients, providing pre- and postmortem care, conflict over symptom control, misunderstandings among staff and families, lack of leadership, futile treatment, and inappropriate family and patient behavior, among others. Recommendations from the study identified that multifaceted conflict-reducing intervention should be designed and evaluated to target the well-being of ICU professionals [1].

Establishing a healthy work environment in the ICU is a priority area to ensure that healthcare professionals have a supportive practice setting. In 2005, the American Association of Critical Care Nurses (AACN) identified six standards for establishing and sustaining healthy work environments based on evidence-based and relationship-centered principles of professional performance [4]. The standards include:

- Skilled Communication
- True Collaboration
- Effective Decision Making
- Appropriate Staffing
- Meaningful Recognition
- Authentic Leadership

The standards align with the core competencies for health professionals recommended by the Institute of Medicine's Committee on Quality Health Care [5].

AACN issued a call for action for ICUs to adopt the healthy work environment standard and was joined by the American College of Chest Physicians (ACCP) in advocating for a number of steps to create healthy work environments including conducting an assessment of the environment and culture in the ICU and developing a clear plan of action to implement the standards.

A number of ICUs have adopted the Healthy Work Environment (HWE) standards and have implemented initiatives to promote a culture which values respectful relationships, interdisciplinary teamwork, and active engagement. At Rush University Medical Center in Chicago Illinois, the Professional Nursing Staff utilized the HWE standards to shape and frame priorities and goals that supported these core philosophies. Education on the healthy work environment standards was provided to clinical staff and committee chairs were encouraged to structure committee goals based on the six standards. A Work Life Committee was formed to evaluate formalizing the HWE standards throughout the organization. As part of the work of the Work Life Committee, a code of conduct was developed to reinforce the emphasis on respectful communication and expected professional behavior (Figs. 10.1a–c and 10.2). Key components of the code of conduct for physicians and nurses identified that professional behavior, integrity, and ethical behavior were an expectation. Truth, honesty, communication, and cooperation with other healthcare providers are expected along with respect and regard for their dignity. Development of the professional code of conduct has helped to reinforce the importance of professional behavior to other healthcare clinicians, patients, and family members.

In response to clinical staff surveys that identified that some staff were not taking rest or meal breaks a Meal Break Guiding Principles statement was created and a toolkit was developed that could assist units in creating a culture that encouraged rest periods (Fig. 10.3). A respite room was also created to provide a dedicated space for clinicians to take breaks away from the clinical care areas. Additional projects included an initiative to address staff resilience, and development of an educational tool to assist staff in resourcing quick, real-time safety and distressing issues (Fig. 10.4). These initiatives have been beneficial in promoting a culture focused on improving the work environment for clinicians including improving communication and promoting collaboration. A number of resources exist for promoting the HWE standards including position statements on respectful behavior expectations, workplace violence prevention, and teamwork training (Table 10.1).

RUSH UNIVERSITY
MEDICAL CENTER

Medical Staff Code of Conduct and Professional Behavior

Professional behavior, ethics and integrity are expected of each individual member of the Medical Staff at Rush University Medical Center. This Code is a statement of the ideals and guidelines for professional and personal behavior of the Medical Staff in all dealings with patients, their families, other health professionals, employees, students, vendors, government agencies, society and among themselves, in order to promote the highest quality of patient care, safety, trust, integrity and honesty.

Each Medical Staff member has a responsibility for the welfare, well-being, and betterment of the patient being served. In addition, the Medical Staff member has responsibility to maintain his/her own professional and personal well-being, in addition to maintaining a reputation for truth and honesty.

Guidelines for Interpersonal Relationships

- Treat all medical staff, hospital staff, housestaff or students, and patients with courtesy and respect
- You will not engage in the following behaviors:
  - Sexual harassment or making sexual innuendoes
  - Using abusive language or repetitive sarcasm
  - Making threats of violence, retribution, litigation, or financial harm
  - Making racial or ethnic slurs
  - Actions that are reasonably felt by others to represent intimidation
  - Using foul language, shouting, or rudeness
  - Criticizing medical staff, hospital staff, housestaff, or students in front of others while in the workplace or in front in patients
  - Shaming others for negative outcomes
  - Physically or verbally slandering or threatening other physicians or health care professionals
  - Romantic and/or sexual relationships with your current or former patients. This extends to key third parties such as spouses, children or parents of patients
  - Revealing confidential patient or staff information to anyone not authorized to receive it.
- Do not treat patients while impaired by alcohol, drugs, or illness. The patient would be placed at risk
- Support and follow hospital policies and procedures; address dissatisfaction with policies through appropriate channels
- Use conflict management skills and direct verbal communication in managing disagreements with associates and staff
- Cooperate and communicate with other providers displaying regard for their dignity

Fig. 10.1 (continued)

- Be truthful at all times
- Wear attire that reflects your professional role and respects your patients
- Develop and institute a plan to manage your stress and promote your personal well being

Guidelines for Clinical Practice

- Respond promptly and professionally when called upon by fellow practitioners to provide appropriate consultation and service
- Respond to patient and staff request promptly ands appropriately
- Respect patient confidentiality and privacy at all times; follow all regulations for release of information
- Treat patient families with respect and consideration while following all applicable laws regarding such relationships (release of information, advance directives, etc,)
- Seek and obtain appropriate consultation
- Arrange for appropriate coverage when not available
- Do one's best to provide the best and efficient care
- Prepare and maintain medical records within established time frames
- Disclose potential conflicts of interests and resolve the conflict in the best interest of the patient
- When terminating or transferring care of a patient to another physician, provide prompt, pertinent and appropriate medical documentation to assure continuation of care

Guidelines for Relationshiops with Hospital & Community

- Abide by all rules, regulations, policies and bylaws of Rush University Medical Center
- Serve on Hospital and medical staff committees
- Assist in the identification of colleagues who may be professionally impaired or disruptive
- Maintain professional skills and knowledge and participate in continuing education
- Refrain from fraudulent scientific practices
- Accurately present data derived from research
- Request appropriate approval from the Institutional Review Board (IRB) prior to human research activities and abide by all laws and regulations applying to these activities
- Follow and obey the law of the land and refrain from unlawful activity at all times
- Cooperate with legal professionals, including Hospital legal counsel, unless such cooperation is prohibited by law
- Participate in clinical outcome reviews, quality assurance procedures and quality improvement programs
- Hold in the strictest confidence all information pertaining to peer review, quality assurance, and quality improvement
- Protect from loss or theft, and not share, log-ins and passwords to any hospital system that contains patient identifiable information or other confidential information.

Fig. 10.1 (**a–c**) Medical staff code of conduct example. Reprinted with permission, Rush University Medical Center, Chicago, IL, USA

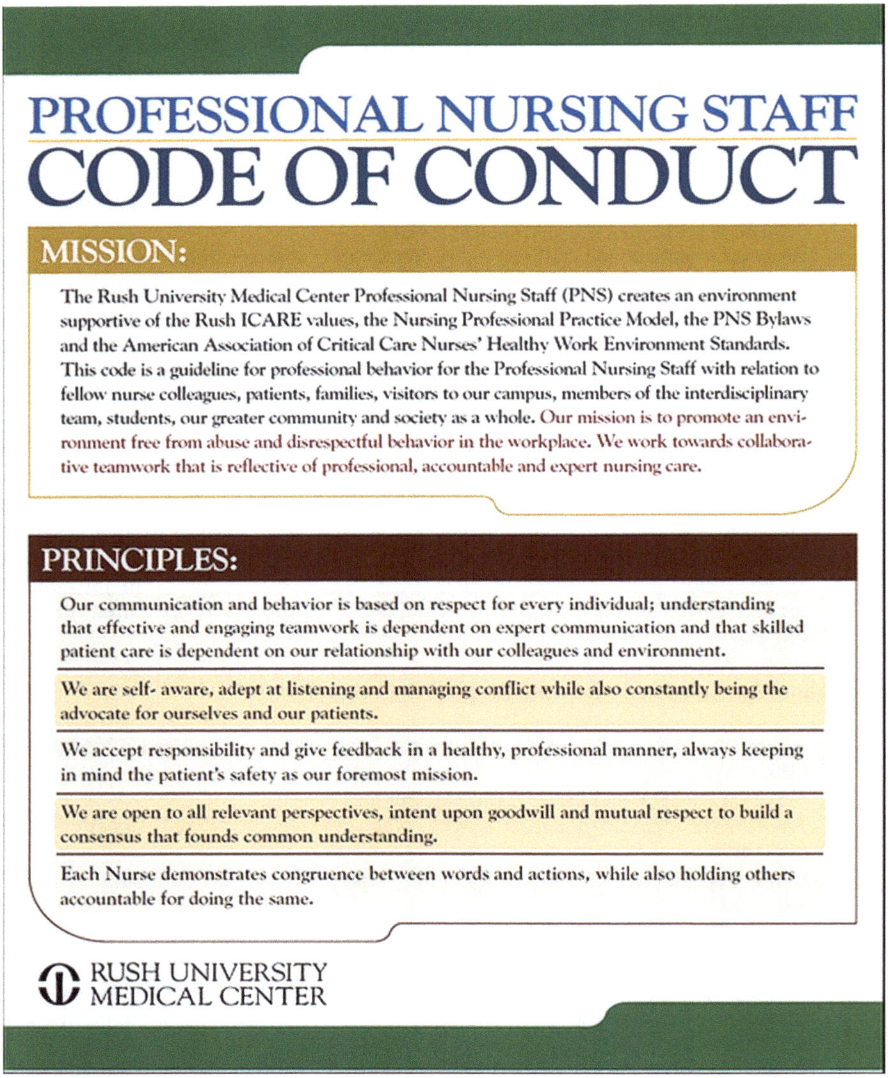

PROFESSIONAL NURSING STAFF
CODE OF CONDUCT

MISSION:

The Rush University Medical Center Professional Nursing Staff (PNS) creates an environment supportive of the Rush ICARE values, the Nursing Professional Practice Model, the PNS Bylaws and the American Association of Critical Care Nurses' Healthy Work Environment Standards. This code is a guideline for professional behavior for the Professional Nursing Staff with relation to fellow nurse colleagues, patients, families, visitors to our campus, members of the interdisciplinary team, students, our greater community and society as a whole. Our mission is to promote an environment free from abuse and disrespectful behavior in the workplace. We work towards collaborative teamwork that is reflective of professional, accountable and expert nursing care.

PRINCIPLES:

Our communication and behavior is based on respect for every individual; understanding that effective and engaging teamwork is dependent on expert communication and that skilled patient care is dependent on our relationship with our colleagues and environment.

We are self- aware, adept at listening and managing conflict while also constantly being the advocate for ourselves and our patients.

We accept responsibility and give feedback in a healthy, professional manner, always keeping in mind the patient's safety as our foremost mission.

We are open to all relevant perspectives, intent upon goodwill and mutual respect to build a consensus that founds common understanding.

Each Nurse demonstrates congruence between words and actions, while also holding others accountable for doing the same.

RUSH UNIVERSITY MEDICAL CENTER

Fig. 10.2 Nursing code of conduct example. Reprinted with permission, Rush University Medical Center, Chicago, IL, USA

Strategies for Enhancing Care for Providers in the ICU

Improving care in the ICU for care providers requires focused efforts at assessing the ICU environment and creating an action plan for improvement. Table 10.2 outlines an example of an assessment to evaluate the healthcare work environment. Addressing communication, collaboration, and teamwork are fundamental to

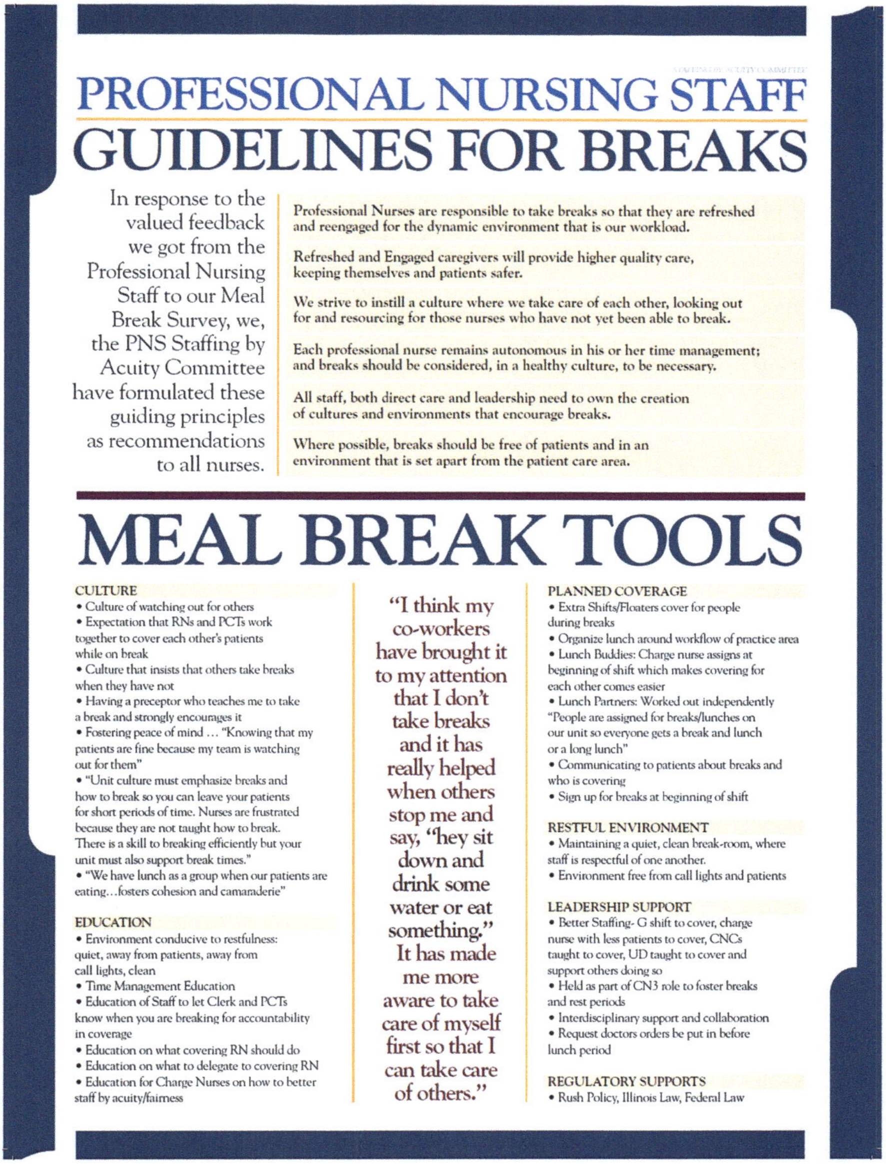

STAFFING BY ACUITY COMMITTEE

PROFESSIONAL NURSING STAFF

GUIDELINES FOR BREAKS

In response to the valued feedback we got from the Professional Nursing Staff to our Meal Break Survey, we, the PNS Staffing by Acuity Committee have formulated these guiding principles as recommendations to all nurses.

Professional Nurses are responsible to take breaks so that they are refreshed and reengaged for the dynamic environment that is our workload.

Refreshed and Engaged caregivers will provide higher quality care, keeping themselves and patients safer.

We strive to instill a culture where we take care of each other, looking out for and resourcing for those nurses who have not yet been able to break.

Each professional nurse remains autonomous in his or her time management; and breaks should be considered, in a healthy culture, to be necessary.

All staff, both direct care and leadership need to own the creation of cultures and environments that encourage breaks.

Where possible, breaks should be free of patients and in an environment that is set apart from the patient care area.

MEAL BREAK TOOLS

CULTURE
- Culture of watching out for others
- Expectation that RNs and PCTs work together to cover each other's patients while on break
- Culture that insists that others take breaks when they have not
- Having a preceptor who teaches me to take a break and strongly encourages it
- Fostering peace of mind … "Knowing that my patients are fine because my team is watching out for them"
- "Unit culture must emphasize breaks and how to break so you can leave your patients for short periods of time. Nurses are frustrated because they are not taught how to break. There is a skill to breaking efficiently but your unit must also support break times."
- "We have lunch as a group when our patients are eating…fosters cohesion and camaraderie"

EDUCATION
- Environment conducive to restfulness: quiet, away from patients, away from call lights, clean
- Time Management Education
- Education of Staff to let Clerk and PCTs know when you are breaking for accountability in coverage
- Education on what covering RN should do
- Education on what to delegate to covering RN
- Education for Charge Nurses on how to better staff by acuity/fairness

"I think my co-workers have brought it to my attention that I don't take breaks and it has really helped when others stop me and say, "hey sit down and drink some water or eat something." It has made me more aware to take care of myself first so that I can take care of others."

PLANNED COVERAGE
- Extra Shifts/Floaters cover for people during breaks
- Organize lunch around workflow of practice area
- Lunch Buddies: Charge nurse assigns at beginning of shift which makes covering for each other comes easier
- Lunch Partners: Worked out independently "People are assigned for breaks/lunches on our unit so everyone gets a break and lunch or a long lunch"
- Communicating to patients about breaks and who is covering
- Sign up for breaks at beginning of shift

RESTFUL ENVIRONMENT
- Maintaining a quiet, clean break-room, where staff is respectful of one another.
- Environment free from call lights and patients

LEADERSHIP SUPPORT
- Better Staffing- G shift to cover, charge nurse with less patients to cover, CNCs taught to cover, UD taught to cover and support others doing so
- Held as part of CN3 role to foster breaks and rest periods
- Interdisciplinary support and collaboration
- Request doctors orders be put in before lunch period

REGULATORY SUPPORTS
- Rush Policy, Illinois Law, Federal Law

Fig. 10.3 Healthy work environment guideline example. Reprinted with permission, Rush University Medical Center, Chicago, IL, USA

improving care in the ICU. The literature on ICU teamwork identifies that communication, leadership, coordination, and decision making are processes that influence performance in the ICU. Effective teamwork has been identified as crucial for

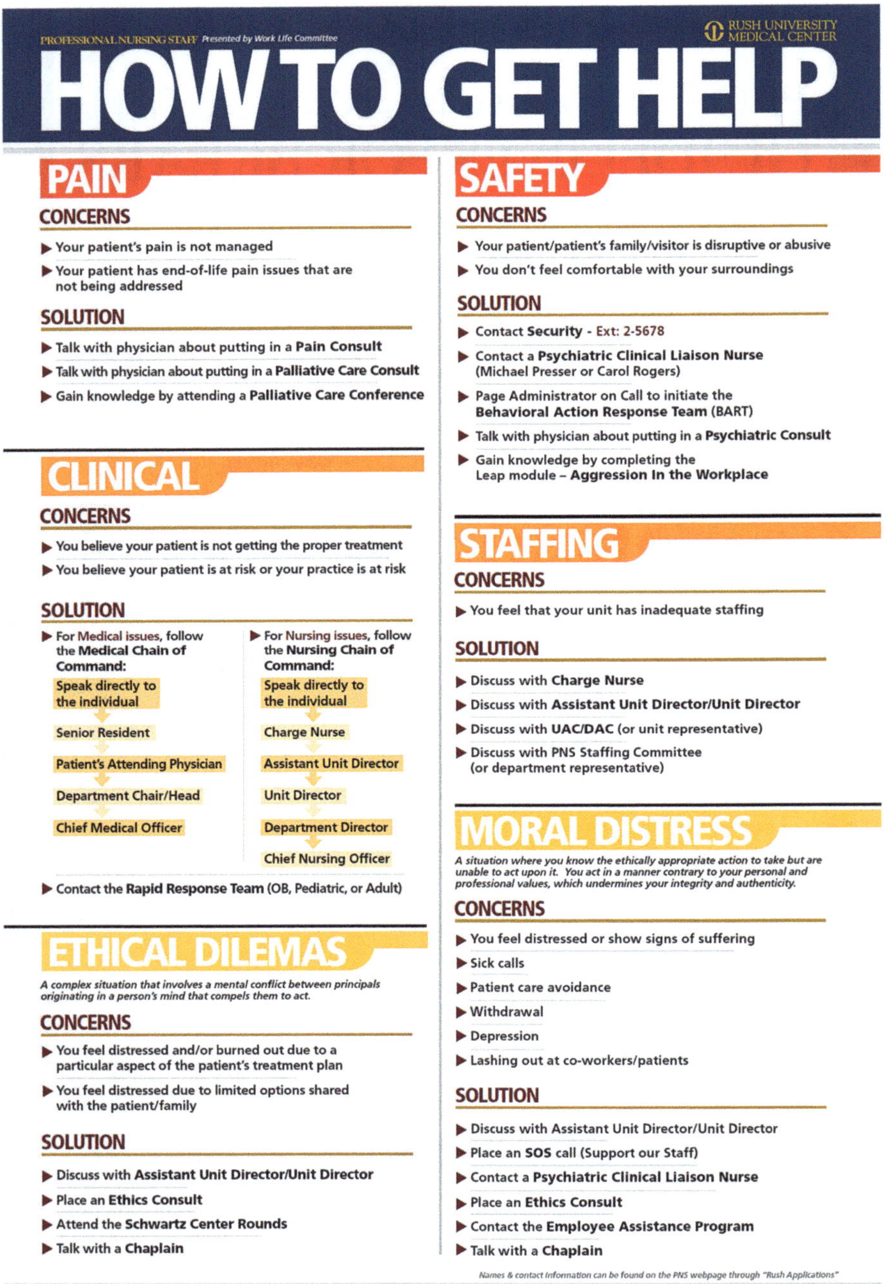

PROFESSIONAL NURSING STAFF Presented by Work Life Committee

RUSH UNIVERSITY MEDICAL CENTER

HOW TO GET HELP

PAIN

CONCERNS

- Your patient's pain is not managed
- Your patient has end-of-life pain issues that are not being addressed

SOLUTION

- Talk with physician about putting in a **Pain Consult**
- Talk with physician about putting in a **Palliative Care Consult**
- Gain knowledge by attending a **Palliative Care Conference**

CLINICAL

CONCERNS

- You believe your patient is not getting the proper treatment
- You believe your patient is at risk or your practice is at risk

SOLUTION

- For Medical issues, follow the **Medical Chain of Command:**
  Speak directly to the individual → Senior Resident → Patient's Attending Physician → Department Chair/Head → Chief Medical Officer
- For Nursing issues, follow the **Nursing Chain of Command:**
  Speak directly to the individual → Charge Nurse → Assistant Unit Director → Unit Director → Department Director → Chief Nursing Officer
- Contact the **Rapid Response Team** (OB, Pediatric, or Adult)

ETHICAL DILEMAS

A complex situation that involves a mental conflict between principals originating in a person's mind that compels them to act.

CONCERNS

- You feel distressed and/or burned out due to a particular aspect of the patient's treatment plan
- You feel distressed due to limited options shared with the patient/family

SOLUTION

- Discuss with **Assistant Unit Director/Unit Director**
- Place an **Ethics Consult**
- Attend the **Schwartz Center Rounds**
- Talk with a **Chaplain**

SAFETY

CONCERNS

- Your patient/patient's family/visitor is disruptive or abusive
- You don't feel comfortable with your surroundings

SOLUTION

- Contact **Security** - Ext: 2-5678
- Contact a **Psychiatric Clinical Liaison Nurse** (Michael Presser or Carol Rogers)
- Page Administrator on Call to initiate the **Behavioral Action Response Team** (BART)
- Talk with physician about putting in a **Psychiatric Consult**
- Gain knowledge by completing the Leap module – **Aggression In the Workplace**

STAFFING

CONCERNS

- You feel that your unit has inadequate staffing

SOLUTION

- Discuss with **Charge Nurse**
- Discuss with **Assistant Unit Director/Unit Director**
- Discuss with **UAC/DAC** (or unit representative)
- Discuss with PNS Staffing Committee (or department representative)

MORAL DISTRESS

A situation where you know the ethically appropriate action to take but are unable to act upon it. You act in a manner contrary to your personal and professional values, which undermines your integrity and authenticity.

CONCERNS

- You feel distressed or show signs of suffering
- Sick calls
- Patient care avoidance
- Withdrawal
- Depression
- Lashing out at co-workers/patients

SOLUTION

- Discuss with Assistant Unit Director/Unit Director
- Place an **SOS** call (Support our Staff)
- Contact a **Psychiatric Clinical Liaison Nurse**
- Place an **Ethics Consult**
- Contact the **Employee Assistance Program**
- Talk with a **Chaplain**

Names & contact information can be found on the PNS webpage through "Rush Applications"

Fig. 10.4 Healthy work environment resource tool example. Reprinted with permission, Rush University Medical Center, Chicago, IL, USA

Table 10.1 ICU healthy work environment resources

- Standards for Establishing and Sustaining Healthy Work Environments: http://www.aacn.org/WD/HWE/Docs/ExecSum.pdf
- Workplace Violence Prevention Position Statement: http://www.aacn.org/WD/practice/docs/publicpolicy/workplace-violence.pdf
- Zero Tolerance for Abuse Position Statement: http://www.aacn.org/WD/practice/docs/publicpolicy/zero-tolerance-for-abuse.pdf
- Moral Distress Position Statement: http://www.aacn.org/WD/Practice/Docs/Moral_Distress.pdf
- TeamSTEPPS™: http://teamstepps.ahrq.gov/abouttoolsmaterials.htm

  TeamSTEPPS™ is an evidence-based teamwork training system aimed at optimizing patient outcomes by improving communication and teamwork skills among health care professionals

Chest physician

- Creating Healthy Work Environments: Introduction (January 2007, p. 18)
- Creating Healthy Work Environments: Skilled Communication (February 2007, p. 16)
- Creating Healthy Work Environments: Authentic Leadership (March 2007, p. 19)
- Creating Healthy Work Environments: Appropriate Staffing (April 2007, p. 18)
- Creating Healthy Work Environments: True Collaboration (May 2007, p. 10)
- Standards for Establishing and Sustaining Healthy Work Environments: Effective Decision Making (June 2007, p. 16)
- Creating Healthy Work Environments: Meaningful Recognition (July 2007, p. 15)

Table 10.2 Sample assessment questions to evaluate healthy work environments

Administrators, nurse managers, physicians, nurses, and other staff maintain frequent communication to prevent each other from being surprised or caught off guard by decisions
Administrators, nurse managers, and physicians involve nurses and other staff to an appropriate degree when making important decisions
Administrators and staff work to ensure there are enough staff to maintain patient safety
The formal reward and recognition systems work to make staff feel valued
Administrators, nurse managers, physicians, nurses, and other staff members speak up and let people know when they've done a good job
Staff feel able to influence the policies, procedures, and bureaucracy around them
Administrators, nurse managers, physicians, nurses, and other staff have zero-tolerance for disrespect and abuse. If they see or hear someone being disrespectful, they hold them accountable regardless of the person's role or position
When administrators, nurse managers, and physicians speak with nurses and other staff, it is not one-way communication or order giving. Instead, they seek input and use it to shape decisions
Administrators, nurse managers, physicians, nurses, and other staff are careful to consider the patient's and family's perspectives whenever they are making important decisions
There are motivating opportunities for personal growth, development, and advancement

Adapted from The AACN Healthy Work Environment Assessment: http://www.aacn.org/dm/hwe/hweviewquestions.aspx?menu=hwe, accessed 3 November 2012

providing optimal care in the ICU [6]. A recent literature review on ICU team performance identified a number of factors that impact ICU performance including communication norms, attitudes and personalities, leadership styles, collaboration, which in turn impact patient and team outcome (Fig. 10.5) [7].

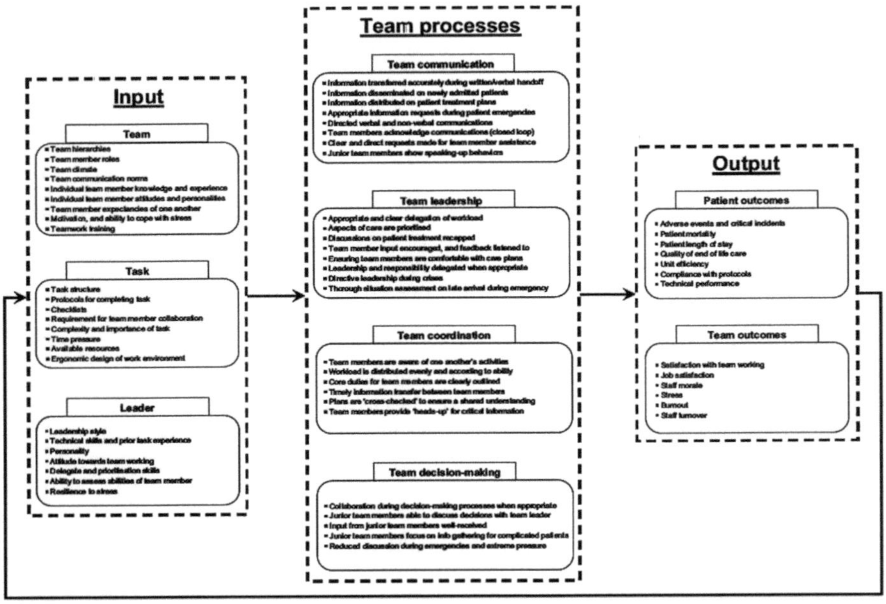

Fig. 10.5 ICU team performance framework. Adapted from Reader et al., Critical Care Medicine 2009 [7]

Effective communication is a component of quality of care and patient safety [8, 9]. An increased emphasis on communication for healthcare professionals has been advocated for optimal patient care [10–15]. This is especially relevant to critically ill patients who often have care needs from multiple services, increasing the risk of communication breakdowns in the ICU [16–19]. A number of resources for improving communication are available including suggested communication formats. The SBAR (Situation–Background–Assessment–Recommendation) [20] communication format provides a framework to promote effective communication between members of the health care team. SBAR allows for an easy and focused way to set expectations for what will be communicated and how between members of the team, which is essential for developing teamwork and fostering a culture of patient safety (Fig. 10.6).

The application of crew resource management (CRM) methods to health care settings has also been proposed as a strategy to improve teamwork and communication and patient safety [21]. At our university medical center, CRM training was integrated into all care areas over a several-year timeline. In the ICUs, all staff attended a 4 h CRM training session, which focused on establishing principles that were deemed important by our specific team members. The CREW training session occurred over a period of 2 days for each adult ICU, emergency department, and operating room. In addition, areas of pediatrics and labor and delivery were included in the sessions as well. During the two-day training session, each section

SBAR report to physician about a critical situation

S	**Situation** **I am calling about** <patient name and location>. **The patient's code status is** <code status> **The problem I am calling about is** ____________________________. I am afraid the patient is going to arrest. **I have just assessed the patient personally:** **Vital signs are:** Blood pressure _____/_____, Pulse ______, Respiration_____ and temperature ______ **I am concerned about the:** Blood pressure because it is over 200 or less than 100 or 30 mmHg below usual Pulse because it is over 140 or less than 50 Respiration because it is less than 5 or over 40. Temperature because it is less than 96 or over 104.
B	**Background** **The patient's mental status is:** Alert and oriented to person place and time. Confused and cooperative or non-cooperative Agitated or combative Lethargic but conversant and able to swallow Stuporous and not talking clearly and possibly not able to swallow Comatose. Eyes closed. Not responding to stimulation. **The skin is:** Warm and dry Pale Mottled Diaphoretic Extremities are cold Extremities are warm **The patient is not or is on oxygen.** The patient has been on ________ (l/min) or (%) oxygen for ______ minutes (hours) The oximeter is reading _______% The oximeter does not detect a good pulse and is giving erratic readings.
A	**Assessment** **This is what I think the problem is:** <say what you think is the problem> **The problem seems to be cardiac infection neurologic respiratory** _____ **I am not sure what the problem is but the patient is deteriorating.** **The patient seems to be unstable and may get worse, we need to do something.**
R	**Recommendation** **I suggest or** request that you <say what you would like to see done>. transfer the patient to critical care come to see the patient at this time. Talk to the patient or family about code status. Ask the on-call family practice resident to see the patient now. Ask for a consultant to see the patient now. **Are any tests needed:** Do you need any tests like CXR, ABG, EKG, CBC, or BMP? Others? **If a change in treatment is ordered then ask:** How often do you want vital signs? How long to you expect this problem will last? If the patient does not get better when would you want us to call again?

This SBAR tool was developed by Kaiser Permanente. Please feel free to use and reproduce these materials in the spirit of patient safety, and please retain this footer in the spirit of appropriate recognition.

Fig. 10.6 SBAR communication tool

met and the first task was introductions. The training session included physicians, nurses, pharmacists, respiratory therapists, and the dietitian (where applicable). The first day of the session included identification of three high priority patient safety initiatives. Once these were agreed upon and approved by the team, the room was divided into groups of three to four individuals. The smaller groups were tasked on how they would best accomplish the three tasks chosen with current resources.

In addition, we were encouraged to suggest resources needed to support the changes. The discussions created a healthy and open environment for all as the moderator was a pilot who utilizes the team and checklist concept on a daily basis. The second day of the session also allowed us to test the process improvement initiatives for patient safety to observe if there were any issues the group did not think of. The training received positive feedback and many of these initiatives are the core of ICU practice today.

Another formal training program is TeamSTEPPS™, an evidence-based teamwork training system aimed at optimizing patient outcomes by improving communication and teamwork skills among health care professionals. TeamSTEPPS, developed by the United States Department of Defense in collaboration with the Agency for Healthcare Research and Quality [22], focuses on developing a cadre of teamwork instructors with the skills to train and coach other staff members and a series of interactive workshops focusing on communication and teamwork skills (http://teamstepps.ahrq.gov/about-2cl_3.htm#TSTP).

Burnout and Moral Distress in the ICU

ICU care providers are at risk for burnout and moral distress in the ICU due to prolonged exposure to job stressors and conflicts related to goals of care for complex critically ill patients. Burnout is a psychological term used to describe the experience of long-term exhaustion. It can lead to emotional instability, fatigue, loss of purpose and energy, absenteeism, and lower job satisfaction [2, 23, 24]. The known factors associated with burnout include end-of-life issues, conflicts, lack of recognition and responsibility overload and the stressors associated with the ICU environment [23, 25–27]. A recent study on burnout in ICU caregivers with 3,052 physicians, nurses, and nursing assistants found several factors that were associated with higher risk of burnout including being a nurse assistant, being male, having no children, and being under age 40 [23].

At our university medical center, anecdotal reports from ICU clinical staff indicated that some staff were experiencing stress and at times distress related to providing care for complex critically ill patients with uncertain prognosis. As part of a quality improvement initiative to further address the staff reports, formal assessment of moral distress was assessed with the use of a descriptive questionnaire study [28]. An established moral distress assessment tool, the Corley Moral Distress scale [29, 30], was used to assess levels of moral distress among 28 ICU staff nurses.

Overall, nurses reported that situations associated with moral distress did not occur frequently, but they indicated that prior situations were associated with a moderate level of moral distress. The highest levels of distress were associated with the provision of aggressive care to patients not expected to benefit from the care. Moral distress was significantly correlated with years of nursing experience. Respondents identified that moral distress adversely affected job satisfaction, retention, psychological and physical well-being, self-image, and spirituality [28]. Additionally, the experience of moral distress influenced attitudes toward advanced directives and participation in blood donation and organ donation, with some identifying they would not donate blood or donate an organ after experiencing futile care for patients who were terminal. The results of the study reinforced that moral distress is experienced by ICU providers, often as a result from providing aggressive care to patients not expected to benefit from critical care. Based on the experience of conducting the study, the ICU began to incorporate a more proactive approach to recognizing difficult patient care situations and integrating additional discussion on rounds. Palliative care consultations were also more readily accepted as an expected component of caring for critically ill patients with complex care needs. In addition, there have been Palliative Care team members who have rounded with the ICU team (e.g., MICU) and following up on past, current, and future cases which helped with giving the nursing and physician staff feedback and allow time to debrief on clinical scenarios. Additionally, a process was created by which any members of the health care team could call a consult to both the ethics consultative serve or the palliative care team directly.

Supporting ICU Providers

A number of coping strategies may assist ICU caregivers in the process of caring for themselves including staff support groups, regular interdisciplinary meetings to discuss difficult cases, and formal staff training in communication and conflict-resolution skills [2]. The use of team workshops and staff education to help ICU staff cope with moral distress has been shown to be effective in reducing moral distress among ICU care providers [31]. Other strategies such as the use of a daily goals worksheet to improve communication about patient care have been demonstrated to also improve ICU clinician satisfaction [32–34].

One successful initiative that has been implemented at our university medical center has been to host Schwartz Center Rounds based on the model proposed by the Schwartz Center for Compassionate Healthcare (www.theschwartzcenter.org), a nationwide nonprofit organization dedicated to strengthening the relationship between patients and their clinical caregivers. Founded by the family of Ken Schwartz who died of lung cancer at age 40, the center promotes the provision of compassionate care. Schwartz Center Rounds allows caregivers to come together on a regular basis to discuss challenging emotional and social issues they have faced in caring for patients. Each session begins with a brief introduction with multiprofessional co-facilitators welcoming participants and sharing background information about the Schwartz Center. A panel representing members of the healthcare team who were involved in the care for a patient speak to the specific case and share their personal experiences. The facilitators promote discussion with the panel and audience, some of whom may have also been involved in the specific case and also share their experiences and thoughts. The rounds have proven to be a successful format for facilitating interprofessional discussion of difficult cases and promote a forum for sharing [35]. By creating an environment in which people could freely discuss their emotions health care providers have found their concerns are not isolated and merit conversation. Regardless of the results of the conversation, the mere discussion often facilitates healing by our health care providers.

The Schwartz Center Rounds format has been adopted by more than 230 healthcare organizations in the USA and UK to promote compassion, improved teamwork and reduce caregiver stress, and is another strategy to address and lessen the effects of moral distress in healthcare professionals and raise awareness of the importance of compassionate care.

Summary

The stressful work environment of the ICU can be taxing to ICU providers, posing risk for ICU burnout and moral distress. Promoting awareness of the importance of teamwork, communication and collaboration, along with adopting strategies to promote a healthy work environment can help to ensure that ICU providers are supported and valued for their commitments to providing patient and family-centered compassionate care.

References

1. Azoulay E, Timsit JF, Sprung CL, et al. Prevalence and factors of intensive care unit conflicts: the conflicus study. Am J Respir Crit Care Med. 2009;180:853–60.
2. Levy MM. Caring for the caregiver. Crit Care Clin. 2004;20(3):541–7.
3. Murphy JF. Providing support to doctors working in intensive care. Ir Med J. 2012;105(5):132.
4. American Association of Critical Care Nurses: Standards for establishing and sustaining healthy work environments. Aliso Viejo California: AACN. http://www.aacn.org/WD/HWE/Docs/ExecSum.pdf (2005). Retrieved 23 Apr 2014.
5. Committee on Quality of Health Care in America. Institute of Medicine. Crossing the quality chasm: a new health care system for the 21st century. Washington, DC: National Academies Press; 2001.
6. Reader TW, Cuthbertson BH, Decruyenaere J. Burnout in the ICU: potential consequences for staff and patient well being. Intensive Care Med. 2008;34:4–6.
7. Reader RW, Flin R, Mearns K, Cuthbertson BH. Developing a team performance framework for the intensive care unit. Crit Care Med. 2009;37:1781–93.
8. Manojlovich M. Nurse/physician communication through a sensemaking lens: shifting the paradigm to improve patient safety. Med Care. 2010;48(11):941–6.
9. Moorman DW. Communication, teams and medical mistakes. Ann Surg. 2007;245:173–5.
10. Bihorac Z. Let the beauty of what you love be what you do: finding balance between work and personal life in critical care medicine. In: Cheng EU, Park PK, editors. Current concepts in adult critical care. Chicago: Society of Critical Care Medicine; 2012. p. 1–11.
11. Curtis JR, Shannon SE. Transcending the silos: toward an interdisciplinary approach to end-of-life care in the ICU. Intensive Care Med. 2006;32:15–7.
12. Lingard L, Espin S, Evans C, Hawryluck L. The rules of the game: interprofessional collaboration on the intensive care unit team. Crit Care. 2004;8(6):R403–8.

13. Shannon DW, Myers LA. Nurse-to-physician communications: connecting for safety. Patient Saf Qual Healthc. 2012;9(20–22):24–6.
14. Azoulay E, Fassier T. Conflicts and communication gaps in the intensive care unit. Curr Opin Crit Care. 2010;16:654–65. doi:10.1097/MCC.0b013e32834044f0.
15. Kleinpell RM, Thompson D, Kelso L, Pronovost PJ. Targeting errors in the ICU: use of a national database. Crit Care Nurs Clin North Am. 2006;18:509–14.
16. Lateef O, Chen E, Darin M. Communication breakdowns in the academic intensive care unit. ICU Director. 2012;3:194–8.
17. Lundgren-Laine H, Kontio E, Perttila J, Korvenranta H, Forsstrom J, Salantera S. Managing daily intensive care activities: an observational study concerning ad hoc decision making of charge nurses and intensivists. Crit Care. 2011;15:R188.
18. Schmalenberg C, Kramer M. Nurse-physician relationships in hospitals: 20 000 nurses tell their story. Crit Care Nurse. 2009;29:74–83.
19. Walton MM. Hierarchies: the Berlin Wall of patient safety. Qual Saf Health Care. 2006;15:229–30.
20. Institute for Healthcare Improvement; SBAR tool for communication: a situational briefing mode. http://www.ihi.org/knowledge/Pages/Tools/SBARTechniqueforCommunicationASituationalBriefingModel.aspx (2011). Retrieved 23 Apr 2014.
21. Pratt SD, Mann S, Salisbury M, Greenberg P, Marcus R, Stabile B, et al. John M. Eisenberg Patient Safety and Quality Awards. Impact of CRM-based training on obstetric outcomes and clinicians' patient safety attitudes. Jt Comm J Qual Patient Saf. 2007;33(12):720–5.
22. Agency for Healthcare Research and Quality: TeamSTEPPS: national implementation. http://teamstepps.ahrq.gov/about-2cl_3.htm (2012). Retrieved 23 Apr 2014.
23. Merlani P, Verdon M, Businger A, Domenighetti G, Pargger H, Ricou B, et al. Burnout in ICU caregivers: a multicenter study of factors associated to centers. Am J Respir Crit Care Med. 2011;184(10):1140–6.
24. American Association of Critical Care Nurses. AACN policy position statement: moral distress. Aliso Viejo California: AACN; 2004.
25. Embriaco N, Papazian L, Kentish-Barnes N, Pochard F, Azoulay E. Burnout syndrome among critical care health-care workers. Curr Opin Crit Care. 2007;13(5):482–8.
26. Poncet MC, Toullic P, Papazian L, et al. Burnout syndrome in critical care nursing staff. Am J Respir Crit Care Med. 2007;175(7):698–704.
27. Raggio B, Malacarne P. Burnout in intensive care unit. Minerva Anestesiol. 2007;73 (4):195–200.
28. Elpern EH, Covert B, Kleinpell R. Moral distress of staff nurses in a medical intensive care unit. Am J Crit Care. 2005;14:523–30.
29. Corley MC, Elswick RK, Gorman M, Clor TR. Development and evaluation of a moral distress scale. J Adv Nurs. 2001;33:250–6.
30. Beumer CM. Innovative solutions: the effect of a workshop on reducing the experience of moral distress in an intensive care unit setting. Dimens Crit Care Nurs. 2008;27(6):263–7.
31. Narasimhan M, Eisen LA, Mahoney CD, Acerra FL, Rosen MJ. Improving nurse-physician communication and satisfaction in the intensive care unit with a daily goals worksheet. Am J Crit Care. 2006;15(2):217–22.
32. Bujak JS, Bartholomew K. Transforming physician-nurse communication. Deteriorating relationships must be reversed for the benefit of patients, staff and the organization. Healthc Exec. 2011;26(56):58–9.
33. Dingley C, Daugherty K, Derieg MK, Persing R. Improving patient safety through provider communication strategy enhancements. In: Henriksen K, Battles JB, Keyes MA, Grady ML, editors. Advances in patient safety: new directions and alternative approaches, Performance and tools, vol. 3. Rockville: Agency for Healthcare Research and Quality; 2008.
34. Joint Commission. The Joint Commission guide to improving staff communication. 2nd ed. Illinois: Oakbrook Terrace; 2009.
35. Zack E. Rush University Medical Center's First Year Experience Hosting Schwartz Center Rounds® (in review).

Part III
Integrating Intensive Care

Chapter 11
Rationing Without Contemplation: Why Attention to Patient Flow Is Important and How to Make It Better

Michael D. Howell and Jennifer P. Stevens

Abstract Inattentiveness to patient flow leads to rationing of critical care without contemplation. Many ICUs today operate at the limits of their capacity, making daily decisions about which patients can receive critical care. Historically, hospitals have dealt with this by building additional ICU beds. However, improving patient flow effectively increases ICU capacity without building additional beds, and problems with patient flow have well-documented, harmful effects on patients both in the ICU and waiting for care in the ICU. A number of tools from manufacturing and operations research allow us to understand, measure, and model patient flow, and to use this understanding to make meaningful improvements in real-world ICUs.

Keywords Communication • Mathematical theory • Patient safety • Efficiency • Interdisciplinary rounds • Protocols • Language

Background

As the United States' population ages, the demand for critical care will continue to increase. Annual costs for intensive care have increased by 44 % over 5 years, culminating in an investment of 0.7 % of the U.S. gross domestic product in 2005 [1]. Our current health care system may not be able to meet this demand. In the first quarter of the twenty-first century, the prevalence of ventilated patients is expected

M.D. Howell (✉)
Center for Quality, University of Chicago Medicine, 850 E. 58th Street, Chicago, IL 60637
e-mail: mdh@uchicago.edu

J.P. Stevens
Center for Healthcare Delivery Science, Division of Pulmonary, Critical Care and Sleep Medicine, Beth Israel Deaconess Medical Center, 330 Brookline Avenue, Boston, MA 02215, USA
e-mail: jpsteven@bidmc.harvard.edu

D.C. Scales and G.D. Rubenfeld (eds.), *The Organization of Critical Care*, Respiratory Medicine 18, DOI 10.1007/978-1-4939-0811-0_11,

to rise 80 % [2] while projections about the future supply of intensivists suggests one-fifth of the demand for critical care services may not be met in 2020 [3]. Further, residents of some parts of the country may face an even greater disparity between supply and demand. Already, geographic variation in intensive care unit (ICU) bed availability per capita varies nearly fivefold [4].

Why should we care about patient flow?

Inattentiveness to patient flow leads to rationing of critical care resources without contemplation, a state detrimental to both patients and providers.

At best, we are barely keeping up with the clinical need for critical care services [3]. But given the extensive investment in training necessary to generate every new intensivist, the field has had to turn to other, creative methods for meeting the demand for critical care. Other chapters of this text discuss some of these methods, such as using telemedicine to extend access to intensivists, regionalizing critical care (e.g., regionalization of sepsis centers), and broadening the use of non-critical-care-boarded physicians and nonphysician extenders in intensive care settings. These strategies are highly valuable as ways to extend the current system. A complementary strategy is the careful measurement, management and improvement of patient flow through current ICUs so as to increase the availability of existing resources to patients and minimize waste and wait. Better patient flow creates more ICU capacity without building more ICU beds.

We use the term "patient flow" to refer to the movement of patients into, through and out of an ICU. The movement of patients through this space is highly integrated in and dependent on other aspects of the hospital environment. Inattentiveness to patient flow leads to rationing of critical care resources without contemplation, a state detrimental to both patients and providers. Conceptualizing patient flow necessitates a deep understanding of the interconnectedness of the ICU to other departments and physical spaces within the hospital (the geographic structure of patient care) and of the directionality and motion of patients within critical care spaces (the temporal and dynamic flow of patient care). This chapter will address why it is valuable for all physicians to contemplate patient flow, several models proposed in the literature for how to measure it, and currently available proposals for what to do about it.

What Is Patient Flow?

Aggregate patient flow involves one complex organizational structure, the ICU, embedded within a larger network of complex organization structures. Figure 11.1 represents an example of how patients move into and out of a hypothetical ICU. Patients arrive in the ICU from a range of locations, including other critical care

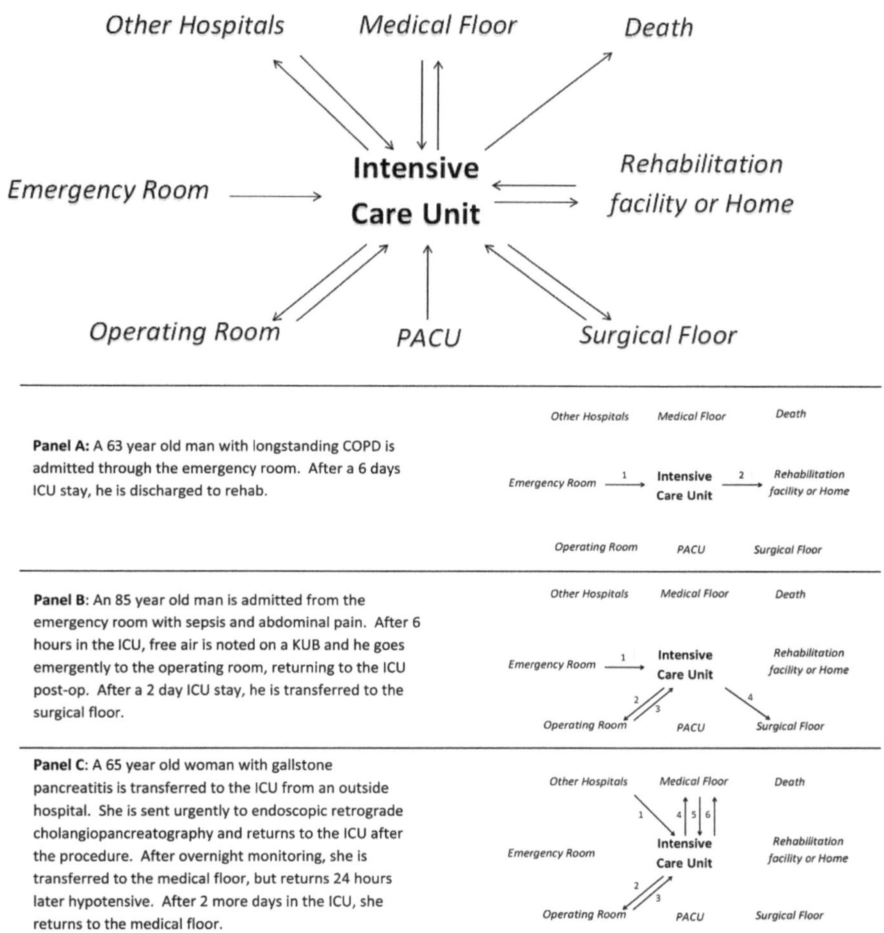

Fig. 11.1 A simplified example of the multiple points of entry and exit into a single intensive care unit at a single hospital with only one medical floor and one surgical floor. Each line represents a potential patient path. Even in this idealized example, measuring and understanding patient flow would need to accommodate the practice patterns of seven different entry sites with differing levels of acuity, predictability, and patient needs. The three panels below describe three different possible paths for individual patients

delivery spaces (e.g., other ICUs, the post-anesthesia care unit, the operating room), other hospitals, and other patient care areas (e.g., the emergency department, the medical or surgical floors). Once in the ICU, patients may stay for a short or long time, they may require ventilation, and they may undergo a series of procedures, both in and outside of the ICU. To leave, they may go to the medical or surgical floors, to another hospital, to a rehabilitation facility or home, or they may die.

Panels A–C describe the paths of three different patients as they flow through this ICU.

The movement of patients into, through and out of the ICU on any given day is affected by different forces at each of these levels. The patient flow in each of the other patient care spaces affects the patient flow in the ICU. For example, the number of patients arriving today in the ICU will be affected by the number of cases booked in the operating room that require an ICU bed (and if those cases are delayed or run on time), the number of patients in the emergency room, and any critically ill patients on non-ICU floors. Whether patients are transferred to the ICU will depend on how many beds are available, which is a marker of, again, multiple system-level forces including the acuity of the ICU itself, how quickly patients can be discharged to less acute levels of the hospital, whether staffing is available to care for those patients or if it is a weekend or holiday when the unit is short staffed, among other forces. This fragile homeostasis of patient flow can quickly unravel with a sudden surge of demand for critical care due to a disaster or other sudden influx of patients.

Each of the interconnected patient units of a hospital may have different and conflicting motivations from one another. An emergency room might be motivated to move a patient quickly to the next area of care. An ICU may be reluctant to accept a patient just as the nurses are changing shift, so as to minimize rework and handoffs. In the absence of system-level thinking, these conflicting motivations will continue to dominate patient flow, with both patient- and physician-level consequences.

Why Patient Flow Matters

Patient-Level Consequences of the Current State

Without a prospective effort to understand and alter patient flow through an ICU, patients and providers are buffeted about by the seemingly random and frustrating daily surges in demand for ICU beds. When demand for beds goes up, the ICU must perform rapid changes in staffing arrangements, consider discharging patients to the floor (potentially prematurely), or, alternatively, turn patients away. Patients with the misfortune to need critical care during high occupancy times in the ICU are left waiting in areas able to accommodate higher levels of patient acuity, such as the emergency room or PACU, or are triaged directly to the medical floor.

None of these choices serve patients well; patients who do not get ICU-level care when needed, whether through delays in the emergency room [5, 6], delays on the floor due to high ICU census [7–15], or premature discharge from the ICU, all appear to be at risk for harm. Chalfin and Trzeciak [14] examined over 50,000 patients transferred to the ICU from the emergency room and found those whose transfer was delayed by 6 or more hours had longer ICU length of stay (7 versus

6 days, $p < 0.001$), greater ICU mortality (10.7 % versus 8.4 %, $p < 0.001$), and greater hospital mortality (17.4 % versus 12.9 %, $p < 0.001$). Cardoso et al. [9] quantified each hour of waiting to be associated with a 1.5 % increased risk of death (HR 1.015, 95 % CI 1.006–1.023, $p = 0.001$). Similarly, Parkhe et al. [15] found that sick patients who were detoured to the medical floor had an increased relative risk of 30-day mortality of 2.46 (95 % CI 1.2–5.2) versus patients directly admitted to the ICU. Robert et al. [16] found that patients admitted to the ICU after initial refusal had higher risk-adjusted odds of mortality at day 60 as compared with those patients admitted initially (OR 1.83, 95 % CI 1.03–3.26, $p = 0.04$; odds of mortality at 28 days also trended in the same direction but was nonsignificant) and Sprung et al. [8] found that those who were never admitted after refusal also had a lower 28-day survival as compared with those patients who were admitted. Discharge at night, an event likely to occur due to inordinately large ICU census or because of inefficient patient flow, was found to independently predict death or ICU readmission among 3,462 ICU patients in France, along with other clinical factors [17]. The failure to align critical care resources with patient need, whether due to delays in transfer, blocked transfers, or premature discharges, can cause actual patient harm and have been described as "preventable adverse events" by healthcare safety advocates [18].

The literature around registered nurse staffing is quite clear—and makes intuitive sense—about another way of examining problems in patient flow, the risk of staffing strain. Needleman et al. [19] found higher nurse-to-patient ratios were associated with lower rates of hospital complications for patients such as urinary tract infections, pneumonia, and upper GI bleeding. Kane et al. [20] found an increase of one registered nurse per day was associated with 30 % lower odds of hospital acquired pneumonia, 50 % decreased odds of unplanned extubation, 60 % decreased odds of respiratory failure and nearly 30 % decreased odds of cardiac arrest, as well as both a decreased risk of patient mortality and shorter ICU lengths of stay. Since nurses are the providers with the greatest amount of time at the bedside delivering care, these studies illustrate the direct link between patient outcomes and availability of nurses for each patient.

The patient-level outcomes that result from busy physicians and decreased physician-to-patient ratios (e.g., when the ICU census is high) are less clear [21]. Admission during rounds, presumably when demands on providers intellectually and physically are greatest, appears to be risky. These patients have more than a 30 % increased odds of risk-adjusted hospital death [22]. But the risk to patients of admission during periods of high occupancy is not as clear. Tarnow-Mordi et al. [10] found a higher mortality rate for patients exposed to periods of higher ICU workload, as measured both through bed occupancy and staffing, while other investigators noted a higher ICU length of stay during periods of strain [11]. However, Iwashyna et al. [23] found that after risk adjustment, patients admitted on highest census days had no difference in mortality rates nor were they at an increased risk of transfer to other hospitals, a result confirmed when they also examined census in the previous 2-week period to admission. Other investigators who have examined the opposite condition, the risk of death from admission during low staffing time (as opposed to high patient volume), whether through nighttime admissions or weekend admissions, also found mixed results [24–26]. A meta-analysis by Cavallazzi et al. [27] reported no difference in mortality during nighttime admissions (OR 1.0, 95 % CI 0.87–1.17) but a small increased risk-adjusted odds of death from weekend admission (OR 1.08, 95 % CI 1.04–1.13). One can imagine that a full ICU places different demands on the intensivist than an admission during the intellectual process of morning rounds. Further, how different institutions manage periods of "high strain" with regard to staffing may vary, leading to the inconsistent conclusions in the literature. At the very least, these authors raise the concern that simply asking intensivists to work harder may not serve patients well, although Iwashyna et al. [23] demonstrated intensivists may be able to pull this off for the short term.

Whether or not patients suffer an increased risk of death, physicians do appear to behave differently during periods of high census. Stelfox et al. [12] examined patients on the floors with sudden clinical instability and found that availability of ICU beds was a driver of transfer to the ICU and of transitions in goals of care, although not of mortality. "Premature" discharge, presumably in response to increased demand for ICU beds, was associated with a higher severity-adjusted risk of death [28]. These findings suggest many physicians have a conscious or unconscious algorithm they use in order to triage patients to critical care beds, an algorithm that changes under external pressure from the scare resource of bed availability, often generated in the absence of formal triaging strategies or recommendations [29]. Put another way, physicians may ration critical care as a result of transient bed availability, either in an effort to adapt to scarce resources or as a way to cope with an intolerable situation. But the entire burden of managing transient surges in patient flow is controlled by the provider left to triage this process by whatever means necessary.

Provider-Level Consequences of the Current State

The demand for greater critical care bed availability [2, 3] and the call for the most experienced providers to deliver care [30] in the absence of more careful consideration of patient flow also will have a detrimental effect on providers. Nighttime and weekend hours was the most common reason cited by physicians in pediatric emergency rooms for 80 % of subjects not believing they would be able to work after 50 years of age [31]. In Ali and colleagues [32] cluster-randomized trial of different ICU staffing strategies comparing a strategy with weekends off versus continuous 14-day coverage, patients fared the same in the arm of the trial with weekends off but intensivists reported less burnout, less work-home life imbalance and less job distress. Burnout is already prevalent among intensivists, including among almost half of French intensivists, and is independently associated with clinical workload rather than only with severity of illness of the patient population [33]. Further, an increase in intensivist workload may limit the time available to teach and increase attending stress, both items that may increase trainee dissatisfaction and decrease the number of individuals going into the field [21, 34].

What Can We Do About It? Understanding Patient Flow

Consider the hypothetical example of a 20-bed ICU at a small, urban, academic hospital. We will return to this hypothetical ICU's dilemma throughout the rest of the chapter. The demand for each ICU bed has increased steadily in the past year. Patients are backing up into the emergency room and physicians and nursing staff are beginning to feel unsafe on the medical floors because they cannot transfer patients to the ICU in a timely way. Further, the ICU is often unable to accept outside hospital transfers to the unit for lack of available beds.

The hospital management has indicated that it wants to build another 10-bed ICU to solve the supply problem. They think the majority of admissions come in at the end of the day or overnight and the new ICU could off-load some of this supply. They suggest staffing can be rearranged to accommodate these new beds in the new ICU, with additional shifts for nurses and physicians and greater coverage demands for pharmacists and respiratory therapists, without hiring new staff. The hospital management believes quality of care with improve if they are able to make critical care resources more available to a larger number of patients.

As a guiding framework, consider that patient flow has a spatial component and a temporal component. The spatial component describes the number of different stops a patient will make through the ICU; in other words, this is the *map* of patient movement. The dynamic components are measurements of the various *rates* of patient movements, from one part of the map to another.

Alternatively, one could approach the question whether a new 10-bed ICU is needed by asking different questions. If we implemented evidence-based quality improvement strategies known to reduce ICU length of stay, would we be able to increase the *rate* of flow of patients enough to accommodate the demand? If, instead, we looked *why* most admissions are admitted to the ICU in the evening, could we make this process safer? If we examined how patients leave the ICU and improve this process, could we increase the timeliness of available, clean ICU beds? Perhaps building a new ICU actually *is* the best approach—but are there ways of testing different staffing arrangements prior to the capital investment of actually breaking ground?

The field of operations research provides us with a number of methods to quantify patient flow, which in turn reveal opportunities for improvement. In this section, we present a number of different approaches to measure and to quantify patient flow. As a guiding framework, consider that patient flow has a spatial component and a temporal component. The spatial component describes the number of different stops a patient will make through the ICU; in other words, this is the *map* of patient movement. The dynamic components are measurements of the various *rates* of patient movements, from one part of the map to another. To make improvements and changes in patient flow, an understanding of both how patients move and the rate at which they move is required.

We will first describe tools from *Lean* manufacturing to map the intricate detail of one's interconnected ICU and to quantify patient or provider time spent in each part of the process, the spatial component. (Chapter 12 of this text describes quality improvement strategies in detail that are also powerful for mapping how, why and when patients flow through the ICU.) We will then provide three different approaches from operations research to quantify the dynamic flow of patient movement. With each method, we will describe how it could be used to address the case study and create an alternative to building a new ICU.

Lean/Toyota Production System

Lean manufacturing, as created by Toyota, burst on the scene of the American car industry in the 1990s, as the industry sought out ways to improve its waste-filled industrial processes in the face of rapid loss of market share to foreign competitors [30, 31]. Health care, a complex industry riddled with waste of its own, has turned to Lean techniques in the past 10 years as a set of tools useful in standardizing processes of care and refocusing activities around adding value for the patient [35, 36].

A full discussion of Lean is beyond the scope of this chapter, but we will describe two tools that are particularly useful for understanding patient flow: process mapping and value-stream mapping. Implementing Lean methods requires that one map out each part of the process in careful detail. For example, in the ICU, if one is interested in understanding the patient flow out of the ICU to a medicine team, one would map out the details of each of the following processes: (1) how are patients triaged in the ICU to stepdown-level care? (2) How is a bed procured through the admitting department? (3) How do physicians communicate between the ICU and the medicine floor? (4) How do nurses communicate between the ICU and the medicine floor? (5) How does the system change if the patient has to make a stop along the way (e.g., in radiology)? (6) How is transport called? (7) What happens once the patient arrives at the medicine floor? For example, at our institution, when we analyzed the process required to administer a first dose of antibiotics in the ICU, we determined that it took 24 meaningful process steps.

After developing a detailed process map, the next step is mapping each step of each process as *value-added* or *non-value-added*. Processes are deemed to add value when the **customer** values the work being done in the particular step.[1] To add value, a step in the process must meet three criteria: (1) Does it transform the service or product? (2) Would someone pay for it? (3) Is it done right the first time? A pragmatically useful question to determine whether a particular step adds value is, "Would someone pay a dollar for this particular action?" Thus, a process step would be considered value-added when a *patient* would actually pay for what's being done. This might be actually *receiving* an antibiotic, actually talking with a doctor, or participating in physical therapy. In contrast, non-value-added processes fail to add value for the patient and represent waste, or "muda." Examples of non-value-added activities might be the time physicians spend writing a note, the transport of patients from one room to another, or the time that providers spend gathering supplies for a procedure. Even though these are all required, they are required because we have an imperfect system of care: no one would actually want to spend a dollar (for example) for a physician to gather up supplies to do a thoracentesis; they would pay for the *procedure* itself. In this kind of analysis, surprisingly little time is spent on value-added processes.

A critical insight of Lean is to direct attention to eliminating non-value-added steps rather than focusing effort on improving value-added steps. At first this seems counterintuitive—don't we want to focus on the things that matter? But it turns out to be a matter of simple math: if your process is 10 % value-added steps, and 90 % non-value-added steps (as is commonly the case), it is much more efficient to improve the overall process by *eliminating* non-value-added steps. Any process can be made more reliable in only two ways: by making each and every step more reliable, or by eliminating steps ... and even perfectly reliable steps still take time. If they don't add value, you should try to get rid of them.

Non-value-added waste can further be subdivided into *over-production, waiting, inventory, transport, motion, rework, and over-processing* [37]. Table 11.1 describes each of these types of non-value-added waste and provides examples from the process of gathering equipment to place a central venous catheter and inserting that catheter into the patient. There are commonly used formalisms to represent a value-stream map, but a simple example suffices. After the decision to give an IV antibiotic, the value-added step is actually receiving the antibiotic—for example, the 30 minute that the antibiotic is actually infusing. But the process might include 3 minute of writing an order in the computer, 2 minute to look up and page the antimicrobial stewardship team, 5 minute waiting for them to call back, 5 minute of discussion, 2 minute for them to approve the order in the computer, 15 minute waiting for the pharmacist to electronically approve the order, 30 minute waiting in queue in the central pharmacy, 15 minute of preparation, 5 minute for a double-check by another pharmacist, 30 minute of waiting to be transported to the ICU, 20 minute

[1] In healthcare, decisions about who the customer is can be complex (e.g., patient, payor, family members, etc.; sometimes another physician is the customer of a service), but we usually adopt the perspective of the patient as the customer. This is both simpler and, usually, clarifying in both a practical and ethical sense.

Table 11.1 Seven types of non-value-added steps in a process ("waste" or *muda*)

Non-value-added category (waste)	Definition	Example
Over-production	Generating an item before it is necessary, "just in case."	The physician who grabs an extra set of sterile gloves for the central line, just in case.
Waiting	Any good or service that is not moving or being processed.	Waiting for a chest X-ray after central line placement.
Transporting	Moving a product from one place to another, increasing risk that the product could be damaged en route.	The physician who must carry a large number of sterile items necessary for a procedure into the patient's room.
Inventory	The result of over-processing and waiting.	The large number of central line kits that sit in storage in the ICU and expire before they are used.
Motion	Unnecessary movements in a process.	The physician who realizes that all equipment is not available in the room and must return to the supply room for additional items
Rework	Required when defective products are made.	The physician who must reestablish a sterile field because sedation and pain control was inadequate and the patient contaminated the field.
Over-processing	Excessive or expensive processes when simpler processes would be just as effective.	The central line procedure is documented on a paper checklist, in an electronic note by the nurse, and in a dictated procedure note by the physician.

Definitions of the seven types of non-value-added waste in Lean and examples of each from the process of obtaining central access in a patient

for the actual transport, 15 minute for the nurse to find that the antibiotic was delivered, and 5 minute to transport and hang the antibiotic—a total of 152 minute of non-value-added time for a process with 30 minute of value-added-time. Put another way, ~84 % of the entire process is non-value-added. This is a typical amount of non-value-added time in many healthcare processes. From a patient or a societal perspective, particularly considering that a delay in antibiotics may increase the risk of death [37, 38], this seems like something we should try to make better. Calling the steps "non-value-added" is not a judgment about providers—these steps are absolutely required by our current system. But the system can be changed. In this example, the importance of focusing on the elimination of non-value-added steps becomes clear, and it suggests a straightforward approach for improvement. If we simply move this particular antibiotic into the ICU's automated dispensing cabinet, we will eliminate many steps in the process. Re-doing the calculation, we will find that the non-value-added time has dropped to 37 minute. We have changed from a process with only 16 % value-added time to one with 45 % value-added time, a near-tripling of efficiency. We could never have achieved this by focusing on improving the actual value-added steps. Can this translate into the real world?

In our own ICU, using Lean methods including the one described here, we reduced the median time to first-dose antibiotics by almost 2 hours, or 61 %, which was sustained for more than a year without ongoing intervention.

Returning to the case of our hypothetical 20-bed ICU, we will start to address management's question of whether we need another ICU by mapping out patient flow in the existing ICU. We are interested in why patients seem to be admitted later in the day and why there is a delay in moving them from the emergency room and floors into the ICU. Figure 11.2 maps the process of discharging a patient from the ICU to the medicine floor to make a new ICU bed clean and available to a new patient who is waiting in the emergency room. This is only one possible map for the discharge process—patients could also go home, to rehabilitation, to the surgical floor or to other hospitals, as described in Fig. 11.1. The process map for the ICU team moves from left to right and then continues on the second half of the diagram; the steps and the ICU patient are highlighted. Because the movement of the ICU patient is dependent on the availability of a floor bed, the process map also includes the floor team's steps for discharging a patient, moving sometimes in tandem and sometimes in sequence. The three patients involved, the ICU patient, the floor patient and the emergency room patient, all are waiting in their beds at each step of the process. At every step that they want to move, an arrow indicates where they would go if they could, but it is blocked by an X if they are unable to move due to the process that is unfolding below them. Despite the 24 steps involved between the two process maps, a patient moves at only three points: once from the floor to home, once from the ICU to the floor, and once from the ER to the ICU.

The process map also highlights the solution: only 3 of 24 steps (12.5 %) could be considered at least partially value-added to the customer, when they move to a new level of care. To improve this process and reduce the wait time of patients, we could drill down on each of these steps to improve them or eliminate them entirely. During six steps in Fig. 11.2, a bed is dirty and unable to be used for any patient. During five steps, a bed is clean but there are other delays in the system that prevents the transfer. These steps are waste. Eliminating even one of these steps—e.g., creating a system whereby the discharge order from the physician in the computer automatically notifies housekeeping to arrive to clean the bed—would reduce delay. Further, this process map only describes the current state. Lean would challenge providers to then take the next step to create the ideal system from scratch, minimizing waste and non-value-added steps.

The tools derived from lean production methods allow for several key tools in measuring and understanding patient flow: (1) what is the true process of patient care in the ICU, including the minutiae of each aspect of patient flow, and (2) what fraction of a patient's time in any given process does not add value. Based on this process, one could return to the hospital administration with the hypothesis that ICU delays are due to discharge delays and recommend a series of improvements to reduce wait times (and thereby decrease length of stay).

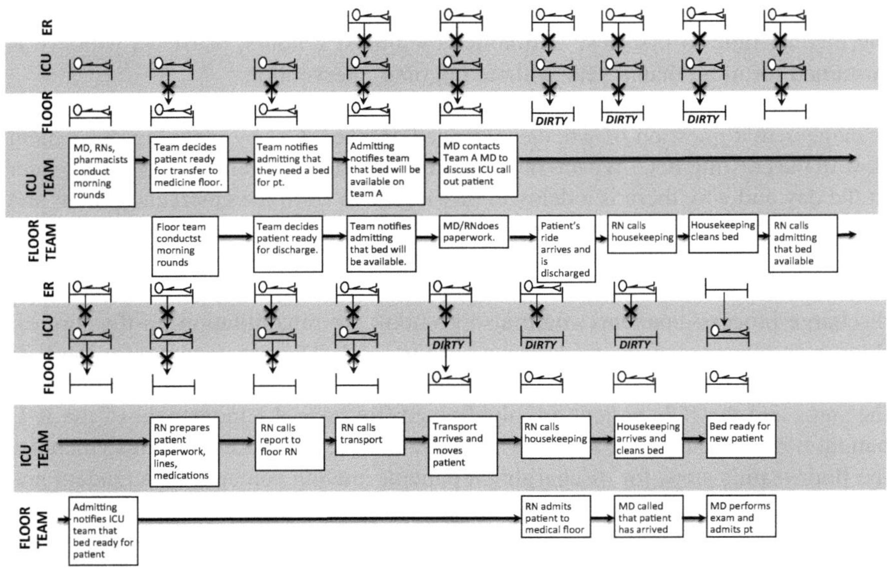

Fig. 11.2 An example of a process map of how a patient is moved from the ICU to the medicine floor to create a clean ICU bed. The process map for the ICU team moves from left to right, and then continues on the second half of the diagram; the steps and the ICU patient are highlighted. However, the movement of an ICU patient is dependent on the availability of a bed on another floor; the process of a medicine patient discharge is therefore included as well. At each step, three patients are illustrated waiting in their beds: the ICU patient (*shaded*), the medicine floor patient, and an emergency room patient who arrives mid-morning and must wait for an ICU bed to become available. Steps where patients want to move to a different bed are indicated by *arrows* between beds; steps where movement is blocked are then marked with an "X"

Operations Research

With the map of where and how patients move through the ICU, the *rate* at which patients moves through this web also becomes critical for changing and improving the process. Tools from operations research are well suited to measuring the dynamic aspects of patient flow. In 2005, the Institute of Medicine and the National Academy of Engineering produced a joint report, "Building a Better Delivery System: A New Engineering/Health Care Partnership" [39]. This report highlighted the usefulness of operations research, a field that developed over the twentieth century, to inform and improve health care. Operations research and queuing theory, the oldest branch of operations research, allows us a mathematical foundation on which to understand, quantify, and alter patient flow through the interconnected parts of the hospital. We will present three different approaches, from least to greatest complexity, and clarify when each might be helpful.

Little's Law

In 1961, John Little proposed a mathematical tautology for calculating the length of time an item remains in any given system. Little's Law suggests that under specific, essential conditions, the average number of items in the queue (the waiting time) is equal to the average rate items arrive multiplied by the average time in the system.

$$L = \lambda W,$$

where $L =$ average items in the queuing system, $W =$ average waiting time in the system, and $\lambda =$ average number of items per unit time arriving. For Little's Law to hold, there must be a conservation of items, that is, all those items that come in must come out [40].

Little offers the straightforward example of email turnaround to explain the law [41]. If one receives 50 emails a day ($\lambda = 50$ messages/day) and the average size of one's inbox is 150 messages ($L = 150$ messages), then the average time to return an email is 150 messages/50 messages/day or 3 days. This presumes that messages are deleted when answered (and all messages are answered and cannot exit the system any other way) [41].

To apply this same concept to the ICU, we will return to our case. After addressing ICU discharge, we now hope to decrease length of stay by implementing spontaneous breathing trials and spontaneous awakening trials in all patients ventilated for more than 2 days. Management wants to know what effect we should expect. To answer this question, we would like to estimate the average patient flow benefit this improvement strategy might provide. Girard et al.'s [42] awakening and breathing controlled trial found a reduction of 3 days median ICU length of stay for subjects in the intervention arm that received both daily spontaneous awakening trials and spontaneous breathing trials. Let's say our ICU has 1,360 admissions a year but only 22 % of patients are intubated with a length of stay of more than 2 days, i.e., could have met criteria for entrance into the ABC trial. Let's assume that these 22 % of patients have an average LOS of 9 days, but that everybody else has an average LOS of 4 days. That means that our average LOS will be $(0.22 \times 9) + (0.78 \times 4)/1{,}000 = 5.1$ days.

What is Little's Law good for? First, it lets us calculate the average daily census as a measure of capacity strain. But more importantly, it lets us understand how changes in length of stay will affect ICU census and throughput.

Little's Law tells us:

- $L = \lambda W \rightarrow$ Average daily census = # of admissions per day × average length of stay
- Average daily census = (1,360 admission per year/365) × 5.1 = 3.73 × 5.1 = 19

No wonder things feel so busy in our 20-bed ICU! An average daily census of 19 in a 20-bed unit is running very full, indeed. It is no surprise that there are many patients whom physicians would like to place in the ICU who cannot get in.

So what would happen to ICU throughput if our ICU institutes the approach of the ABC trial and drops the average length of stay for those 22 % of patients by 3 days—from 9 days to 6 days? Our new average LOS becomes $(0.22 \times 6) + (0.78 \times 4)/1{,}000 = 4.44$ days. This will drop our average daily census to 16.5 ($L = \lambda W \rightarrow \text{ADC} = (1{,}360/365) \times 4.44 = 3.73 \times 4.44 = 16.5$). Alternatively, if ICU demand has been higher than capacity (as is often the case), we will see an increase in ICU admissions until we are back at an average daily census of ~19. How many admissions would that be?

$L = \lambda W$
Average daily census = # admissions/day × average LOS
19 = # admissions/day × 4.44
# admissions/day = 4.28 (up from 3.73)
In a year: 1,561 admissions, up from 1,360 admissions per year previously

That's right: this single quality improvement intervention would let us care for ***201 additional patients every year***, without building additional ICU beds.

What can this surprisingly simple calculation tell us about patient flow through the ICU? We can see that wait time (i.e., length of stay) and arrival rate (i.e., number of admissions per day) provide the driving factors of ICU census. If we are to alter patient flow, these will be the two major levers to pull to alter patient flow without adding more beds. We have demonstrated that implementing an evidence-based strategy that makes the ICU safer would increase the number of admissions per year by about 15 % through decreasing length of stay and length of mechanical ventilation, which in turn may decrease rates of hospital-associated complications.

Queuing Theory

Unfortunately, Little's Law falls short when considering the details of any given day, rather than the average total capacity of the ICU, limiting its utility for solving problems such as managing staffing. To model the day-to-day changes in patient flow rather than average patient flow, we must build increasingly complex models that can accommodate the fluctuations in patient demand for ICU services. Queuing theory helps address some of these complexities of patient flow by calculating how much time customers (or patients) spend waiting. Originally derived at the turn of the last century around wait times and queuing for telephone exchanges [43], it has been applied to a range of health care concepts, including organ allocation [44], infectious diseases [45], operating room scheduling practices [46], and modeling of wait time management and changes in workforce due to surges in demand for diagnostic imaging [47]. The mathematical models used in queuing theory require assumptions that are simpler than the real world, such as all patients are triaged using the same method. Despite this shortcoming—that is present with any set of modeling assumptions—queuing theory does allow one to model the specific aspects of the process that can often derail patient flow, such as the randomness of patient arrivals and surges.

Queuing theory uses models that are broken down in terms of the *customer* and the *server* (e.g., vehicles waiting to go through a toll booth or patients waiting for admission to the ICU), the *input process* or *arrival process* (e.g., do patients arrive to the ICU as single patients or in large groups), the *service mechanism* (e.g., the number of physicians and nurses able to admit patients to the ICU at once), the *system capacity* (e.g., the size of the emergency room and waiting room), and *queue discipline* (e.g., how patients are triaged) [48]. This allows one to make different assumptions for each of these interactions. For example, one could model that the arrival time of patients to the ICU is random (e.g., the arrival rate of patients follows a Poisson distribution) while modeling that the system capacity, the size of the ICU, is a constant [48].

A helpful worked example is provided by Foster et al. [49] who demonstrate queuing theory in the context of developing capacity for a drug treatment facility. The authors argue that a hypothetical drug treatment facility can be modeled assuming: (1) arrivals come in a random but constant way (using a Poisson distribution), (2) if a bed is available, they will undergo treatment and otherwise will wait, (3) and that services require a predetermined time to complete. The number of "servers" in this example represents the number of beds. Other assumptions include that the wait list is infinitely large, the arrival rate and the number of clients treated is independent, and clients are not triaged but cared for on a first come first served basis.

Queuing theory output is in the form of distributions of events, rather than summative averages, as we obtain using Little's Law. This allows one to ask complicated questions of the output, such as the distribution of wait times, the longest potential wait time, or the number of arrivals who had to wait more than a certain unacceptable length of time. In Foster et al.'s worked example, they demonstrate that with an arrival time of 1 patient per day, a length of treatment of 28 days and 32 beds available, about one-third of the time the facility is full, two-thirds of patients do not have to wait and among those who do wait, the expected wait time is about 4 days. Only about 6 % of patients wait more than 1 week for treatment [49]. Foster et al. [49] also provide MatLab programming to build this model.

In our case, the hospital administrators are responding to the emergency room's concern that patients are waiting too long to be transferred. Under current conditions, we could use queuing theory to answer questions about our ICU patient flow and alternative arrangements. For example, we could estimate what proportion of emergency room patients must wait more than 1 h for a bed and at what times of day. We could calculate what proportion of patients would have a similar wait under the length of stay benefit from the worked example of the spontaneous breathing trial/spontaneous awakening trial in the previous section. We could also calculate whether an increase in the capacity to 30 beds from 20 beds would change this. Queuing theory provides tools to begin to flesh out more complicated models for understanding how patients arrive, interact, and move through the ICU.

Simulation

Queuing theory's utility begins to decrease when the initial modeling assumptions start to fall apart. For example, consider how patients are triaged in the ICU and the interconnectedness of triaging decisions to the acuity and volume of other patients in the ICU. The same discharge process may take 30 minute or 3 h, depending on how critically a bed is needed. Assuming all patients are triaged the same way in a queuing theory model (e.g., first come-first serve, a common assumption made in queuing theory) may be very inappropriate when attempting to understand the nuances of patient flow in the ICU. Simulation allows for even greater complexity in modeling patient flow, such as varying patient acuity. Approaches include static models, such as Monte Carlo models that generate a result in a specific point in time, dynamic models that are able to evolve over time, stochastic models that have probabilistic variables, and models that make use of time in a discrete or continuous way [50]. Our experience is that simulation models, particularly approaches like discrete event simulation, are also easier to explain to clinicians and administrators, having less of a "black box" component than approaches that rely more heavily on equations. Examples of different models in health care include examining the staffing and workflow changes in two hospital-based pharmacies [51], a model of ICU capacity and operative wait times for surgeries necessitating an ICU stay [52], and operating room scheduling designs [53].

Costa et al. [54] describe a helpful model of ICU bed capacity, relevant to our case example. The details of their model are beyond the scope of this chapter, but provide an example of how one may build a simulated environment that reliably reproduces real-world outcomes. Prior to physically building additional ICU beds, they used their simulation to understand the effects of each additional bed. Their model used classification and regression tree (CART) analysis [55] and queuing theory in combination. They concluded that increasing the number of ICU beds from five to ten would drop hospital transfer and ICU denial rates down meaningfully [54]. Just as important, however, they found that if they built 12 or more beds, this expansion would be at the expense of reasonable occupancy rates [54]. One could conduct similar analyses in our case example, creating a model that asked exactly how many additional beds are needed in our ICU (and how many is too many)—before committing the capital to actually build beds.

Other authors have used models to level variation in ICU admissions by understanding elective surgical cases that require ICU care postoperatively [56, 57]. Kolker [56] modeled the effect of smoothing the number of elective surgical cases across days of the week and found that they could reduce the number of surgical cases that were diverted to other days due to unavailable ICU beds from 10 to 1.5 %. Of interest, they found queuing theory to be inadequate to their task as they believed the distributional assumptions necessary for the model did not allow for the hour-to-hour variation in ICU admissions. Another pediatric team who also targeted elective surgical cases to smooth variability in ICU admissions used discrete event simulation to develop and understand the problem [57]. From a patient's perspective, once the organization smoothed the number of elective surgical cases to five cases per day, patients nearly ceased having their surgery cancelled due to lack of ICU bed: in 2 years' time, only 10 cases were cancelled while 55,000 cases were completed [57].

Conclusion

Inattentiveness to patient flow leads to rationing without contemplation. Providers in ICUs should carefully contemplate patient flow and its interconnectedness to other aspects of the hospital. Failure to appropriately measure and improve patient flow has well-documented, harmful effects on patients both in the ICU and waiting for care in the ICU. Tools exist from manufacturing and operations research allow us to understand, measure, and model patient flow, and to use this understanding to make meaningful improvements in real-world ICUs.

Case Study: Using Patient Flow to Improve Patient Care Without Building Beds

Beginning in 2006, our institution, an urban, tertiary care teaching hospital in Boston, Massachusetts, with 77 ICU beds and about 600 hospital beds, tackled a number of challenges to improve patient quality and flow. We worked sequentially on improving care for patients with sepsis [58], preventing central line infections, preventing ventilator-associated pneumonia, and implementing a rapid response team [59], along with other quality interventions. Additionally, we collaborated with other services in our hospital, particularly the emergency department and the medical floors, to reduce delays in the length of time ICU patients waited for beds on non-ICU floors [60].

The result was an improvement in ICU length of stay, ICU throughput and mortality (Fig. 11.3a–c). Earlier efforts to meet the clinical and patient level demand for ICU care had revolved around building additional beds, as seen in Fig. 11.3d, between 2004 and 2006. With the interventions described above, we were able to care for more than 1,000 additional ICU admissions per year, without building any additional ICU beds. In fact, our hospital had planned and budgeted for a capital expense of several million dollars to build a new ICU, but was able to avoid this expenditure entirely.

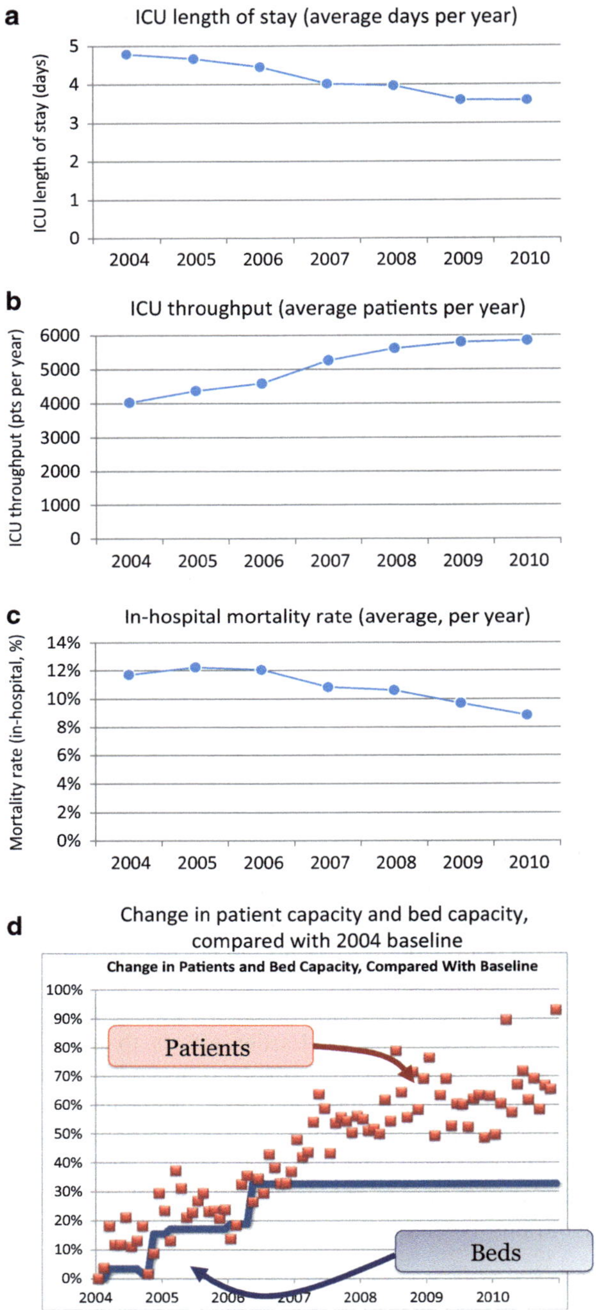

Fig. 11.3 (**a**) ICU length of stay (average days per year). (**b**) ICU throughput (average patients per year). (**c**) In-hospital mortality rate (average, per year). (**d**) Change in patient capacity and bed capacity, compared with 2004 baseline

References

1. Halpern NA, Pastores SM. Critical care medicine in the United States 2000–2005: an analysis of bed numbers, occupancy rates, payer mix, and costs. Crit Care Med. 2010;38(1):65–71.
2. Needham DM, Bronskill SE, Calinawan JR, Sibbald WJ, Pronovost PJ, Laupacis A. Projected incidence of mechanical ventilation in Ontario to 2026: preparing for the aging baby boomers. Crit Care Med. 2005;33(3):574–9.
3. Angus DC, Kelley MA, Schmitz RJ, White A, Popovich Jr J. Caring for the critically ill patient. Current and projected workforce requirements for care of the critically ill and patients with pulmonary disease: can we meet the requirements of an aging population? JAMA. 2000;284(21):2762–70.
4. Carr BG, Addyson DK, Kahn JM. Variation in critical care beds per capita in the United States: implications for pandemic and disaster planning. JAMA. 2010;303(14):1371–2.
5. Pines JM, Pollack Jr CV, Diercks DB, Chang AM, Shofer FS, Hollander JE. The association between emergency department crowding and adverse cardiovascular outcomes in patients with chest pain. Acad Emerg Med. 2009;16(7):617–25.
6. Bernstein SL, Aronsky D, Duseja R, et al. The effect of emergency department crowding on clinically oriented outcomes. Acad Emerg Med. 2009;16(1):1–10.
7. Young MP, Gooder VJ, McBride K, James B, Fisher ES. Inpatient transfers to the intensive care unit: delays are associated with increased mortality and morbidity. J Gen Intern Med. 2003;18(2):77–83.
8. Sprung CL, Geber D, Eidelman LA, et al. Evaluation of triage decisions for intensive care admission. Crit Care Med. 1999;27(6):1073–9.
9. Cardoso LT, Grion CM, Matsuo T, et al. Impact of delayed admission to intensive care units on mortality of critically ill patients: a cohort study. Crit Care. 2011;15(1):R28.
10. Tarnow-Mordi WO, Hau C, Warden A, Shearer AJ. Hospital mortality in relation to staff workload: a 4-year study in an adult intensive-care unit. Lancet. 2000;356(9225):185–9.
11. Dara SI, Afessa B. Intensivist-to-bed ratio: association with outcomes in the medical ICU. Chest. 2005;128(2):567–72.
12. Stelfox HT, Hemmelgarn BR, Bagshaw SM, et al. Intensive care unit bed availability and outcomes for hospitalized patients with sudden clinical deterioration. Arch Intern Med. 2012;172(6):467–74.
13. Renaud B, Santin A, Coma E, et al. Association between timing of intensive care unit admission and outcomes for emergency department patients with community-acquired pneumonia. Crit Care Med. 2009;37(11):2867–74.
14. Chalfin DB, Trzeciak S, Likourezos A, Baumann BM, Dellinger RP. Impact of delayed transfer of critically ill patients from the emergency department to the intensive care unit. Crit Care Med. 2007;35(6):1477–83.
15. Parkhe M, Myles PS, Leach DS, Maclean AV. Outcome of emergency department patients with delayed admission to an intensive care unit. Emerg Med. 2002;14(1):50–7.
16. Robert R, Reignier J, Tournoux-Facon C, et al. Refusal of intensive care unit admission due to a full unit: impact on mortality. Am J Respir Crit Care Med. 2012;185(10):1081–7.
17. Ouanes I, Schwebel C, Francais A, et al. A model to predict short-term death or readmission after intensive care unit discharge. J Crit care. 2012;27(4):422.e1–9.
18. Kaboli PJ, Rosenthal GE. Delays in transfer to the ICU: a preventable adverse advent? J Gen Intern Med. 2003;18(2):155–6.
19. Needleman J, Buerhaus P, Mattke S, Stewart M, Zelevinsky K. Nurse-staffing levels and the quality of care in hospitals. N Engl J Med. 2002;346(22):1715–22.
20. Kane RL, Shamliyan TA, Mueller C, Duval S, Wilt TJ. The association of registered nurse staffing levels and patient outcomes: systematic review and meta-analysis. Med Care. 2007;45 (12):1195–204.

21. Ward NS, Afessa B, Kleinpell R, et al. Intensivist/patient ratios in closed ICUs: a statement from the Society of Critical Care Medicine Taskforce on ICU Staffing. Crit Care Med. 2013;41 (2):638–45.
22. Afessa B, Gajic O, Morales IJ, Keegan MT, Peters SG, Hubmayr RD. Association between ICU admission during morning rounds and mortality. Chest. 2009;136(6):1489–95.
23. Iwashyna TJ, Kramer AA, Kahn JM. Intensive care unit occupancy and patient outcomes. Crit Care Med. 2009;37(5):1545–57.
24. Barnett MJ, Kaboli PJ, Sirio CA, Rosenthal GE. Day of the week of intensive care admission and patient outcomes: a multisite regional evaluation. Med Care. 2002;40(6):530–9.
25. Laupland KB, Shahpori R, Kirkpatrick AW, Stelfox HT. Hospital mortality among adults admitted to and discharged from intensive care on weekends and evenings. J Crit Care. 2008;23(3):317–24.
26. Morales IJ, Peters SG, Afessa B. Hospital mortality rate and length of stay in patients admitted at night to the intensive care unit. Crit Care Med. 2003;31(3):858–63.
27. Cavallazzi R, Marik PE, Hirani A, Pachinburavan M, Vasu TS, Leiby BE. Association between time of admission to the ICU and mortality: a systematic review and metaanalysis. Chest. 2010;138(1):68–75.
28. Goldfrad C, Rowan K. Consequences of discharges from intensive care at night. Lancet. 2000;355(9210):1138–42.
29. Teres D. Civilian triage in the intensive care unit: the ritual of the last bed. Crit Care Med. 1993;21(4):598–606.
30. Pronovost PJ, Needham DM, Waters H, et al. Intensive care unit physician staffing: financial modeling of the Leapfrog standard. Crit Care Med. 2004;32(6):1247–53.
31. Losek JD. Characteristics, workload, and job satisfaction of attending physicians from pediatric emergency medicine fellowship programs. Pediatric Emergency Medicine Collaborative Research Committee. Pediatr Emerg Care. 1994;10(5):256–9.
32. Ali NA, Hammersley J, Hoffmann SP, et al. Continuity of care in intensive care units: a cluster-randomized trial of intensivist staffing. Am J Respir Crit Care Med. 2011;184(7):803–8.
33. Embriaco N, Azoulay E, Barrau K, et al. High level of burnout in intensivists: prevalence and associated factors. Am J Respir Crit Care Med. 2007;175(7):686–92.
34. Ward NS, Read R, Afessa B, Kahn JM. Perceived effects of attending physician workload in academic medical intensive care units: a national survey of training program directors. Crit Care Med. 2012;40(2):400–5.
35. Jimmerson C, Weber D, Sobek 2nd DK. Reducing waste and errors: piloting lean principles at Intermountain Healthcare. Jt Comm J Qual Patient Saf. 2005;31(5):249–57.
36. Shannon RP, Frndak D, Grunden N, et al. Using real-time problem solving to eliminate central line infections. Jt Comm J Qual Patient Saf. 2006;32(9):479–87.
37. Eaton M. Lean for practitioners: an introduction to lean for healthcare organisations. Hertfordshire: Ecademy Press; 2009.
38. Gaieski DF, Mikkelsen ME, Band RA, et al. Impact of time to antibiotics on survival in patients with severe sepsis or septic shock in whom early goal-directed therapy was initiated in the emergency department. Crit Care Med. 2010;38(4):1045–53.
39. Reid PP, Compton WD, Grossman JH, Fanjiang G, editors. Building a better delivery system: a new engineering/health care partnership. Washington (DC): National Academy Press; 2005.
40. Little JDC, Graves SC. Little's law. In D. Chhajed and TJ. Lowe (eds.) Building Intuition: Insights From Basic Operations Management Models and Principles. New York: Springer Science and Business Media; 2008.
41. Little JDC. A proof of the queuing formula: $L = \lambda W$. Oper Res. 1961;9:383–7.
42. Girard TD, Kress JP, Fuchs BD, et al. Efficacy and safety of a paired sedation and ventilator weaning protocol for mechanically ventilated patients in intensive care (awakening and breathing controlled trial): a randomised controlled trial. Lancet. 2008;371(9607):126–34.

43. Erlang AK. Solution of some problems in the theory of probabilities of significance in automatic telephone exchanges. Post Office Electrical Eng J. 1912;10:189–97.
44. Alagoz O, Maillart LM, Schaefer AJ, Roberts MS. Choosing among living-donor and cadaveric livers. Manag Sci. 2007;49(12):1702–15.
45. Basu S, Galvani AP. The transmission and control of XDR TB in South Africa: an operations research and mathematical modelling approach. Epidemiol Infect. 2008;136(12):1585–98.
46. Gerchak Y, Gupta D, Henig M. Reservation planning for elective surgery under uncertain demand for emergency surgery. Manag Sci. 1996;42:321–34.
47. Patrick J, Puterman ML. Reducing wait times through operations research: optimizing the use of surge capacity. Healthc Policy. 2008;3(3):75–88.
48. Bhat UN. An introduction to queueing theory: modeling and analysis in applications. Boston: Birkhauser; 2008.
49. Foster EM, Hosking MR, Ziya S. A spoonful of math helps the medicine go down: an illustration of how healthcare can benefit from mathematical modeling and analysis. BMC Med Res Methodol. 2010;10:60.
50. Sobolev BG, Sanchez V, Vasilakis C. Systematic review of the use of computer simulation modeling of patient flow in surgical care. J Med Syst. 2011;35(1):1–16.
51. Reynolds M, Vasilakis C, McLeod M, et al. Using discrete event simulation to design a more efficient hospital pharmacy for outpatients. Health Care Manag Sci. 2011;14(3):223–36.
52. Troy PM, Rosenberg L. Using simulation to determine the need for ICU beds for surgery patients. Surgery. 2009;146(4):608–17. discussion 617–620.
53. Dexter F, Macario A, Traub RD, Hopwood M, Lubarsky DA. An operating room scheduling strategy to maximize the use of operating room block time: computer simulation of patient scheduling and survey of patients' preferences for surgical waiting time. Anesth Analg. 1999;89(1):7–20.
54. Costa AX, Ridley SA, Shahani AK, Harper PR, De Senna V, Nielsen MS. Mathematical modelling and simulation for planning critical care capacity. Anaesthesia. 2003;58(4):320–7.
55. Breiman L, Friedman JH, Olshan RA, Stone CJ. Classification and regression trees. London: Chapman & Hall; 1993.
56. Kolker A. Process modeling of ICU patient flow: effect of daily load leveling of elective surgeries on ICU diversion. J Med Syst. 2009;33(1):27–40.
57. Ryckman FC, Yelton PA, Anneken AM, Kiessling PE, Schoettker PJ, Kotagal UR. Redesigning intensive care unit flow using variability management to improve access and safety. Jt Comm J Qual Patient Saf. 2009;35(11):535–43.
58. Shapiro NI, Howell MD, Talmor D, et al. Implementation and outcomes of the Multiple Urgent Sepsis Therapies (MUST) protocol. Crit Care Med. 2006;34(4):1025–32.
59. Howell MD, Ngo L, Folcarelli P, et al. Sustained effectiveness of a primary-team-based rapid response system. Crit Care Med. 2012;40(9):2562–8.
60. Howell MD. Managing ICU, throughput and understanding ICU census. Curr Opin Crit Care. 2011;17(6):626–33.

Chapter 12
Rapid Response Systems

Ken Hillman and Jack Chen

Abstract A rapid response system (RRS) is a way of identifying a seriously ill or deteriorating patient and linking it to a rapid response by clinicians with the appropriate skills and knowledge necessary to manage the patient. Like ICUs, the widespread implementation of RRSs is simply another intervention, developed around the needs of seriously ill or deteriorating patients. It is no coincidence that many of the systems are operated by clinicians trained in intensive care medicine. The level of illness and outcomes for patients in intensive care and those subject to rapid response calls is comparable. In other words, whether in the ICU or outside it, these patients require clinicians with high levels of skills, experience, and knowledge. There is, as yet, no conclusive data on the most accurate triggering criteria, or on the ideal responding staff. There is some early evidence that hospitals with RRSs significantly reduce the mortality and cardiac arrest rates and the concept has now been adopted in many hospitals around the world.

Keywords Rapid response systems • Medical emergency team • Early intervention • Patient safety • Hospital mortality rates • Intensive care • Cardiac arrest rates • Hospital outcome indicators

---

K. Hillman (✉)
Intensive Care, South Western Sydney Clinical School, University of New South Wales, Liverpool Hospital, Locked Bag 7103, Liverpool, NSW 1871, Australia

Simpson Centre for Health Services Research, South Western Sydney Clinical School, University of New South Wales, Kensington, NSW, Australia
e-mail: k.hillman@unsw.edu.au

J. Chen
Simpson Centre for Health Services Research, South Western Sydney Clinical School, University of New South Wales, Kensington, NSW, Australia

Australian Institute of Health Innovation, University of New South Wales, Kensington, NSW, Australia
e-mail: jackchen@unsw.edu.au

D.C. Scales and G.D. Rubenfeld (eds.), *The Organization of Critical Care*,
Respiratory Medicine 18, DOI 10.1007/978-1-4939-0811-0_12,

Acute hospitals have been around for centuries. Until about the time of the Second World War, they mainly provided bed rest and convalescence for the poor [1]. Then began an explosion of medical advances including complex surgery and procedures, safe anesthesia, the increased availability of drugs as well as sophisticated diagnostic and monitoring equipment. In order to support patients with high levels of illness and monitoring, the first intensive care unit (ICU) was established in Copenhagen in the early 1950s [2]. Artificial ventilation was used to support patients with poliomyelitis. As a result, the mortality was reduced from 89 to 40 %. The concept of intensive care quickly spread to other parts of the world. Firstly, as a distinct geographical site, then with specialized and formally trained medical and nursing staff. Intensive care medicine is now recognized as a distinctive and independent specialty with its own societies, textbooks, journals and conferences.

At the same time, the nature of acute hospitals was rapidly changing [1] and sub-specialization of medicine and surgery resulted in great advances in what we could offer patients in terms of complex diagnostic and therapeutic procedures. The ageing population could be kept alive for much longer as a result of better public health as well as modern medical drugs and interventions. Thus the nature of the hospital population also changed. There were no longer many younger patients with single acute disease states. They were older, often had significant chronic illness, and were being subject to complex interventions and powerful drugs with many potential side effects. Similarly, the population of patients managed in ICUs changed. Within a decade or two after the development of ICUs, we had moved from managing a small number of seriously ill patients in intensive care environments, who were usually young with a large potentially reversible disease component, to large ICUs that mainly treated older patients with a large chronic disease component.

At the same time, and almost imperceptibly, there were other changes. Hospital bed numbers decreased; the length of stay decreased; and patients on the general floors had a high level of illness, having interventions with a high rate of complications.

Failure to Match Level of Illness with Appropriate Care

The changing nature of the hospital population was not matched with more appropriate systems of care. In most cases, patients were still admitted "under" a single specialist who worked with a team of nursing staff, paramedical ancillary staff and usually the 24 h presence of medical cover of varying degrees. It could be a hierarchy of doctors in training or hospital employed doctors with more general, rather than specialized skills. This coincided with even greater sub-specialization of admitting practitioners.

We soon found ourselves with a specialist, in say neurology, having a patient admitted under them who had developed line-related sepsis. Suddenly he and his trainees are confronted with a seriously ill patient who they may not even recognize as seriously ill, let alone be familiar with the latest guidelines for treating sepsis as well as having the necessary procedural skills to support the patient's level of illness. Not wishing to isolate this problem to neurologists, the same applies to other hospitalized patients under the care of different specialists. Compounding the problem, patients now usually had multiple chronic problems or co-morbidities. During hospitalization, any of these may suffer an acute exacerbation. Patients, particularly elderly "medical" patients, may be randomly admitted under a specialist familiar with that organ; whereas the other organs contribute to the total level of illness. Similarly, with surgery. The technical aspects of the surgery are usually carried out in a competent way. However, the major risk for surgical patients is often their multiple co-morbidities. As a result, the best that can often be offered to a patient with multiple co-morbidities is a committee-type approach with the admitting specialist requesting consultations for all the other medical problems outside his area of specialization. The expertise to care for the seriously ill or at-risk patients remained largely in places where physicians with these skills practiced such as in emergency rooms (ERs) or ICUs.

Hospitals Are Dangerous Places

There was little in the way of systems operating across the whole organization to deal with the changing nature of the hospital population. The level of complexity of illness in hospital patients was not matched by appropriate medical skills and expertise. It is not surprising then that an unacceptable rate of potentially preventable deaths and serious adverse events were beginning to be reported [3–5]. These events were system related [6]. A system developed in the nineteenth century on the general floors of hospitals was being used to manage a very different and at-risk population of patients.

Many deteriorating patients were unrecognized and remained untreated on the general floors of acute hospitals. The basic principles of acute medicine were not available for at-risk patients. Up to 40 % of admissions to ICUs were found to be potentially avoidable because of sub-optimal care related to lack of organization, lack of knowledge, and failure to seek advice [7]. It is also not surprising that delays before admission to the ICU were responsible for an increase in mortality [8, 9]. Many even failed to survive to ICU admission. As early as 1978 it was noted that vital sign disturbances preceded many patients who suffered an in-hospital cardiac arrest [10]. Up to 84 % of patients who had a cardiac arrest on general floors had documented deterioration within the 8 h before the arrest [11].

Approximately half of all patients who died in hospital, and who did not have a do-not-attempt resuscitation (DNAR) order, had severe vital sign abnormalities before they died which were not responded to appropriately [12].

Early Intervention in the Seriously Ill

It became obvious that the problem was the delay in recognizing and treating seriously ill and at-risk patients. The wrong people with the wrong skills at the wrong time. In the 1980s and early 1990s this was overlooked. Intensivists were still practicing within the four walls of their ICU [13]. It was hypothesized that if seriously ill patients were given supranormal levels of oxygen delivery and aggressive resuscitation after their admission to the ICU that their outcome would improve [14]. This was later proved to be incorrect [15, 16]. Careful reading of these studies suggests that many patients admitted to both the treatment and control groups had prolonged untreated hypotension and delayed admission to the ICU.

Tissue ischemia often begins outside the ICU environment. It is the basis of the "golden hour" concept which emphasizes one of the most important principles of acute medicine—to rapidly restore oxygenated blood flow to tissues. Ischemia and hypoxia are known to initiate the cytokine cascades which eventually result in multiorgan failure [17].

Initially research on the specialty of intensive care was confined to patients within the four walls of the ICU. We are now increasingly evaluating improvement in patient outcomes as a result of early intervention [18]. Patient-centered system change before admission to the ICU is often more effective than magic bullets administered to the seriously ill after admission to the ICU [19].

The Limitations of the Cardiac Arrest Team Concept

In spite of the increasing number of vulnerable patients in acute hospitals, the compelling data showed that there were many potentially preventable deaths and serious adverse events, and the fact that it was mainly a systems issue. The only patient-centered, organization-wide system for many years was the cardiac arrest team. Up until the mid-1990s, and despite the obvious data about patients deteriorating on general floors, practice in intensive care was confined to procedures within the ICU such as inserting a pulmonary artery catheter and supporting patients with powerful drugs and machines. Perhaps some units also participated in the delivery of cardiopulmonary resuscitation (CPR) on the general floors of hospitals [20].

While CPR was an advance after a patient's heart had stopped, the initially reported high success rates were mainly in young, otherwise fit patients whose heart had stopped while being anesthetized [21]. This was at a time when anesthesia was considered dangerous and not the specialty it is now where deaths under anesthesia are a rare event requiring intense investigation. Moreover, patients in the operating rooms were being closely monitored on a 1:1 basis. Nevertheless, the concept of CPR soon caught on and was delivered "anywhere and anytime" where a heart was thought to have stopped. Unfortunately, most patients who have in-hospital CPR die before they leave hospital and the prognosis has changed little since CPR was first introduced [22], despite huge sums being spent on researching the best ways to perform it and prolonged discussions by national bodies on the best way to deliver it.

Unfortunately in the excitement of delivering CPR, it is sometimes overlooked that for many patients it is simply the final event of the dying process [22]. Nevertheless, CPR became a medical icon. Many medical dramas on television reported success rates of about 70 % as opposed to the reality of less than 15 % [23]. It has also been estimated to cost up to $600,000 per survivor, one of the most expensive interventions in health [24]. One also has to question why we spend so much time on designating patients as DNAR, when the procedure itself is almost universally unsuccessful in patients who are naturally dying.

The Need for an Improved System

Silo delivered health care can be a strength in a hospital. Individual doctors taking responsibility for individual patients; the pride in organizing a well-run ICU; and the feeling of belonging to a team within its safe hierarchies. Unfortunately silos can also be a weakness in patients with complex problems outside the expertise of individual organ-based specialties, where the patients are deteriorating and beginning to fall between the cracks. For many years the only response to seriously ill patients was the cardiac arrest team after their heart had stopped. It is not difficult to construct a new system around the needs of patients.

The first system to be constructed around a patient's needs was developed at Liverpool Hospital, Sydney, Australia in the early 1990s [25, 26]. An at-risk patient was defined from data available from studies around the antecedents before death and cardiac arrest. The urgent response was simply provided by the old cardiac arrest team which changed its name to the Medical Emergency Team (MET).

The system thus consisted of two major components—the calling criteria which defines a seriously ill, at-risk patient and a rapid response to that emergency [27].

The Calling Criteria: Or Afferent Limb

The first reports of a rapid response system (RRS) included many diagnostic, metabolic as well as vital sign abnormalities [25]. These criteria were soon refined to simple vital sign and observational abnormalities [26] which remain the basis of all RRSs to this day.

The criteria usually include vital sign measurements considered outside a range that would be considered "safe." There is little research on the exact sensitivity and specificity of these levels but interestingly there has been almost universal agreement on the approximate levels that are considered to indicate a patient at-risk [28] such as a pulse rate (low 40–50; high 120–140), respiratory rate (low 4–6; high 25–35), and blood pressure (low 80–90).

Not many calling criteria include temperature or high blood pressure as being immediately life-threatening. Oxygen saturation is also often added as a criteria. It is important to recognize that serious illness is not only defined in terms of abnormal numbers. Abnormal observations are equally important. These include airway obstruction and a sudden fall in the level of consciousness. The only diagnostic category that seems to indicate an immediate and life-threatening criteria and perhaps not identified by other abnormal criteria is seizures.

Urine output is also sometimes included but is subject to inaccuracies in a general floor environment. Finally, and arguably the most important criteria is "concern." In mature RRSs, the "worried" or "concerned" criteria is the most common reason for urgent assistance [29, 30]. This is not surprising as clinical impression remains an important part of the practice of medicine. Sometimes numbers do not define the level of illness and consequent concern by a clinician. Nursing staff account for most rapid response interventions and experienced nursing staff develop the same clinical impressions around serious illness that experienced doctors do. Moreover, the presence of the "worried" criteria empowers nursing staff to call for immediate help in a way that was not possible when there was only a cardiac arrest team.

Apart from the high percentage of calls for "worried," the order of frequency in the largest study on RRS calls [30] were for decreased level of consciousness, decreased systolic blood pressure, changes in respiratory rate, and changes in pulse rate. The rates for airway obstruction and seizures were lower but obviously can have immediate fatal consequences if not attended to appropriately.

Vital Signs: Their Role in Guaranteeing Patient Safety

The recording of vital signs is the most common intervention in hospital health care. It has been an important part of health care in hospitals for over 150 years [31]. Despite that, there has been almost no research on its utility or cost. One of the early studies challenged the routine measurement of respiratory rate suggesting that it was an unreliable, largely useless routine, which has been continued wholly because of tradition [32]. It went on to suggest that the elimination of erroneous information would save 3.5 million hours of nursing time in US hospitals.

The introduction of RRSs attracted overdue attention to the measurement of vital signs as they were an important part of the criteria for triggering an urgent call.

In the largest study on RRS [33] it was shown that there were failures in the measurement, documentation, understanding and communication of vital sign abnormalities. There was marked variability across the 23 hospitals involved ranging from 0 to 64 % of any vital signs not being measured before death, cardiac arrest or admission to the ICU [34]. Respiratory rate was three times more likely to be missing than heart rate or blood pressure. Other studies have also shown incomplete and infrequent documentation of vital signs [35–38].

Obviously urgent responses to abnormal vital signs cannot be made if they are inaccurately measured or not measured at all.

The Most Appropriate Criteria for Triggering a Rapid Response

While there is general agreement around the use of abnormal vital signs and observations as triggers for urgent responses, there is little knowledge around what is the most appropriate [27]. Apart from abnormal vital signs and observations, there are studies which are beginning to also use laboratory tests to improve the power of predicting at-risk patients [39].

The only extensive evaluation of RRSs have used single criteria triggering [40, 41]. However, problems with specificity and sensitivity have prompted some to use complex composite scoring systems. Many studies have shown improved sensitivity and specificity when correlating abnormal criteria with specific end-points but none have demonstrated that these improve patient outcome [42–46]. Moreover, the use of scoring systems rather than single criterion triggers are inaccurate in their calculation [47, 48]; as well as introducing significant intra and interrater reliability error [46].

Not only can they be complex and inaccurate but they focus on a number rather than observations (e.g. seizures and airway obstruction) and ignore the most important trigger—clinician concern [29, 30]. Scoring systems reinforce the traditional nursing role as a passive recorder of numbers rather than encouraging and emphasizing their clinical judgment. In the same way that reducing a physician's judgment of the seriously ill to a score and ignoring their clinical judgment would be unacceptable.

Some centers are now expanding on the concept of calling when clinicians are concerned to encouraging patients and their families to also activate an urgent response when they have serious concerns [49]. While it is early days, there does not appear to be a high rate of trivial calls.

Concentrating on the perfect score or single trigger probably overlooks the most important impact of a RRS—the change in the culture of an organization which moves from a traditional hierarchical and silo-based system to one where there is universal awareness that there are at-risk patients and there is a system where urgent help can be summoned at any time by any member of the organization.

The Rapid Response

As with developing the most appropriate criteria for defining a seriously ill patient, there are many forms of a rapid response. Some systems simply change the name of the cardiac arrest team to a rapid response team (RRT). The advantage is that presumably the RRT would require the same advanced resuscitation skills, knowledge and experience as most cardiac arrest teams. Moreover, as the RRS develops, the incidence of cardiac arrests decreases and there is less need for a specific cardiac arrest team [41].

Other systems maintain a separate cardiac arrest team and have a separate RRT. There are also reports of separate teams for issues such as a threatened airway [50]. In specific geographical environments such as ERs, the team may consist of local staff [51]. There is even a report from a patient who called for emergency paramedical ambulance assistance from his hospital bed [52].

In a project where over 250 hospitals in one health jurisdiction has had a standardized RRS implemented, there is the challenge of using available resources for the rapid response [53]. In the smaller hospitals, the responding doctor is a local family practitioner. In even smaller hospitals where there was no doctor in the town, nursing staff or local ambulance staff are the first responders. They have specific advanced resuscitation training enabling them to resuscitate and stabilize seriously ill patients until an appropriate medical team arrives.

The same project uses a two-tiered response, where certain levels of vital signs and observations, lower than the usual triggers for a rapid response, are used as triggers for a "home" team response. The appropriately trained RRT is always available as a back-up to the home team if they request it or when more serious triggers are met [54].

The largest study describing the nature of interventions by the responding team demonstrated that of the 2,376 interventions, all but five required critical care procedures such as intubation, central line insertion, and administration of vasopressors [55]. Obviously, in this case most "home" teams would not have all those skills.

The nature of the responding team would vary for each hospital but the principle behind the composition of the team is the same in each case. The nature of the patient's illness needs to be defined first and this determines the appropriate skills, knowledge, and experience needed to address the needs of those patients. Then at least one member of the responding team needs to possess all of those attributes and needs to be available 24/7 [54]. It is not surprising then that most response teams have focused on ICU-based teams [41].

There have been suggestions that widespread education programs to train all hospital-based medical staff may be appropriate. In theory, this may be feasible but it would require enormous resources in terms of time and funding to continually train the rapidly changing population of hospital clinicians to a level of competence where they could deal with all aspects of serious illness. Moreover, in a time of increasing medical specialization it is hard to imagine that trainees could spend so much time training in a specialty very different from their own. It is estimated that the cost to organizations of widespread training of CPR is at least $600,000 (US) per survivor [24]. Obviously, the training of personnel for all aspects of advanced resuscitation would be more challenging than simply training in CPR.

Implementation of a RRS

Implementing a new system has many different challenges compared to introducing a new drug or procedure. The implementation of an RRS is almost always done on an organization-wide basis. In countries such as Holland, the United Kingdom and Australia and in health regions such as Copenhagen in Denmark and Ontario in Canada, the implementation process is on a much larger scale and involves many more hospitals.

The largest implementation project so far has been in NSW, Australia [53]. A standardized system has been introduced in over 250 different hospitals ranging from large urban teaching hospitals to less than 10 bed hospitals in small towns without a doctor.

The implementation process was based on a framework of five pillars.

1. **Standardized Chart**
   A standardized patient vital signs chart was introduced into every hospital. On the chart in the areas where pulse rate, respiratory rate, blood pressure, and temperature are graphed, there is a red horizontal line at levels requiring an urgent rapid response call and a yellow horizontal line at levels where the "home" team needs to review the patient within half-an-hour. When the nurse records vital signs within the colored zones an appropriate action must occur. The chart also contains instructions about abnormal observations such as airway, oxygen saturation, seizures, level of consciousness, and staff concern as triggers for an urgent response.
2. **Standard Response**
   Each hospital must have 24/7 availability of at least one person who has the appropriate advanced resuscitation skills to manage every possible level of patient illness in that hospital.
3. **Education**
   Educational strategies are aimed at three different levels. Firstly, every staff member in the hospital must be aware that such a system exists and that they may have occasion to activate it. Approximately 5 % of all calls can be for staff or visitors in areas such as the car park or cafeteria (unpublished observation). The education program is a simple one and part of everyone's orientation. A second level of education is aimed at frontline clinicians—doctors and nurses [56]. Unfortunately undergraduate education around the management of the seriously ill is often poor [57, 58] and education of trainee medical staff also needs improvement [59]. A universal program aimed at frontline staff can

concentrate on issues such as the importance of recognizing serious illness early and how to deliver some of the less complex interventions until personnel with appropriate training arrive. Education programs supporting RRSs have been shown to reduce mortality [60]. The third educational strategy aims to teach a small group of staff the appropriate advanced resuscitation skills necessary to deal with all possible levels of illness within each organization. Specific training is often not required in larger hospitals as they have resources such as staff in ICUs. However, smaller hospitals have to identify appropriate staff (e.g. family practitioners, nurses, local ambulance personnel) and arrange appropriate training and maintenance of skills enabling them to resuscitate and support a patient until support arrives.

4. **Governance**
   The implementation of a patient-centered, organizational-wide system is a relatively novel challenge and involves the whole hospital in various ways. A senior person, such as the Chief Executive Officer of an organization, should be made responsible for the implementation and effective maintenance of the RRS. This usually involves establishing an overseeing committee structure, support for the extra infrastructure and resources necessary to maintain the system as well as the collection, analysis and targeting of key performance indicators (KPIs) which evaluate the effectiveness of the system.
5. **Key Performance Indicators**
   Health systems often pay nominal attention to the importance of KPIs. They are often no more than collated administrative data which tells us how many patients are admitted to hospital; their demographics; what procedures occurred; the average length of stay; and waiting times for various procedures. They tell us little about the clinical performance of a hospital; how systems are performing; and how safe the hospital is.

   Clinical outcome indicators are crucial to ensure quality clinical practice [61]. Unfortunately the lack of reliable patient outcome data makes it difficult to improve practice or implement "quality improvement" strategies as there is no benchmark to work with [62, 63]. The lack of reliable patient outcome data and reliance on administrative data leads to cynicism in the workforce and defines our health system in a distorted way. This is exacerbated by whatever data is collected locally being sent up the system to distant administrative outposts who have little clinical and contextual knowledge and who interpret the data in terms of business models.

An RRS gives us a unique opportunity to evaluate not only how well the system is working but also the safety of the hospital. An RRS can be looked at as a safety net. No matter what clinical course or complications the patient suffers, they will always deteriorate in a predictable and generic way. No matter what the cause of the clinical situation, eventually it will be detected in the form of abnormal observations or vital signs. The level of illness detected will depend on the levels at which the vital signs and observations are set. In other words, we have a system which not only defines the patient problem but also reacts to it. This is different to research which concentrates on defining the problem without connecting it to an answer [3, 64].

An RRS is designed to improve patient safety and specifically to prevent potentially preventable deaths and serious adverse events. Even without an RRS there are important patient events that the health care system should be aware of. Having a system that not only defines an at-risk patient but has a built-in action or efferent arm enables us to measure these incidents in a way that previously has not been possible.

Crude death rates expressed in per 1,000 hospital admissions have been utilized for many years as a way of comparing hospitals. It has the obvious shortcomings of being related to the nature of the patient population. A hospital that only deals with complex cardiothoracic surgery and advanced cancer will have a higher death rate than a hospital dealing with elective orthopedics in young patients.

The use of standardized mortality rates can deliver more meaningful data on patient outcome but has many shortcomings [65]. One of the most important shortcomings when interpreting mortality is the highly variable incidence of designating patients as DNAR and the fact that these patients are not excluded from mortality data despite the fact that systems are not designed to keep these patients alive and their death is not a marker of patient safety except as ensuring that they die without pain and suffering [66]. An RRS is obviously not aimed at prolonging the life of patients where it is deemed futile. Patients who have died without a DNAR are defined as "unexpected." This not only makes death rates more useful but becomes a useful tool for evaluating rates of DNAR orders. The next step is to define "potential preventability." This is arbitrarily done by examining the notes of the last 24 h in patients who have died and determining whether they had any calling criteria that were not responded to or where the call was delayed. Thus we now have a powerful agent for evaluation and change in a system—the rate of *unexpected, potentially preventable deaths*, expressed in terms of per 1,000 admissions [62, 67]. The same definitions can be used to define "unexpected, potentially preventable cardiac arrest." In a well-functioning RRS, the occurrence of a cardiac arrest is a sentinel patient safety event which deserves thorough investigation. The arrest may have been in a patient who should have been made DNAR and was not; or in a patient where it was *potentially preventable*. This leaves a small minority of patients who have had a sudden cardiac event, not preceded by any warning and who was in an unmonitored area.

Admission to the ICU from the general floors has been used to evaluate the effectiveness of an RRS [34, 68]. Unfortunately it is difficult to interpret. While early calls with an efficient response may reduce admission to an ICU, delayed calls may prevent deaths and cardiac arrests but may increase admission rates to the ICU [69].

The use of these indicators can also be extended to better define concepts such as the *placement failure*. For example, patients who have been initially admitted from the ER to a general floor and are the subject of a RRS resulting in admission to ICU. Or even more serious, patients who are admitted to a general floor from the ER who die or have a cardiac arrest.

Death audits can be conducted in a way which enables the crude death rate to be refined and actually used as a tool which informs the system of areas for improvement. For example, all deaths can be separated into those with and without DNAR orders. Those with DNAR orders can then be examined for *potential preventability* and be used as a basis for rapid review and adjustment to the system.

An important finding has been the strong relationship between the *number of calls per 1,000 admissions* and the reduction in the number of deaths and cardiac arrests [40, 70–72]. This becomes a powerful indicator of the effectiveness of implementation of the RRS in an organization. Mature systems achieve at least 40 calls per 1,000 admissions.

It is crucial that data collected by clinicians involved in the system have access to that data in order to identify weak points and to continuously improve the quality of care [62]. The data around the RRS encounter should be entered at the time of the call, e.g. place of call, reason for call, interventions performed and immediate outcomes [67]. Similarly, the information could be entered in real time around whether DNAR orders had been made and noting any criteria within 24 h of the call that had not resulted in a response. This data should be entered, analyzed, and targeted to all levels of the organization in a format that is easy to understand and that facilitates change [62]. Data entry could be facilitated by software with drop-down boxes enabling the responder to immediately enter the data in the easiest way and eliminating the need for a paper-based system and separate data entry and analysis.

Acceptance of System Change

It is hard to imagine why a system, which is constructed around the pressing needs of deteriorating patients, would not be readily accepted. After all, the introduction of a new drug or procedure is often embraced by clinicians. Perhaps this is because it fits in with the traditional doctor: patient relationship, where the doctor makes a final decision in the interest of the patient to utilize the new drug or procedure. Whereas acceptance of a new system which is organization-wide is relatively foreign to clinicians. Cardiac arrest teams have been accepted because there is not much to lose once the heart has stopped but for admitting physicians to give up the management of their patient before their heart stops is more difficult. Clinicians had traditionally managed every aspect of their patient's care unless they sought a formal consultation from another specialist. One of the problems was that the admitting physician and their team had difficulty recognizing the deteriorating patient [7, 11, 12, 73] and even then, they often did not have the necessary advanced resuscitation skills required to manage the seriously ill patient. This was not necessarily a shortcoming, just a predictable result of medical specialization and the difficulty in maintaining skills, knowledge and experience in specialties outside their own.

Another issue is that hospital-wide systems which usurp part of their patient's management had to be organized by other medical specialists, hospital administrators or, at a wider level, by governments and patient safety organizations. All of these present a potential threat to patient ownership and imply a dictate from outside and a threat to the traditional doctor: patient relationship. These factors were a great impediment for many years in the adoption of RRSs. As well as threats to professional silos and professional control over individual patient care, other barriers to the implementation of an RRS include a failure to view errors as products of the system rather than individual mistakes [74, 75].

In summary, medicine is relatively resistant to system change. For example, it took trauma systems 10 years before they demonstrated a decrease in mortality [76–78].

It would be fair to say that health has little knowledge or experience on how to implement a new system as opposed to introducing a new drug or procedure. There are other interesting factors that we are only just beginning to analyze. For example, the results of the largest study of the implementation of an RRS showed a large variability in the success of implementation across the interventional hospitals [33, 79]. Some made remarkable improvements in reducing deaths and serious adverse events between baseline and the study's end. This large variability was the main reason why the study was inconclusive. We have little knowledge about what are the characteristics or culture of organizations which facilitated the impressive implementation compared to ones that failed. Because health has little experience with organization-wide system implementation, it may simply be related to the time necessary to successfully implement. For example, one hospital which showed no statistical improvement in patient outcome during the MERIT trial [80] experienced gradual improvement over time [81]. Other drivers to change come from societal expectations and national safety bodies [82–84].

Perhaps the greatest driver for change is by the nursing staff directly caring for the patients [85]. Nurses no longer have to wait for the patient's heart to stop before calling for urgent assistance. Most calling criteria in RRSs now include "nursing concern." This accounts for approximately half of all calls. After almost 150 years, nursing staff are now empowered to translate the concern they have for their patient into urgent action.

Finally, there needs to be much more work around optimal implementation strategies; the effect of organizational culture on the success of implementation; as well as the influence of the implementation of systems across the whole hospital on the culture of the organization.

Moving to a Patient-Centered Approach

A RRS is one of the first patient-centered, organization-wide systems. Its implementation occurred as a result of urgent patient needs without being subject to the usual hierarchical and silo-based practice that occurs in hospital. It exposed the reality that a clinician specializing in one area does not necessarily have the knowledge, skills and experience to practice outside that specialty. Moreover, it exposed the similarly inadequate medical hierarchy working within the usual single doctor: patient construct. While medical trainees may have a broader range of skills and knowledge than the specialist they are working with, most studies demonstrate that these skills are not adequate to deal with the complexities of a seriously ill patient. Similarly, the need and implementation of RRSs exposed the passive role of nursing staff where, for many years, they had been reduced to documenting serious patient deterioration but were not empowered to act effectively. They were constrained to referring to a slow and inappropriate hierarchy of medical practitioners.

A similarly potentially dangerous situation exists for patients being managed at the end-of-life (EOL) in acute hospitals [66, 86]. Not only is it often performed poorly but is one of the most important challenges facing critical care and health generally [87].

The presence of an RRS exposes the weakness in our management of patients at the EOL [88, 89] where up to one-third of all rapid response calls are for issues around EOL care associated with limitations of medical therapy [90]. RRSs have, in many cases, become the surrogate dying team. Thus not only is there a problem around inappropriate management of deteriorating patients who have a potentially reversible cause of their illness but an RRS also exposes the inappropriate recognition and management of patients at the EOL.

There is early work on developing similar patient-centered systems to deal with this issue, employing the same generic components used in the implementation of an RRS. Firstly, defining those patients at the EOL, using agreed criteria; constructing an efferent response such as placement on a palliative care pathway; implementation in a multidisciplinary way across the organization; educating those involved in the system; and finally developing KPIs which accurately reflect the effectiveness of the system and empowering those responsible for the system to make the necessary adjustments and improvements.

Do RRSs Work?

An RRS is simply a system to manage seriously ill patients, the same as an ICU. The major difference, of course, is that an ICU is a geographical construct [13]. Both identify and treat patients who have life-threatening illnesses. In fact the level of illness and mortality rates of patients who are subject to an RRT is much the same as those in an ICU [91, 92]. The boundaries between whether a patient is seriously ill on the general floor and in an ICU have blurred. The hospital population has become older with more chronic health issues and the criteria for admission to, and discharge from, an ICU are extremely variable between countries or even within ICUs in the same city. Some hospitals have many ICU beds and a relatively low number of general floor beds and vice versa. And some hospitals have a high proportion of seriously ill patients compared to others. In the largest study on RRSs, of the 2,500 urgent calls only five did not require advanced resuscitation interventions delivered by skills usually confined to places like ICUs [54].

Even so, RRSs have been subject to more evaluation than ICUs. Most of single-center, before and after studies have shown a marked reduction in cardiac arrest rates [60, 70–72, 93, 94] and a significant relationship between the number of calls (dose) and reduction in deaths and cardiac arrests [40, 95] (response). The largest cluster randomized controlled trial was inconclusive and underpowered [33], but it did demonstrate a reduction in death rates in the adult intervention hospitals [40]. The most extensive meta-analysis demonstrated a significant reduction in cardiac arrest rates in adult hospitals as well as a reduction in cardiac arrest and death rates in pediatric hospitals with a RRS [41]. These reductions were around the 30 % rate. While there are always problems with how to interpret research, it is difficult to imagine any other intervention of any kind achieving such an effect in acute hospitals.

Just as a randomized control trial evaluating the effectiveness of admitting seriously ill patients to an ICU would almost certainly not be ethical, it is hard to imagine that ethics committees would allow a comparison of patients between those who have an early intervention by appropriately skilled personnel compared to those with no intervention. Nevertheless, there needs to be further research around the most appropriate triggering criteria; the most appropriate skills, knowledge and experience of those who respond; and the most effective way of implementing organization-wide systems designed around patient needs.

References

1. Hillman K. The changing role of acute-care hospitals. Med J Aust. 1999;170:325–8.
2. Lassen HC. A preliminary report on the 1952 epidemic of poliomyelitis in Copenhagen with special reference to the treatment of acute respiratory insufficiency. Lancet. 1953;1:37–41.
3. Brennan TA, Leape LL, Laird NM, et al. Incidence of adverse events and negligence in hospitalized patients: results from the Harvard Medical Practice Study I. N Engl J Med. 1991;324:370–6.
4. Wilson RM, Runciman WB, Gibberd RW, Harrison BT, Newby I, Hamilton JD. The quality in Australian Health Care Study. Med J Aust. 1995;163:458–71.
5. Vincent C, Neale G, Woloshynowych M. Adverse events in British hospitals: preliminary retrospective record review. BMJ. 2001;322:517–9.
6. Kohn LT, Corrigan JM, Donaldson MS, editors. To err is human: building a safer health system. Washington, DC: National Academy Press; 2000.
7. Goldhill DR, Sumner A. Outcome of intensive care patients in a group of British intensive care units. Crit Care Med. 1998;26(8):1337–45.
8. Rapoport J, Teres D, Lemeshow S, Harris D. Timing of intensive care unit admission in relation to ICU outcome. Crit Care Med. 1990;18(11):1231–5.
9. Dragsted L, Jorgenson J, Jensen N-H, et al. Interhospital comparisons of patient outcome from intensive care: importance of lead time bias. Crit Care Med. 1989;17(5):418–22.
10. Castagna J, Weil MH, Shubin H. Factors determining survival in patients with cardiac arrest. Chest. 1974;65:527–9.

11. Schein RMH, Hazday N, Pena M, Ruben BH, Sprung CL. Clinical antecedents to in-hospital cardiopulmonary arrest. Chest. 1990;98:1388–92.
12. Hillman KM, Bristow PJ, Chey T, et al. Antecedents to hospital deaths. Intern Med J. 2001;31:343–8.
13. Hillman K. Critical care without walls. Curr Opin Crit Care. 2002;8:594–9.
14. Bishop MH, Shoemaker WC, Appel PL, et al. Prospective, randomized trial of survivor values of cardiac index, oxygen delivery, and oxygen consumption as resuscitation endpoints in severe trauma. J Trauma. 1995;38:780–7.
15. Hayes MA, Timmins AC, Yau EHS, et al. Elevation of systemic oxygen delivery in the treatment of critically ill patients. N Engl J Med. 1994;330:1717–22.
16. Hayes MA, Yau EH, Timmins AC, et al. Response of critically ill patients to treatment aimed at achieving supranormal oxygen delivery and consumption. Chest. 1993;103:886–95.
17. Rush Jr BF. The bacterial factor in hemorrhagic shock. Surg Gynecol Obstet. 1992;175:285–92.
18. Rivers E, Nguyen B, Havstad S, et al. Early goal-directed therapy in the treatment of severe sepsis and septic shock. N Engl J Med. 2001;345:1368–77.
19. Oxman AD, Thomson MA, Davis DA, et al. No magic bullets: a systematic review of 102 trials of interventions to improve professional practice. Can Med Assoc J. 1995;153:1423–31.
20. Ayres SM. Preventing cardiac arrest. Crit Care Med. 1994;22(2):189–91.
21. Kouwenhoven WB, Jude JR, Knickerbocker GG. Closed chest cardiac massage. JAMA. 1960;173:1064–7.
22. Sandroni C, Nolan J, Cavallaro F, Antonelli M. In-hospital cardiac arrest: incidence, prognosis and possible measures to improve survival. Intensive Care Med. 2007;33:237–45.
23. Diem SJ, Lantos JD, Tulsky JA. Cardiopulmonary resuscitation on television. Miracles and misinformation. N Engl J Med. 1996;334:1578–82.
24. Lee KH, Angus DC, Abramson NS. Cardiopulmonary resuscitation: what cost to cheat death? Crit Care Med. 1996;24:2046–52.
25. Lee A, Bishop G, Hillman KM, Daffurn K. The medical emergency team. Anaesth Intensive Care. 1995;23:183–6.
26. Hourihan F, Bishop G, Hillman KM, Daffurn K, Lee A. The medical emergency team: a new strategy to identify and intervene in high risk patients. Clin Intensive Care. 1995;6:269–72.
27. DeVita MA, Bellomo R, Hillman K, et al. Findings of the first consensus conference on medical emergency teams. Crit Care Med. 2006;34(9):2463–78.
28. DeVita MA, Smith GB, Adam SK, et al. "Identifying the hospitalised patient in crisis" – a consensus conference on the afferent limb of rapid response systems. Resuscitation. 2010;81:375–82.
29. Santiano N, Young L, Hillman K, et al. Analysis of medical emergency team calls comparing subjective to "objective" call criteria. Resuscitation. 2009;80:44–9.
30. Chen J, Bellomo R, Hillman K, Flabouris A, Finfer S, The MERIT Study Investigators for the Simpson Centre and the ANZICS Clinical Trials Group. Triggers for emergency team activation: a multicenter assessment. J Crit Care. 2010;25:359.e1–7.
31. Shepard K, Lawrence CH. Textbook of attendant nursing. 2nd ed. New York: The Macmillan Company; 1942.
32. Kory RC, Wood W. Routine measurement of respiratory rate. An expensive tribute to tradition. JAMA. 1957;165(5):448–50.
33. Hillman K, Chen J, Cretikos M, Bellomo R, Brown D, Doig G, Finfer S, Flabouris A. MERIT Study Investigators. Introduction of the medical emergency team (MET) system: a cluster-randomised controlled trial. Lancet. 2005;365(9477):2091–7.
34. Chen J, Hillman K, Bellomo R, Flabouris A, Finfer S, Cretikos M, The MERIT Study Investigators for the Simpson Centre and the ANZICS Clinical Trials Group. The impact of introducing medical emergency team system on the documentation of vital signs. Resuscitation. 2009;80:35–43.

35. Hillman KM, Bristow PJ, Chey T, et al. Duration of life-threatening antecedents prior to intensive care admission. Intensive Care Med. 2002;28:1629–34.
36. Cioffi J, Salter C, Wilkes L, Vonu-Boriceanu O, Scott J. Clinicians' responses to abnormal vital signs in an emergency department. Aust Crit Care. 2006;19(2):66–72.
37. Cuillinane M, Findlay G, Hargraves C, Lucas S. An acute problem? London: A report of the National Confidential Enquiry into Patient Outcome and Death; 2005.
38. Cretikos MA, Bellomo R, Hillman K, Chen J, Finfer S, Flabouris A. Respiratory rate: the neglected vital sign. Med J Aust. 2008;188(11):657–9.
39. Loekito E, Bailey J, Bellomo R, et al. Common laboratory tests predict imminent death in ward patients. Resuscitation. 2013;84(3):280–5. Available on-line 31st July 2012 http://dx.doi.org/10.1016/j.resuscitation.2012.07.025.
40. Chen J, Bellomo R, Flabouris A, Hillman K, Finfer S, Cretikos M, The MERIT Study Investigators for the Simpson Centre and the ANZICS Clinical Trials Group. The relationship between early emergency team calls and serious adverse events. Crit Care Med. 2009;37(1):148–53.
41. Chan PS, Jain R, Nallmothu BK, Berg RA, Sasson C. Rapid response teams. A systematic review and meta-analysis. Arch Intern Med. 2010;170(1):18–26.
42. Cuthbertson BH, Smith GM. A warning on early-warning scores! Br J Anaesth. 2007;98(6):704–6.
43. Gao H, McDonnell A, Harrison DA, et al. Systematic review and evaluation of physiological track and trigger warning systems for identifying at-risk patients on the ward. Intensive Care Med. 2007;33:667–79.
44. Smith GB, Prytherch DR, Schmidt PE, Featherstone PI. Review and performance evaluation of aggregate weighted 'track and trigger' systems. Resuscitation. 2008;77:170–9.
45. Cuthbertson BH. Optimising early warning scoring systems. Resuscitation. 2008;77:153–4.
46. Subbe CP, Gao H, Harrison DA. Reproducibility of physiological track-and-trigger warning systems for identifying at-risk patients on the ward. Intensive Care Med. 2007;33:619–24.
47. Smith AF, Oakley RJ. Incidence and significance of errors in a patient 'track and trigger' system during an epidemic of Legionnaires' disease: retrospective case note analysis. Anaesthesia. 2006;61:222–8.
48. Prytherch D, Smith GB, Schmidt P, et al. Calculating early warning scores – a classroom comparison of pen and paper and hand-held computer methods. Resuscitation. 2006;70:173–8.
49. Lavelle BE. Patient and family activation of rapid response teams. Society of Critical Care Medicine Update. Critical Connections April/May 2011; pp. 18–19.
50. Afifi S, Ault M, Morris LL, Smith BL. Benefits of a separate airway emergency response team. ICU Manag. 2006;6(3):17–9.
51. Considine J, Lucas E, Wunderlich B. The uptake of an early warning system in an Australian emergency department: a pilot study. Crit Care Resusc. 2012;14(2):135–41.
52. Keene N. War veteran calls triple-0 from own hospital bed. The Daily Telegraph, Sydney, 5 April2010.
53. Between the Flags. Keeping patients safe. A statewide initiative of the Clinical Excellence Commission, Sydney. The Way Forward, October 2008. http://www.cec.health.nsw.gov.au/_documents/programs/between-the-flags/the-way-forward.rtf.
54. Hillman KM. Run, don't walk. Crit Care Med. 2012;40(9):2712–3.
55. Flabouris A, Chen J, Hillman K, Bellomo R, Finfer S, The MERIT study investigators from the Simpson Centre and the ANZICS Clinical Trials Group. Timing and interventions of emergency teams during the MERIT study. Resuscitation. 2010;81(1):25–30.
56. Jacques T, Fisher M, Hillman K, Fraser K, editors. DETECT Manual. Detecting deterioration, evaluation, treatment, escalation and communicating in teams. 1st edn. NSW Health Department; 2009. ISBN: 978-0-9806896-0-0.
57. Perkins GD, Barrett H, Bullock I, et al. The Acute Care Undergraduate TEaching (ACUTE) initiative: consensus development of core competencies in acute care for undergraduates in the United Kingdom. Intensive Care Med. 2005;31:1627–33.

58. Harrison GA, Hillman KM, Fulde GW, Jacques TC. The need for undergraduate education in critical care. (Results of a questionnaire to year 6 medical undergraduates, University of New South Wales and recommendations on a curriculum in critical care. Anaesth Intensive Care. 1999;27(1):53–8.
59. Bunch TJ, White RD. Education is what remains after medical emergency teams are trained. Crit Care Med. 2009;37(12):3174–5.
60. Sebat F, Musthafa AA, Johnson D, et al. Effect of a rapid response system for patients in shock on time to treatment and mortality during 5 years. Crit Care Med. 2007;35(11):2568–75.
61. Berwick DM. Continuous improvement as an ideal in health care. N Engl J Med. 1989;320:33–6.
62. Hillman K, Alexandrou E, Flabouris M, et al. Clinical outcome indicators in acute hospital medicine. Clin Intensive Care. 2000;11(2):89–94.
63. Hillman KM. Rapid response systems: you won't know there is a problem until you measure it. Crit Care. 2011;15:1001.
64. Leape LL, Brennan TA, Laird NM, et al. The nature of adverse events in hospitalized patients: results from the Harvard Medical Practice Study II. N Engl J Med. 1991;324:377–86.
65. Lilford R, Pronovost P. Using hospital mortality rates to judge hospital performance: a bad idea that just won't go away. BMJ. 2010;340:c2016.
66. Hillman K. Dying safely. Int J Qual Health Care. 2010;22:339–40.
67. Cretikos M, Parr M, Hillman K, et al. Guidelines for the uniform reporting of data for medical emergency teams. Resuscitation. 2006;68(1):11–25.
68. Bristow PJ, Hillman KM, Chey T, et al. Rates of in-hospital arrests, deaths and intensive care admissions: the effect of a medical emergency team. Med J Aust. 2000;173(5):236–40.
69. Calzavacca P, Licari E, Tee A, et al. The impact of rapid response system on delayed emergency team activation patient characteristics and outcomes – a follow-up study. Resuscitation. 2010;81:31–5.
70. Jones D, Bates S, Warrillow SF, et al. Long term effect of a medical emergency team on cardiac arrests in a teaching hospital. Crit Care. 2005;9:R808–15.
71. Buist M, Harrison J, Abaloz E, Van Dyke S. Six year audit of cardiac arrests and medical emergency team calls in an Australian outer metropolitan teaching hospital. BMJ. 2007;335:1210–2.
72. Foraida MI, DeVita MA, Braithwaite RS, et al. Improving the utilization of medical crisis teams (condition C) at an urban tertiary care hospital. J Crit Care. 2003;18:87–94.
73. McQuillan P, Pilkington S, Allan A, et al. Confidential inquiry into quality of care before admission to intensive care. BMJ. 1998;316(7148):1853–8.
74. Schneider EC, Lieberman T. Publicly disclosed information about the quality of health care: response of the US public. Qual Saf Health Care. 2001;10:96–103.
75. DeVita MA, Hillman K. Potential sociological and political barriers to medical emergency team implementation. In: Hillman K, Bellomo R, DeVita MA, editors. Medical Emergency Teams. Implementation and outcome measurement. New York: Springer; 2006. p. 91–103.
76. Nathens AB, Jurkovich GJ, Cummings P, Rivara FP, Maier RV. The effect of organized systems of trauma care on motor vehicle crash mortality. JAMA. 2000;283:1990–4.
77. Lecky F, Woodford M, Yates DW. Trends in trauma care in England and Wales 1989–97. The UK Trauma Audit Research Network. Lancet. 2000;355:1771–5.
78. Mullins RJ, Veum-Stone J, Helfand M, Zimmer-Gemback M, Trunkey D. Outcome of hospitalized patients after institution of a trauma system in an urban area. JAMA. 1994;27:1919–24.
79. Cretikos MA, Chen J, Hillman KM, Bellomo R, Finfer SR, Flabouris A, The MERIT Study Investigators. The effectiveness of implementation of the medical emergency team (MET) system and factors associated with use during the MERIT study. Crit Care Resusc. 2007;9 (2):205–12.
80. Santamaria J, Tobin A, Holmes J. Changing cardiac arrest and hospital mortality rates through a medical emergency team takes time and constant review. Crit Care Med. 2010;38(2):445–50.

81. Jones D, Opdam H, Egi M, et al. Long-term effect of a medical emergency team on mortality in a teaching hospital. Resuscitation. 2007;74:235–41.
82. Beyea SC. Implications of the 2004 National Patient Safety Goals. AORN J. 2003;78:834–6.
83. National Institute for Health and Clinical Excellence (UK). Acutely ill patients in hospital. Recognition of and response to acute illness in adults in hospital. NICE clinical guideline 50; July 2007.
84. Australian Commission on Safety and Quality in Health Care (Australia). National Consensus Statement: essential elements for recognising and responding to clinical deterioration. Sydney: ACSQHC; 2010 ISBN: 978-0-9806298-8-0.
85. Jones D, Baldwin I, McIntyre T, et al. Nurses' attitudes to a medical emergency team service in a teaching hospital. Qual Saf Health Care. 2006;15:427–32.
86. Lorenz KA, Lynn J, Dy SM, et al. Evidence for improving palliative care at the end of life: a systematic review. Ann Intern Med. 2008;148:147–59.
87. Angus DC, Barnato AE, Linde-Zwirble WT, Weissfeld LA, Watson RS, Rickert T, Rubenfeld GD, on behalf of the Robert Wood Johnson Foundation ICU End-of-Life Peer Group. Use of intensive care at the end of life in the United States: an epidemiologic study. Crit Care Med. 2004;32:638–43.
88. Parr MJA, Hadfield JH, Flabouris A, Bishop G, Hillman K. The medical emergency team: 12 month analysis of reasons for activation, immediate outcome and not-for-resuscitation orders. Resuscitation. 2001;50:39–44.
89. Chen J, Flabouris A, Bellomo R, Hillman K, Finfer S, The MERIT Study Investigators for the Simpson Centre and the ANZICS Clinical Trials Group. The medical emergency team system and not-for-resuscitation orders: results from the MERIT study. Resuscitation. 2008;79:391–7.
90. Jones D, Bagshaw SM, Barrett J, et al. The role of the medical emergency team in end-of-life care: a multicentre prospective observational study. Crit Care Med. 2012;40(1):98–103.
91. Buist M, Bernard S, Nguyen TV, et al. Association between clinically abnormal observations and subsequent in-hospital mortality: a prospective study. Resuscitation. 2004;62:137–41.
92. Jones DA, McIntyre T, Baldwin I, et al. The medical emergency team and end-of-life care: a pilot study. Crit Care Resusc. 2007;9:151–6.
93. Bellomo R, Goldsmith D, Uchino S, et al. A prospective before-and-after trial of a medical emergency team. Med J Aust. 2003;179:283–7.
94. Sharek PJ, Parast LM, Leong K, et al. Effect of rapid response team on hospital-wide mortality and code rates outside the ICU in a children's hospital. JAMA. 2007;298:2267–74.
95. Jones D, Bellomo R, DeVita MA. Effectiveness of the medical emergency team: the importance of dose. Crit Care. 2009;13:313. doi:10.1186/cc7996.

Chapter 13
The Chronically Critically Ill

Shannon S. Carson and Kathleen Dalton

Abstract Chronic critical illness is a condition that affects an increasing number of patients who suffer an acute illness or injury. Patients require prolonged weaning from mechanical ventilation which is best achieved by daily periods of unassisted breathing. They are at high risk of infectious complications, so infection control measures are essential elements of their care. Hospital mortality for chronically critically ill (CCI) patients is similar to that of patients who require mechanical ventilation for shorter periods; however, 1-year mortality is greater than 50 %. Fragmentation of care presents significant organizational challenges as hospital survivors cycle between multiple post-acute care institutions. Associated healthcare costs are significant, and the majority of those costs are covered by public programs. Patients and their surrogate decision makers should be made aware of long-term outcomes and care needs and be engaged in a discussion of patient values and appropriate goals of care.

Keywords Critical care • Critical illness • Critically ill • Mechanical ventilation • Mechanical ventilator weaning • Outcomes assessment • Costs • Costs analysis • Long-term care • Sub-acute care

In any intensive care unit, the majority of patients either survive their hospitalization or die from their acute illness within a few days of ICU admission. However between 10 and 20 % of patients will survive the early days of their ICU stay but fail to recover enough to be discharged from the ICU. This is because they remain

S.S. Carson (✉)
Division of Pulmonary and Critical Care Medicine, University of North Carolina School of Medicine, 4125 Bioinformatics Building, CB# 7020, Chapel Hill, NC 27599, USA
e-mail: scarson@med.unc.edu

K. Dalton
Rural Health Research and Policy Analysis Center, University of North Carolina, Chapel Hill, NC, USA

D.C. Scales and G.D. Rubenfeld (eds.), *The Organization of Critical Care*, Respiratory Medicine 18, DOI 10.1007/978-1-4939-0811-0_13,

dependent on life-sustaining therapies and the high level nursing of the ICU setting. For some patients, this dependence on life-sustaining therapies can last weeks or months. These patients have become recognized as the chronically critically ill (CCI) [1, 2].

CCI patients can be found in all types of ICUs, and risk factors are broad. Prolonged mechanical ventilation for persistent ventilatory or hypoxemic respiratory failure is a common feature, so acute exacerbations of chronic respiratory conditions such as COPD or obesity hypoventilation syndrome are risk factors. However multiorgan failure due to severe illness or injury is a more common cause of CCI than an exacerbation of chronic respiratory failure [3, 4]. The risk of CCI increases with the number of organ failures such as renal failure or cardiac dysfunction that often complicate ventilator weaning. ARDS and multilobar pneumonia are common risk factors as is persistent sepsis. Severe head trauma or multiple traumas are common, as is multiorgan failure following cardiac surgery or cardiac arrest. Nearly half of CCI patients are elderly [5]. This is a result of increased susceptibility to acute respiratory failure beginning at age 65 and higher risk of weaning failure in the elderly [6].

Regardless of what leads to their ICU admission, CCI patients usually develop a common phenotype [2]. They are profoundly weak as a result of systemic inflammatory processes and disuse atrophy during weeks of being bedbound. A prolonged catabolic state and feeding limitations contribute to weakness and general edema [7], which in turn predisposes patients to persistent skin wounds. Delirium or coma are present in as many as 62 % of patients and often persists beyond their ICU admission [8]. Since most CCI patients require prolonged mechanical ventilation, tracheostomies are usually required which limit swallowing and communication. All of these clinical problems demand careful nursing attention. Even after liberation from mechanical ventilation and ICU discharge, patients require further prolonged care in step-down units or specialized facilities. There they remain susceptible to recurrent episodes of nosocomial infections and respiratory failure necessitating subsequent ICU admissions.

Since comorbidities and multiorgan failure are key risk factors for CCI, the yearly incidence CCI has increased over the past decade as patients live longer with chronic illnesses and critical care clinicians are more successful in resuscitating patients with acute illness and injury [9]. With advanced age as the other key risk factor, the incidence of CCI is expected to increase even more dramatically in the next decade as the baby boom generation of North America advances beyond age 65. In one study, the number of patients requiring at least 4 days of mechanical ventilation will exceed 600,000 by 2020, many of whom will proceed to CCI [10].

Data from the Agency for Healthcare Research and Quality (AHRQ) national inpatient sample of U.S. hospitals (AHRQ National Inpatient Sample, 2010. Accessed at http://hcupnet.ahrq.gov) indicate that out of 39 million admissions to general acute care hospitals in 2010, 1.6 million underwent some form of respiratory intubation and mechanical ventilation, of which nearly one-half million received mechanical ventilation for 96 h or more (Table 13.1). Of these, roughly 116,000 patients received tracheostomies or ECMO for respiratory failure

Table 13.1 Increase in discharges with ventilation procedures

	2000	2010	10-year increase (%)
Any intubation and mechanical ventilation	952,083	1,638,210	72
Prolonged acute mechanical ventilation (96+ hours)	298,168	447,285	50
Tracheostomy, excluding those for head and neck procedures	86,911	116,491	34
All hospitalizations	36,417,565	39,008,298	7

Rows defined by presence of ICD-9 procedure codes
Source: AHRQ National Inpatient Sample for 2010

following surgery or medical complications. Between 2000 and 2010 the number of general hospital discharges increased by only 7.1 %, while discharges for PMV patients increased by 50 %, and those with tracheostomies increased by 34 %. Management of patients with CCI thus account for a growing share of hospital resources.

Clinical Challenges

On a day-to-day basis, the clinical challenges of managing CCI patients are no different than for any other patient in the ICU. The goal is to provide life support as needed, to reduce support as tolerated, while limiting injury to other organ systems by preventing complications in a deliberate and systematic way. The unique aspects of management of the CCI patient relate to the significant extent of muscle atrophy and weakness, including the respiratory muscles, and the greater length of time that patients remain at risk for complications.

For patients requiring PMV, standard measures of readiness for spontaneous breathing trials may not apply. After weeks of mechanical ventilation, they may be able to achieve a reasonable frequency to tidal volume ratio on minimal support for 30 min, but this does not guarantee the endurance required to support extended unsupported breathing. This lack of endurance can also complicate standard pressure support weaning protocols. For this reason, weaning protocols relying on work rest cycles with daily periods of T-piece or tracheostomy collar trials followed by complete support with mandatory ventilation are advocated [11]. Results of a recent clinical trial indicate that daily periods of spontaneous breathing result in shorter weaning times than do weaning protocols using gradual decrements in pressure support ventilation [12].

The optimal timing of tracheostomy placement remains a point of debate [13, 14]. It is a decision that can best be guided by individual patient circumstances. Early tracheostomy might be advocated for a younger patient with severe lung injury for whom prolonged ventilation is anticipated and likely to be accepted by the patient and surrogate decision makers. Later consideration of tracheostomy may be more reasonable for a patient for whom the need or desire for prolonged ventilation is less certain.

A tracheostomy will also facilitate efforts in ICU-based physical and cognitive therapy. The benefits of mobility interventions in mechanically ventilated patients have been demonstrated in one randomized trial and several cohort studies [15, 16]. The benefits of cognitive therapy to improve long-term cognitive function are currently being studied. Given that long-term cognitive and physical limitations are worse in CCI patients than in the general population of mechanically ventilated patients, these ICU-based interventions may benefit CCI patients the most.

The approach to nutrition in CCI patients should also differ from other ICU patients. If sepsis and other catabolic processes have resolved, their overall caloric needs may have decreased, yet adequate protein replacement will remain a priority [7]. Indirect calorimetry may be more useful in CCI patients than in the general ICU population to help avoid overfeeding and needless demands for CO_2 elimination. Prolonged limitations in gut motility can greatly limit calories in an insidious way through frequent holding of enteral nutrition. Routine calorie counts should be performed with provision of some level of parenteral nutrition when necessary.

Infectious complications are the most common cause of death in CCI patients, with central line-related blood stream infections being particularly problematic [17]. As with any ICU patient, central venous catheters should be removed as soon as they are no longer necessary [18]. When patients are hemodynamically stable and courses of intravenous antibiotics are completed, intravenous catheters of any type should be removed unless needed for hemodialysis. ICU directors should recognize that CCI patients are more likely to die from catheter infections than sudden arrhythmias, so policies demanding intravenous access just because a patient is in an ICU bed should not apply.

Outcomes

Despite their prolonged hospital course and complex clinical condition, hospital mortality for CCI patients is similar to or better than that of patients who require mechanical ventilation for shorter periods [19]. This reflects the fact that by definition, CCI patients survived the initial acute course of their critical illness, patients and families have opted for continued invasive care, and ICU technologies have been available to provide that support. However cohort studies that enroll consecutive patients in the acute hospital setting consistently demonstrate poor 1-year survival, ranging from 30 to 50 % [4, 19–22]. CCI patients who are discharged alive from their index hospital stay are very high users of post-discharge care. Discharge disposition codes in the national inpatient sample data show that they have higher transfer rates to other general hospitals (7 % compared to 2 % for all hospital discharges) and are far more likely to be discharged directly into specialized post-acute care facilities (70 % compared to 13 %) (Table 13.2).

Table 13.2 Resource use and discharge disposition, by type of insurance

		Disposition at index hospitalization			
			Share of live discharges		
	Index Hospital operating costs	In-house death (%)	General hospital transfer (%)	Nursing home or specialized post-acute care (%)	Home, hospice or other (%)
All general hospital discharges	$392.7 billion	2	2	13	85
All tracheostomy discharges	$12.6 billion	16	8	70	22
Tracheostomy discharges by payer					
Medicare	41 %	19	7	82	12
Medicaid	22 %	15	8	59	34
Private insurance	27 %	14	8	68	24
Uninsured	5 %	15	7	44	49
Other or missing	4 %	13	14	60	26

Source: AHRQ National Inpatient Sample for 2010, MS-DRGs 003 and 004. Definitions exclude cases with tracheostomies performed for face, mouth, and neck diagnoses

In recent years the Medicare program has funded several projects to identify the elderly CCI population and review their patterns of care. These projects have generated several detailed analyses of the hospital claims submitted for Medicare patients with extended ICU stays, with a special focus on those with PMV and tracheostomy. In 2010 there were nearly 35,000 Medicare discharges from general acute care hospitals that were assigned to the two main tracheostomy DRGs, of which 88 % had spent at least 10 days in ICU or ICU step-down units and 60 % had spent more than 3 weeks (Unpublished data from Kennel & Associates, "Determining medical Necessity and Appropriateness of Care for Medicare Long-Term Care Hospitals," HHSM-500-2006-0081, reproduced with permission from authors). By linking the tracheostomy admission claims to subsequent hospital or skilled nursing claims and to data from the national death index, the Medicare analyses were able to provide more accurate information on discharge disposition than is available through the national inpatient samples (Table 13.3). Twenty percent of these Medicare patients died during the hospitalization in which the tracheostomy occurred, another 2 % were discharged to hospice care. Two-thirds of the patients were confirmed as having transferred to an inpatient post-acute care facility of some type, and of this group, 26 % died within 60 days of the transfer and 55 % had died within 1 year of the transfer. The most common transfer destination was to specialty facilities called long-term care hospitals (LTCHs), which are specialized acute care hospitals that focus on ventilator weaning and the care of other complex medical patients. The second most common disposition was to a skilled nursing facility (SNF), which usually occurs either after the patient is

Table 13.3 Discharge disposition and mortality for Medicare tracheostomy patients in general acute care hospitals (2010)

		Post-discharge mortality	
Disposition at discharge	Cases (*N* = 34,479) (%)	At 60 days (%)	At 1 year (%)
Died in-house	20	100	100
Home, no subsequent readmission	7	12	32
Hospice	2	91	97
Transfers			
Other general acute hospital	2	33	60
Long-term care hospital	41	29	60
Inpatient rehabilitation facility	8	9	28
Skilled nursing facility	16	24	55
Subtotal, transfers	67	26	55
Other or Unknown	4	25	61
All	100 %	41 %	64 %

Note: Tracheostomy patients include those assigned to MS-DRGs 003 and 004
Source: Unpublished data from Kennel & Associates, "Determining medical Necessity and Appropriateness of Care for Medicare Long-Term Care Hospitals", HHSM-500-2006-0081, reproduced with permission from authors. Index and follow-up care constructed from MedPAR claims files, FY 2010–2011

weaned or as a transfer to a chronic ventilator care unit. Transfer to acute rehabilitation hospitals was less common and would occur only after weaning. Only 7 % were discharged to home or community without a readmission within 60 days. One-year post-discharge mortality was considerably lower for both the rehab transfers and the home discharges.

The high mortality rate following hospital discharge can be attributed to the continued presence of chronic comorbidities such as COPD or vascular disease, accumulation of new comorbidities associated with their acute illness such as renal failure or congestive heart failure, functional limitations that often require post-acute institutional care, and limited resources to cope with all of those risk factors. A 1-year follow-up study of 126 CCI patients discharged from a major academic hospital identified extraordinarily complex care trajectories [23]. Of the 99 patients discharged alive within the follow-up period, there were 457 transitions of care that included post-acute hospital transfers, SNF transfers, and multiple readmissions following home discharge and/or following the post-acute transfers. Patients cycled back and forth between different levels of care as they met administrative discharge goals, developed new complications requiring higher levels of care, or encountered reimbursement limitations. One half of the study population had four or more care transitions.

Functional independence is an unusual outcome for the CCI patient. Cohort studies have been consistent in finding that only 10 % of patients achieve functional independence after a year [23–25]. Physical function after CCI is effectively measured by independence in completing activities of daily living such as bathing or feeding oneself. CCI patients require assistance with an average of 6 ADLs 3 months after onset of mechanical ventilation and 2 ADLs after a year [19]. This compares to dependence in 1 ADL for survivors of short-term mechanical ventilation. Preexisting physical limitations are common in patients who develop CCI, but most survivors develop additional limitations. Ongoing severe cognitive limitations are also a common outcome of CCI. In one cohort of patients admitted to an inpatient weaning unit, 68 % of hospital survivors were still experiencing delirium or coma 6 months after hospital discharge [8].

The lower proportion of patients requiring assistance with ADLs at 1 year compared to 3 or 6 months can give the impression that most patients improve over time and regain some functional capabilities. That certainly is the goal of services provided at many post-acute care facilities such as LTCHs and SNFs, and some patients succeed. However these results reflect some degree of survival bias. Patients with more limitations in ADLs are less likely to survive for 12 months, so 1-year survivors reflect fewer limitations in ADLs. In fact, when followed over time, the proportion of CCI hospital survivors who experience a decline in functional capabilities exceeds the proportion that experience improvement [23].

The prolonged illness, interventions, and institutionalization experienced by CCI patients are understandably associated with a significant symptom burden. A comprehensive assessment of symptoms in CCI patients at an acute hospital weaning unit documented an extremely high prevalence of a range of symptoms including pain, anxiety, dyspnea, thirst, frustration with inability to communicate, and fear [26]. In a different LTAC hospital study, 42 % of CCI patients met criteria for clinical depression [27], and 12 % had significant symptoms of post-traumatic stress disorder 3 months after weaning [28].

All of these data regarding long-term outcomes of CCI patients highlight the organizational challenges of providing care. Even after liberation from mechanical ventilation, lasting medical issues, functional limitations, and limited physiologic reserve leave patients susceptible to new acute and critical illnesses. Their acute hospitalizations are significantly longer than other patients, and the majority cannot survive for long periods outside of acute care or subacute care institutions. Their conditions are often too complex for them to be able to go directly to rehabilitation facilities or skilled nursing facilities, and when they can, they have high readmission rates and long stays before discharge home. Care at home is often too challenging for family members without significant outside help. As outliers in every system, reimbursement rules do not match their needs, which can prompt transitions in care that are not dictated by medical need [29].

Costs and Resource Use

Nearly all definitions of CCI found in the clinical literature include the need for prolonged mechanical ventilation. All ICU stays are expensive, but mechanical ventilation is associated with significant increases in the variable cost per ICU day as well as longer ICU stays [30]. Tracheostomy placement for PMV has been suggested as one way to identify CCI patients from insurance claim files

Table 13.4 Inpatient resource use for ventilator care discharges, 2010

	Percent national discharges (%)	Percent national inpatient costs (%)	Mean charge per discharge ($)	Estimated mean cost per discharge ($)
All general hospital patients			33,037	10,067
Tracheostomy cases only (a)	0.30	3.21	355,912	108,249
Other MV for respiratory dx, without tracheostomy (b)	0.64	1.87	94,721	29,235

Source: AHRQ National Inpatient Sample for 2010
Rows defined by assigned Medicare severity diagnosis related group (MS-DRG):
(a) MS-DRGs 003 and 004
(b) MS-DRGs 207 and 208

[31]. These are among the most expensive patients in the general acute hospital setting, with an average charge per discharge that is more than ten times the average charge across all patients (Table 13.4). The Medicare program pays for hospitalizations on a per-discharge basis, using payment weights that are derived from average resource use associated with all Medicare discharges in the patient's major diagnostic category (MDC) and diagnosis-related group (DRG). Several years ago the Medicare program recognized that tracheostomy patients are uniquely high-cost subsets within any one of a number of possible DRGs. To make payments more accurate, hospital payment rules were altered to separate patients receiving this procedure from other patients, placing them in distinct payment groups irrespective of the underlying conditions that necessitated the procedure. This change effectively set special payment rates for CCI patients. Under the new Medicare severity-adjusted DRGs that have been used for payment since 2007, post-surgical patients needing tracheostomy that is not related to head and neck procedures (MS-DRG 003) have an expected stay of 44 days and a relative resource weight of 18.386—second only to heart transplant/implant cases. The equivalent group for non-surgical tracheostomy patients (MS-DRG 004) is slightly less resource intensive, with a mean stay of 26 days and weight of 11.704, but it is still among the ten highest paid Medicare severity-adjusted DRGs.

Public programs pay for the largest share of all hospitalizations where a tracheostomy occurs (Fig. 13.1a, b). Medicare's share of tracheostomy admissions has declined over the last decade from 51 to 45 %, while Medicaid's share has increased from 13 to 20 %, reflecting in part a change towards a younger age distribution. AHRQ estimates that in 2010, hospital operating costs for discharges during which a tracheostomy was performed totaled $12.6 billion, with Medicare patients accounting for 41 % of the costs, Medicaid patients 22 %, and privately insured patients 27 % (Table 13.5).

Another Medicare project constructed episodes of care for 27,000 Medicare discharges in 2009 during which (a) a tracheostomy was performed and (b) the patient spent 4 or more days in a critical care unit [32] (Table 13.6). Episodes began

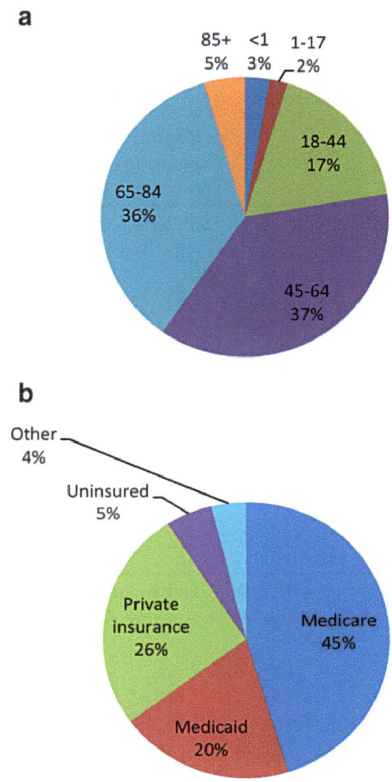

Fig. 13.1 (**a**) 2010 tracheostomy discharges, by age group. (**b**) 2010 tracheostomy discharges, by insurance

with the first (index) stay identified in an episode of illness, and followed each patient until death or until there was a 60-day period without any admission or institutionalization. The median stay for the index discharge in this sample was 25 days, for which Medicare paid the hospital an average of $105,000 per stay. Forty-six percent of all of the tracheostomy patients in the episode sample were transferred to an LTCH, and among these, the average Medicare payment for the index hospitalization was only $92,000, but additional payments to the LTCH averaged another $63,000 per transfer. Across all patients in the study sample, the median hospitalized days over the defined episodes (including the index stay, transfers, and any readmissions) was 49. Among those transferred to an LTCH, however, median total hospitalized days was 66, or one-third higher. Some but by no means all of the increased utilization and costs have been shown to reflect selection of sicker patients for transfer to LTCHs. The Medicare-sponsored studies strongly suggest that transfer to specialized long-term care hospitals is independently associated with longer total hospitalization and higher overall cost of care.

A recent independent study of Medicare beneficiaries also examined costs associated with LTCH transfer of CCI patients [33]. They confirmed that Medicare payments were higher if patients were transferred to LTCHs during their episode of

Table 13.5 Resource use and discharge disposition, by type of insurance

	Index Hospital operating costs	Disposition at index hospitalization	Share of live discharges		
		In-house death (%)	General hospital transfer (%)	Nursing home or specialized post-acute care (%)	Home, hospice or other (%)
All general hospital discharges	$392.7 billion	2	2	13	85
All tracheostomy discharges	$12.6 billion	16	8	70	22
Tracheostomy discharges by payer					
Medicare	41 %	19	7	82	12
Medicaid	22 %	15	8	59	34
Private insurance	27 %	14	8	68	24
Uninsured	5 %	15	7	44	49
Other or missing	4 %	13	14	60	26

Source: AHRQ National Inpatient Sample for 2010, MS-DRGs 003 and 004. Definitions exclude cases with tracheostomies performed for face, mouth and neck diagnoses

illness, but overall healthcare costs were actually lower because LTCH admission was associated with fewer days in skilled nursing facilities and fewer acute hospital readmissions. The higher Medicare payments may be a reflection of reimbursement structure rather than higher costs.

While the costs of mechanical ventilation have been relatively well studied, economic evaluations of the costs versus benefits of long-term mechanical ventilation have received only a moderate amount of attention [34]. One analysis modeled the cost-effectiveness of PMV for a 65-year-old critically ill patient with a history of 7–21 days of MV, where the principal base care option was continued PMV with tracheostomy, and the comparison option was a decision to provide comfort care only [35]. The authors used Markov modeling with patient data obtained from a large cohort of ventilated patients and expected mortality drawn from the medical literature, with costs defined as Medicare payment. For the 65-year-old base case, providing the extended PMV care was estimated to add only 1.75 quality-adjusted life years (QALYs), at an added cost to the Medicare program in 2005 dollars of approximately $144,000, or $82,000 per QALY gained. Estimates of the incremental costs per quality-adjusted year gained were sensitive to patient age (increasing to $206,000 per QALY gained for an 85-year old, holding other factors constant) and to predicted life expectancy (ranging from $61,000 per QALY gained among those with <50 % probability of death to $102,000 for those with ≥ 50 % probability of death). These estimates place continued provision of prolonged ventilator support for the very elderly and/or very ill well beyond the generally accepted range for cost-effective interventions. Given the increasing incidence of PMV and tracheostomy

Table 13.6 Medicare program payments and hospital stays for tracheostomy and PMV patients (2009)

	Two types of CCI as identified from claims data:	
	Tracheostomy patients, w/4+ critical care days	Other PMV patients, w/8+ days of critical care
Number of episodes	26,931	40,868
Median stay, index hospitalization	25 days	16 days
Average Medicare payment for index stay	$105,013	$41,881
Percent of index stays that are high-cost outliers	28 %	42 %
Average Medicare payment for outlier index stays	$150,064	$51,738
Percent of index stays transferred to an LTCH	46 %	8 %
Among those transferred to LTCHs		
Average Medicare payment for index stay	$92,159	$42,057
Average Medicare payment for LTCH stay	$62,045	$43,079
Median total hospital days in the episode		
All episodes	49 days	19 days
High-cost outliers in index stay	64 days	25 days
Episodes NOT transferred to LTCH	33 days	18 days
LTCH transfers	66 days	48 days

Source: Unpublished data from Kennel & Associates, "Chronically Critical Ill Population Payment Reform" HHSM-500-2006-00081, reproduced with permission from authors. Episodes of care constructed from Medicare index discharges in federal year 2009

among the elderly, however, the authors' discussion and conclusions from this work focused on the need to improve quality of life and survival for these patients in order to reduce the cost per adjusted life-year gained, rather than on review of the decisions to provide continued intervention.

Models of Care Delivery

There are a limited number of care venues for complex CCI patients. By definition the initial care site is the critical care unit of a general acute hospital, and in 2010, two-thirds of all patients receiving a tracheostomy were in teaching hospitals. At one time complex CCI patients were expected to remain in the ICU, but the high opportunity costs of occupying a critical care bed for several weeks has led hospitals to look for alternatives such as use of progressive or intermediate care units and/or specialized weaning units, or transfers to long-term care hospitals [29]. There are some skilled nursing facilities that specialize in medically complex patients including those on vents, but these are primarily chronic ventilator care sites and they tend to be limited to states where the Medicaid programs allow extra payments for "sub-acute" level care. For the CCI, choices among care venues depend on both the patient's clinical status and on local access (i.e., whether or not beds of these types are available in the area). They are, however, also heavily influenced by reimbursement policies by payers such as Medicare and Medicaid.

In the 1990s the federal government sponsored demonstration programs to develop specialized weaning units within tertiary care hospitals as a way to lower the costs of treatment and free up intensive care beds for acute critical illness. Several of these models continue today, including dedicated weaning units at the Mayo Clinic, the Cleveland Clinic and Mount Sinai Hospital [36, 37]. Specialized weaning units generally admit patients only after they are hemodynamically stable (off vasopressors) and after the presenting acute problems have been addressed. Weaning units tend to have lower costs per-day than ICUs because they can be staffed more like an intermediate than an intensive care unit. Adherence to weaning protocols and use of multidisciplinary rehabilitation teams are thought to lead to faster weaning, and it is the expectation of shorter overall hospital stays that provides the main incentive for hospitals to operate such units. While there is ample evidence in the literature that specialized PMV units have lower daily costs and reduce utilization of the more expensive ICU beds, the evidence is mixed on whether or not they lead to faster weaning and shorter overall stays at the hospitals where they are operated, due primarily to limitations in non-experimental study design [29]. A consensus conference in 2004 identified the clinical advantages of specialized PMV-focused units, citing among other factors, improved coordination care from multidisciplinary teams, better rehabilitation services, and the expectation of improved clinical outcomes that is associated with higher volumes [38]. The panel recommended that ICU care teams begin planning for transition to a dedicated weaning or other PMV-focused setting, either within the hospital or in a different specialized facility, as soon as possible after a tracheostomy has been performed.

For patients whose care is paid using a facility-specific fixed amount per discharge (such as the DRG system) hospitals face a strong incentive to choose a separate facility rather than an in-house unit for this phase of CCI care. This is because transfer to an in-house unit results in continued hospital costs, but unless the patient becomes an outlier case, there is no increase in the DRG payment. As a result of these financial incentives, in most parts of the USA LTCHs have become the preferred transfer destination [39]. LTCHs are defined simply as licensed acute care hospitals that have an average length of stay of 25 days or more, but they have many other characteristics that distinguish them from general acute care hospitals. They do not perform major surgeries and they rarely have emergency rooms, because they are designed as transfer destinations. Ninety percent of their patients come as transfers from a general acute care hospital, and the remaining patients are generally readmissions from nursing facilities or other care settings within an episode of illness that has already had a long care trajectory [32]. Virtually all LTCHs include ventilator weaning among their specialty services.

Medicare pays LTCHs using the same set of MS-DRGs that it uses for general acute care hospitals, but each LTCH DRG is associated with a much higher payment rate (reflecting the longer expected stays). Most LTCHs are small (very few have more than 100 beds) and are privately owned. They operate in a highly competitive environment with frequent mergers, acquisitions, and reorganizations. About one half of them are freestanding facilities, and the other half lease space from a floor in a "host" hospital. Unlike the specialized psychiatric and rehabilitation units that are both located within and operated by their general hospitals, co-located LTCHs are required by law to be independently owned. They are called "hospitals-within-hospitals," and to prevent de facto dependence on their host hospital, they are penalized if more than 25 % of their admissions are from the hospital where they lease space. The number of LTCHs grew rapidly between 1996 and 2006, after which Congress placed a moratorium on any new licensure pending a review of reasons for transfer and appropriateness of payment.

LTCHs in the USA have an uneven geographic distribution and are most heavily concentrated in southern states including Texas, Oklahoma, and Louisiana. In these areas LTCH transfer rates for Medicare PMV patients can be as high as 70 %. In other parts of the country—for example, in Oregon, northern New York, and northern New England—LTCHs are nearly nonexistent. CCI care in these areas therefore continues to occur in the hospital ICUs and intermediate or progressive care units, with dedicated weaning units operating in a few large teaching hospitals. One recent study showed that LTCH transfer rates for post-ICU patients vary considerably across hospitals, even within areas that have LTCH beds [40]. This suggests that local practice preferences continue to influence choice of setting for CCI patients, independent of access issues or hospital financial incentives.

LTCHs focus on rehabilitation and recovery, and rarely admit for end-of-life care. CCI patients who are sent to LTCHs tend to be those with better prognosis, including those with higher functioning prior to the onset of the illness that led to respiratory failure. A multi-center ventilator outcomes study conducted in 2002 documented characteristics of 1,419 ventilated patients who were transferred for weaning to 23 different LTCHs [41]. The median age of the study sample was 71.2 years, and prior to the precipitating acute illness, 86.5 % of them had been at home or in assisted living, with 77 % assessed in "good" premorbid functional status. The median hospital stay prior to transfer was 27 days, with a median of 25 ventilated days. Ninety-five percent of transfers already had a tracheostomy, and while they were identified as stable, the level of nursing acuity was still quite high: 95 % came to the LTCH directly from an ICU and 4 % came from a step-down unit; 94 % had in-dwelling urinary catheters; 65 % had a gastrostomy tube; 6 % were on TPN, and 42 % had pressure ulcers with broken skin. The reported nurse-to-patient ratios for the PMV patients were roughly 1:4, which is similar to the in-house dedicated weaning units described above. The study did not include a control group of ventilated patients *not* transferred to LTCHs, so it could not provide insights into how patients in the LTCH model of care differ from those that remain at the initial admitting hospital.

In partial response to a request by the U.S. Congress for a review of LTCH care and payment, the Medicare program contracted for a series of site visits to be conducted at LTCHs across the country and at critical care services located within general or academic hospitals in their same geographic areas [42]. In the LTCHs that were visited, nurse staffing for the overall patient population was described as similar to what might be found in a telemetry or intermediate care unit (four to five patients per RN), but was reported as two or at most three per RN for a newly admitted ventilator patient. All of LTCH sites had additional wound nurses or specialist wound care teams. Many of them operated dedicated ICUs with anywhere from 4 to 12 beds, allowing them to accept more complex patients and helping to minimize readmissions. Attending physician coverage at all of the study LTCHs was provided by generalists with heavy use of specialist consultants, and at all sites pulmonary consultants were said to participate in the care of all ventilator patients. Use of weaning protocols was standard, as was intensive rehabilitation through teams of respiratory, physical, speech and occupational therapists. All LTCH sites followed weaning protocols, and most were led by respiratory therapists under the supervision of consultant pulmonologists.

Critical care physicians both at the referring hospitals and at the receiving LTCHs were asked to distinguish the type of ventilated patients that were suitable for LTCH transfer from the type that should remain in the hospital critical care service. Responses from both groups were similar: patients should be hemodynamically stable, acute problems should have been diagnosed and be under treatment, and there should be reasonable prognosis for improved function if not recovery. In LTCHs that operated dedicated ICUs, ventilated patients were often admitted directly from the hospital ICU or progressive care unit into the LTCH ICU for at least an initial observation period. LTCH clinicians frequently commented that referring ICUs hold the PMV patients too long before transfer. Some LTCH clinicians revealed a somewhat more aggressive transfer policy than was recommended by the consortium conference [38] and also than was originally envisioned by the in-house special care units developed under the demonstration projects of the 1990s. In larger LTCHs with ICU capability, for example, staff were comfortable accepting patients who were still on vasopressors provided the doses were not still being titrated, and some sites reported that if an admitted patient became unstable, they would feel comfortable retaining the patient in the LTCH ICU and attempting to titrate the vasopressors before readmitting the patient to the referring hospital.

Results of a recent observational study suggest that CCI patients who are transferred to an LTCH have similar survival to patients who remain in ICUs [33]. Otherwise, there is very limited literature available to compare outcomes for PMV patients across the three major treatment venues of ICU, in-house weaning unit, or LTCH. Key clinical measures to be compared at the patient level should include percent weaned, time to weaning, percent discharged to home or community, functional status at discharge, severity adjusted survival and quality-adjusted survival. Key cost measures to be compared should include total institutional costs per episode, costs or Medicare payments per patient, and costs or Medicare payments per quality-adjusted life year gained. Although clinical trials could be organized to compare continued ICU care with in-house weaning units [43], financial incentives and organizational barriers make it virtually impossible to organize a randomized trial of LTCH transfer. This limits investigators to observational studies of a treatment decision that is highly influenced by clinical factors that are hard to identify retrospectively even from a medical record, let alone from more widely available administrative data.

One single-institution study of LTCH outcomes used historical controls from a period 2 years prior to the opening of a co-located LTCH [44]. The study sample included 196 LTCH admissions between 2004 and 2006 and 187 control cases from 2002 that had been retrospectively identified by clinicians as appropriate LTCH transfers using medical record review and length of stay. Use of historical controls means that the cost data for one group had to be updated for inflation, making the results potentially sensitive to economic assumptions. Both groups were said to be composed of "a majority" of PMV patients, but no statistics were offered, and it is possible that the sample size was not sufficient to control for this factor or for any other case-mix differences in applying the statistical tests. Although they found no significant difference in mortality between the two groups, the authors did find that the LTCH study group had lower per-day and per-patient costs, were more likely to be discharged to home, and less likely to be discharged into an SNF.

This study highlights two major challenges in studying comparative effectiveness or cost-effectiveness of LTCHs for the CCI, which are the need for multicenter studies due to the small number of PMV patients from any one institution, and the difficulty of controlling for the effects of patient selection into PMV-focused settings. To obtain sufficient sample size a well-designed multicenter study would be preferable to a national study using administrative data (such as the Medicare claims files), because administrative data often cannot provide important clinical variables such as time on a ventilator or key lab results. There is also no Medicare administrative data source for information on current or prior functional status for general hospital patients. In the recent comparative cost studies conducted for Medicare [32, 45], propensity-score matching was used to define control groups from the claims files, where clinically similar non-LTCH referrals were chosen based on interactions of ICU use, comorbidities, major organ failures, and age. Results from these models suggest higher per-patient costs for LTCH transfers. These data directly contradict earlier studies, but the results could be biased due to lack of functional status information and other limitations of the claims data. Adequate evaluation of alternative venues of care for CCI patients will depend on access to a large sample of geographically and demographically diverse patients, where the investigators also have access to detailed medical records data and patient or family interviews.

Continuity of Care

It is difficult to begin a discussion of continuity of care for CCI patients when all of the data indicate that care is anything but consistent. The fragmented nature of their care begins in the acute hospital ICU if the ICU is a closed system model covered by weekly or monthly shifts of intensivists. As the patient progresses, they transition to care by one or more medical/surgical ward services followed by the array of post-acute care institutions described above. At each transition, the receiving care team is usually operating on summaries of information from the referring institution, and relevant information from previous care may be two institutions removed. Outpatient-based primary care physicians have often lost contact with the institutionalized patient and are not current on their latest complex issues. Meanwhile, families and patient advocates are challenged to keep up with a bewildering array of events, clinicians, and environments. Whenever a patient does get to go home, it often is not apparent who among the recent treating physicians the family should contact about problems.

In response to this clinical problem of long-term fragmented care, a group of investigators developed an intervention to coordinate care for patients requiring at least 4 days of mechanical ventilation following hospital discharge [46]. They followed outcomes compared to usual care in a randomized trial. In the intervention group, nurse practitioners made regular calls to patient's homes to assess their status and screen for new issues that could lead to readmission. They then directed patients to relevant clinics or other resources in hopes of preventing readmission. They found that the intervention did not decrease the rate of readmissions; however, the length of stay for readmissions was decreased. Unfortunately, the intervention did not decrease mortality. These somewhat disappointing results of interventions to coordinate care may indicate that the complex condition of CCI patients defies preventive intervention, or that intensive interventions involving more direct outpatient care are necessary. A number of trials evaluating the benefit of post-ICU clinics on outcomes of patients with severe critical illnesses such as ARDS are underway. Many of these clinics will include physical and cognitive assessments and rehabilitation plans in addition to care coordination. It will be important to evaluate the benefit of these interventions for CCI patients as a subgroup.

Communication and Prognosis

The communication needs for families and other CCI patient advocates are similar to those of other ICU patients. Families should be informed of daily events and changes in status and receive periodic multidisciplinary review of the patient's condition and discussion of goals of care. As with any ICU patient, this process is often complicated by physician availability, family availability, and limitations in communication skills of the provider. For CCI patients, the process can be further complicated by provider fatigue, fragmentation in care, and prolonged family distress. Some of these communication barriers can be overcome by arranging for scheduled and protocolized family meetings. However a recent clinical trial comparing scheduled family meetings to usual care in patients requiring more than 4 days of mechanical ventilation showed no benefit in ICU length of stay or indicators of aggressiveness of care [47].

One potential barrier to adequate communication may be difficulties in assessing prognosis for CCI patients. They have survived the initial or "worst" phase of their critical illness, yet their rate of recovery has plateaued. Clinicians and providers gain hope from the initial survival and often are uncertain of the implications of the stalled progress. If clinicians are not confident of their prognostic assessments, they will not likely communicate a prognosis very clearly. Qualitative studies of family members of CCI patients confirm that families do not receive much prognostic information about hospital survival, and they receive virtually no information about long-term prognosis for survival or functional outcomes [48].

In response to this problem, investigators have developed and validated a simple clinical prediction rule to help clinicians assess long-term survival in patients with CCI [4, 20]. The ProVent score consists of 4 clinical variables—age, platelet count, and requirement for vasopressors and hemodialysis. When measured on day 21 of mechanical ventilation, the presence of each additional risk factor signifies increasing risk for death at 1 year. Similar scores are being developed for use on day 14 of mechanical ventilation. It is hoped that a simple prognostic score will increase the confidence of clinicians in providing a prognosis for CCI patients, especially when the prognosis is poor. A prognostic rule should not replace clinical judgment when considering prognosis; however, it can provide a starting point for the evaluation and support clinical intuition.

The gap in physician and family perceptions of prognosis is likely to be related to more than clinical uncertainty. There may also be problems with how information is communicated or understood. Many ICU clinicians are not formally trained in communication of prognosis or elicitation of goals of care. In other ICU settings, some clinical trials have demonstrated benefit on family-centered outcomes from providing information brochures, ethics consults, or palliative care consults [49, 50]. In order to enhance the communication of information for CCI patients, investigators for the family care committee of the Society of Critical Care Medicine have developed and validated an information brochure for families of patients with CCI [51]. Two clinical trials are underway to further enhance communication in CCI. One trial randomizes families to meet with palliative care physicians who are trained in communication and family support in addition to usual care and communication by the primary team. The other trial randomizes families to review an electronic decision aid versus usual care. The decision aid explains CCI, provides a long-term prognosis based on the patient's ProVent score, elicits patient values, and reviews general options for continued care. It is hoped that these interventions will enhance the communication process and in turn improve family-centered outcomes such as symptoms of depression and post-traumatic stress disorder. These interventions can be further enhanced by better prognostic systems for long-term function, which is as important for many patients as long-term survival. This will be a challenge for the future.

Summary

CCI is an increasingly common condition affecting 10 to 20 % of patients who receive mechanical ventilation for acute illness or injury. Patients present a number of clinical challenges related to their severe physical deconditioning, persistent delirium, and recurring complications. Costs of care are exceedingly high during the index hospitalization and after discharge due to a high requirement for institutionalized care and frequent transitions in care. Specialized weaning units and LTCHs are alternative sites of care that reduce costs for the index hospital and may reduce costs for the overall episode of illness. Given the poor long-term outcomes for elderly CCI patients and for patients with ongoing multiple organ failure, clinicians should actively engage patients and surrogate decision makers in discussions of the patient's values and preferred goals of care.

References

1. Carson SS. Definitions and epidemiology of the chronically critically ill. Respir Care. 2012;57 (6):848–56. discussion 856–8.
2. Nelson JE, Cox CE, Hope AA, Carson SS. Chronic critical illness. Am J Respir Crit Care Med. 2010;182(4):446–54.
3. Estenssoro E, Reina R, Canales HS, et al. The distinct clinical profile of chronically critically ill patients: a cohort study. Crit Care. 2006;10(3):R89.
4. Carson SS, Kahn JM, Hough CL, et al. A multicenter mortality prediction model for patients receiving prolonged mechanical ventilation. Crit Care Med. 2012;40(4):1171–6.
5. Carson SS, Bach PB. The epidemiology and costs of chronic critical illness. Crit Care Clin. 2002;18(3):461–76.
6. Behrendt CE. Acute respiratory failure in the United States: Incidence and 31-day survival. Chest. 2000;118:1100–5.
7. Hollander JM, Mechanick JI. Nutrition support and the chronic critical illness syndrome. Nutr Clin Pract. 2006;21(6):587–604.
8. Nelson JE, Tandon N, Mercado AF, Camhi SL, Ely EW, Morrison RS. Brain dysfunction. Another burden for the chronically critically ill. Arch Intern Med. 2006;166:1993–9.
9. Cox CE, Carson SS, Holmes GM, Howard A, Carey TS. Increase in tracheostomy for prolonged mechanical ventilation in North Carolina, 1993–2002. Crit Care Med. 2004;32 (11):2219–26.
10. Zilberberg MD, de Wit M, Prirone JR, Shorr AF. Growth in adult prolonged acute mechanical ventilation: implications for healthcare delivery. Crit Care Med. 2008;36(5):1451–5.
11. Scheinhorn DJ, Chao DC, Stearn-Hassenpflug M, Wallace WA. Outcomes in post-ICU mechanical ventilation: a therapist-implemented weaning protocol. Chest. 2001;119 (1):236–42.
12. Jubran A, Grant BJ, Duffner LA, et al. Effect of pressure support vs unassisted breathing through a tracheostomy collar on weaning duration in patients requiring prolonged mechanical ventilation: a randomized trial. JAMA. 2013;309(7):671–7.
13. Scales DC, Ferguson ND. Early vs late tracheotomy in ICU patients. JAMA. 2010;303 (15):1537–8.
14. Freeman BD, Morris PE. Tracheostomy practice in adults with acute respiratory failure. Crit Care Med. 2012;40(10):2890–6.

15. Schweickert WD, Pohlman MC, Pohlman AS, et al. Early physical and occupational therapy in mechanically ventilated, critically ill patients: a randomised controlled trial. Lancet. 2009;373 (9678):1874–82.
16. Morris PE, Goad A, Thompson C, et al. Early intensive care unit mobility therapy in the treatment of acute respiratory failure. Crit Care Med. 2008;36(8):2238–43.
17. Kalb TH, Lorin S. Infection in the chronically critically ill: unique risk profile in a newly defined population. Crit Care Clin. 2002;18(3):529–52.
18. Pronovost P, Needham D, Berenholtz S, et al. An intervention to decrease catheter-related bloodstream infections in the ICU. N Engl J Med. 2006;355(26):2725–32.
19. Cox CE, Carson SS, Lindquist JAH, Olson MK, Govert JA, Chelluri L. Differences in one-year health outcomes and resource utilization by definition of prolonged mechanical ventilation: a prospective cohort study. Crit Care. 2007;11:R9.
20. Carson SS, Garrett J, Hanson LC, et al. A prognostic model for one-year mortality in patients requiring prolonged mechanical ventilation. Crit Care Med. 2008;36(7):2061–9.
21. Combes A, Costa MA, Trouillet JL, et al. Morbidity, mortality, and quality-of-life outcomes of patients requiring > or = 14 days of mechanical ventilation. Crit Care Med. 2003;31 (5):1373–81.
22. Engoren M, Arslanian-Engoren C, Fenn-Buderer N. Hospital and long-term outcome after tracheostomy for respiratory failure. Chest. 2004;125(1):220–7.
23. Unroe M, Kahn JM, Carson SS, et al. One-year trajectories of care and resource utilization for recipients of prolonged mechanical ventilation: a cohort study. Ann Intern Med. 2010;153 (3):167–75.
24. Carson SS, Bach PB, Brzozowski L, Leff A. Outcomes after long-term acute care. An analysis of 133 mechanically ventilated patients. Am J Respir Crit Care Med. 1999;159(5 Pt 1):1568–73.
25. Nasraway SA, Button GJ, Rand WM, Hudson-Jinks T, Gustafson M. Survivors of catastrophic illness: outcome after direct transfer from intensive care to extended care facilities. Crit Care Med. 2000;28(1):19–25.
26. Nelson JE, Meier DE, Litke A, Natale DA, Siegel RE, Morrison RS. The symptom burden of chronic critical illness. Crit Care Med. 2004;32(7):1527–34.
27. Jubran A, Lawm G, Kelly J, et al. Depressive disorders during weaning from prolonged mechanical ventilation. Intensive Care Med. 2010;36(5):828–35.
28. Jubran A, Lawm G, Duffner LA, et al. Post-traumatic stress disorder after weaning from prolonged mechanical ventilation. Intensive Care Med. 2010;36(12):2030–7.
29. Donahoe MP. Current venues of care and related costs for the chronically critically ill. Respir Care. 2012;57(6):867–86. discussion 886–8.
30. Dasta JF, McLaughlin TP, Mody SH, Piech CT. Daily cost of an intensive care unit day: the contribution of mechanical ventilation. Crit Care Med. 2005;33(6):1266–71.
31. Kahn JM, Angus DC, Linde-Zwirble WT, Iwashyna TJ. Development and validation of an algorithm for identifying prolonged mechanical ventilation in administrative data. Health Serv Outcomes Res Methodol. 2009;9(2):117–32.
32. Dalton K, Kandilov AMG, Kennel D, Wright A. Final report: determining medical necessity and appropriateness of care for Medicare long-term care hospitals (LTCHs), CMS Contract No. HHSM-500-2006-0008I-T003. 2012; http://www.rti.org/reports/cms.
33. Kahn JM, Werner RM, David G, Ten Have TR, Benson NM, Asch DA. Effectiveness of long-term acute care hospitalization in elderly patients with chronic critical illness. Med Care. 2013;51(1):4–10.
34. Cooke CR. Economics of mechanical ventilation and respiratory failure. Crit Care Clin. 2012;28(1):39–55, vi.
35. Cox CE, Carson SS, Govert JA, Chelluri L, Sanders GD. An economic evaluation of prolonged mechanical ventilation. Crit Care Med. 2007;35(8):1918–27.

36. Gracey DR, Naessens JM, Viggiano RW, Koenig GE, Silverstein MD, Hubmayr RD. Outcome of patients cared for in a ventilator-dependent unit in a general hospital. Chest. 1995;107 (2):494–9.
37. Dasgupta A, Rice R, Mascha E, Litaker D, Stoller JK. Four-year experience with a unit for long-term ventilation (respiratory special care unit) at the Cleveland Clinic Foundation. Chest. 1999;116(2):447–55.
38. MacIntyre NR, Epstein SK, Carson S, et al. Management of patients requiring prolonged mechanical ventilation: report of a NAMDRC consensus conference. Chest. 2005;128 (6):3937–54.
39. Kahn JM, Benson NM, Appleby D, Carson SS, Iwashyna TJ. Long-term acute care hospital utilization after critical illness. JAMA. 2010;303(22):2253–9.
40. Kahn JM, Werner RM, Carson SS, Iwashyna TJ. Variation in long-term acute care hospital use after intensive care. Med Care Res Rev. 2012;69(3):339–50.
41. Scheinhorn D, Hassenpflug M, Votto J, et al. Ventilator-dependent survivors of catastrophic illness transferred to 23 long-term care hospitals for weaning from prolonged mechanical ventilation. Chest. 2007;131:76–84.
42. Dalton K, Kennel D, Bernard S, Kane H, Wright A. Report on site visits to IPPS critical care services and long term care hospitals, CMS Contract No. HHSM-500-2006-00081-T003. 2012; http://www.rti.org/reports/cms.
43. Rudy EB, Daly BJ, Douglas S, Montenegro HD, Song R, Dyer MA. Patient outcomes for the chronically critically ill: special care unit versus intensive care unit. Nurs Res. 1995;44 (6):324–31.
44. Votto JJ, Scalise PJ, Barton RW, Vogel CA. An analysis of clinical outcomes and costs of a long term acute care hospital. J Med Econ. 2011;14(2):141–6.
45. Kandilov AMG, Dalton K. Utilization and payment effects of Medicare referrals to long-term care hospitals (LTCHs). Final Report. 2011; www.rti.org/reports/cms.
46. Daly BJ, Douglas SL, Kelley CG, O'Toole E, Montenegro H. Trial of a disease management program to reduce hospital readmissions of the chronically critically ill. Chest. 2005;128 (2):507–17.
47. Daly BJ, Douglas SL, O'Toole E, et al. Effectiveness trial of an intensive communication structure for families of long-stay ICU patients. Chest. 2010;138(6):1340–8.
48. Nelson JE, Mercado AF, Camhi SL, et al. Communication about chronic critical illness. Arch Intern Med. 2007;167(22):2509–15.
49. Scheunemann LP, McDevitt M, Carson SS, Hanson LC. Randomized, controlled trials of interventions to improve communication in intensive care: a systematic review. Chest. 2011;139(3):543–54.
50. Lautrette A, Darmon M, Megarbane B, et al. A communication strategy and brochure for relatives of patients dying in the ICU. N Engl J Med. 2007;356(5):469–78.
51. Carson SS, Vu M, Danis M, et al. Development and validation of a printed information brochure for families of chronically critically ill patients. Crit Care Med. 2012;40(1):73–8.

Chapter 14
Regionalization of Critical Care

Theodore J. Iwashyna and Jeremy M. Kahn

Abstract Recent efforts to improve the outcomes of intensive care emphasize not only quality improvement at the local level but also better organization and management of health care systems at the regional and national level. Central to this notion is the concept of regionalization, whereby selected critically ill patients are systematically triaged and transported to regional centers of excellence. Regionalization might improve quality and efficiency by improving access to scarce resources, increasing clinical experience in the care of complex patients, and creating economies of scale. At the same time, there are number of potential risks, including adverse events in the transport of critically ill patients, worsening of crowding at already overburdened referral ICUs, reducing clinical skill at referring hospitals, and creating a non-patient-centered system that values regional care at the expense of receiving care close to the patients' homes. Future research and demonstration should provide insight into these tensions and lay the groundwork for regionalized critical care systems that are both effective and patient-centered.

Keywords Intensive care • Intensive care units • Mechanical ventilation • Regional hospital planning • Health policy

T.J. Iwashyna
Division of Pulmonary and Critical Care Medicine, Department of Internal Medicine, University of Michigan School of Medicine, 2800 Plymouth Road, NCRC, Building 16, Room 332W, Ann Arbor, MI 48109, USA

Veterans Affairs Center for Clinical Management Research, Ann Arbor, MI, USA
e-mail: tiwashyn@umich.edu

J.M. Kahn (✉)
Department of Critical Care, University of Pittsburgh School of Medicine, Scaife Hall, Room 602-B, 3550 Terrace Street, Pittsburgh, PA 15221, USA

Department of Health Policy and Management, University of Pittsburgh Graduate School of Public Health, Pittsburgh, PA, USA
e-mail: kahnjm@upmc.edu

D.C. Scales and G.D. Rubenfeld (eds.), *The Organization of Critical Care*, Respiratory Medicine 18, DOI 10.1007/978-1-4939-0811-0_14,

Introduction

At the completion of this chapter, the reader should be able to:

- Describe what is meant by a regionalized system of critical care;
- Identify the key potential benefits and drawbacks of implementing critical care regionalization;
- Assess the potential metrics by which the success of regional critical care systems might be measured.

Recent efforts to improve the outcomes of intensive care emphasize not only quality improvement at the local level but also better organization and management of health care systems at the regional and national level [1]. In the information age, hospitals and health systems are increasingly interconnected: critically ill patients are frequently transferred between hospitals [2]; expertise for complex therapies such as extracorporeal membrane oxygenation (ECMO) are located at just a few centers [3]; and the threat of pandemics means that hospitals must work together to ensure equitable access to critical care in times of crisis [4]. Given the growing importance of regional cooperation in critical care delivery, it is appealing to harness these interhospital connections as mechanism to improve intensive care unit (ICU) quality [5].

One approach to improving quality at the health care system level is regionalization. Under a regionalized system, pre-hospital providers and hospitals would systematically transport selected critically ill patients to designated regional referral centers, analogous to the trauma systems of many developed nations [6]. As in trauma, regionalization of critical care has the potential to significantly improve the outcomes of the critically ill. However, there are many important challenges to the successful implementation of regionalized critical care as well. ICU clinicians, hospital administrators, and health policy makers must address these issues before attempting to introduce regionalized critical care in their health system. In this chapter, we review the concept of regionalization as a strategy for ICU quality improvement, discuss the potential benefits and risk of such a system, and highlight the key organizational elements of successful regionalized critical care.

Defining Regionalization

Regionalization is the systematic concentration of selected patients in a subset of centers of excellence [7]. The goal of regionalization is to provide higher value care—better care for more patients by ensuring those patients get care at the hospitals best able to care for them.

Regionalization thus depends for its success on four conditions. First, there must be heterogeneity in quality—if every hospital is able to provide the same level of care, then there is no need for regionalization. Note that this may be true not only because all hospitals are equally capable but also because a disease is either uniformly treatable or uniformly terminal. Second, there must be some scarce resources that prevent the highest quality of care from being diffused to lower performing hospitals. Often that scarce resource will either be the lack of sufficient highly skilled providers to staff every hospital [8], although it may also be the financial barrier of providing the equipment needed. Third, the centers of excellence must be identifiable, either by direct measurement of outcomes or, more commonly, by a certification process based on equipment and capabilities. Finally, the patients to be regionalized must be identifiable and transportable.

Note that this definition of regionalization does not require de jure, or even formal, regionalization. Formal regionalization is the process that the term "regionalization" normally brings to mind, a system of officially designated centers of excellence and mandated referral patterns. De jure regionalization occurs when compliance with these referral patterns is legally mandated. Legally regulated systems offer important benefits of transparency and may bring new resources into the system. But formal regionalization does not, in and of itself, insure effective patient triage [9], and it runs the risk of ossification in the presence of evolving technologies of patient care. The absence of a formal system of regionalization does not mean that no regionalization occurs. A 2010 Academy of Emergency Management report [10] defined informal regionalization as "the concentration of select patient populations at specific local centers as a result of selective, historic, or de facto referral patterns to those centers by providers and EMS systems. Such regionalization is informal primarily because selective referral is based on decentralized decisions by individual providers and is not mandated by formal legal or administrative organizations." Informal regionalization, albeit incomplete, maybe quite common for many serious illnesses, although hampered by lack of good data to identify centers of excellence and poor incentives to insure appropriate transfer [11, 5, 12, 13].

Potential Benefits of Regionalized Critical Care

There are numerous potential benefits of regionalization. These relate to both health care outcomes, access to scarce resources and costs (Table 14.1).

Better Care by Access to Scarce Expertise

If there are not enough care experts able to provide the highest level of care, then regionalization increases the likelihood that eligible patients will be cared for by those teams. In the setting of resource scarcity, it is often more efficient to concentrate on the scarce resource in a small number of centers. Regionalization may improve access to high quality care, reducing the morbidity and mortality

Table 14.1 Potential benefits and risks of regionalized critical care

Benefits	Increased access to scarce expertise
	Greater clinical experience leading to improved outcomes
	Acceleration of innovation
	Creation of economies of scale
	Motivation for performance improvement through public recognition
Risks	Adverse events during transport
	Overcrowding of regional referral centers
	Treatment delays due to travel distances
	Worsened family outcomes due to travel distances
	Cascade iatrogenic
	Loss of skill at non-referring hospitals

associated with regionalized problems and/or improving timely referral to palliative care. There is evidence that this has occurred with the introduction of trauma systems [14, 15].

Learning by Doing and Accelerating Innovation

As in many areas of health care, volume-outcome relationships are both prevalent and reproducible [16]. An important hope is that by concentrating on the care of particularly sick patients, it will make possible greater individual provider skill (as they do more of such cases). But it is also hoped that regionalization would lead to greater institutional investment to support excellence. This might take the form of greater development of protocols, of specialized positions (e.g., ICU pharmacists) and of ongoing education and training.

It is also hoped that regionalization makes possible greater generalizable knowledge. For example, the trauma system supports a national trauma registry that has allowed significant study of trauma patients. Repeatedly seeing high acuity patients, it is hoped, will make it more likely that novel therapies and approaches to their problems can be developed. The concentration of such patients then also makes careful testing of new therapies easier with focused enrollment in clinical trials. As such, regionalization would offer not just better care for current patients, but more rapidly improving care for future patients. The extent to which these hopes are born out has not been subjected to significant empirical scrutiny to date.

Economies of Scale

Critical care involves substantial fixed costs, particularly in terms of equipment [17]. By concentrating the care of critically ill patients in a smaller numbers of regional centers, the expensive equipment is more likely to be utilized, distributing the fixed costs over more patients and allowing lower average costs [18]. In a similar vein, regionalization can ensure that the smaller number of providers most able to care for certain specialized cases devote almost all of their time to those specialized cases—rather than spending their valuable time on cases requiring lower or different skill sets.

Social Recognition of Centers of Excellence

Although rarely acknowledged, it seems likely that part of the motivation of regionalization may be self-designated centers' of excellence desire to be recognized as such. Such recognition may bring quite palpable benefits in terms of increased revenues, investments, and donations in addition to the pride and prestige it may instill. The potential magnitude of this benefit may be mitigated by the oft-documented disconnect between critical care practitioners self-assessed expertise and their objectively verifiable levels of competence [19–21].

Potential Risks of Regionalized Critical Care

Although there are many potential benefits to regionalized critical care, there are also potential risks that may negate any hoped for quality improvement. Health policy makers must consider these issues when designed regionalized critical care (Table 14.1).

Adverse Events During Transport

Regionalization would involve large-scale transport of critically ill patients over large distances. Such transports are not only costly but also entail risks of physiological deterioration and other complications. Among the complications are refractory hypoxemia, pneumothorax, hypotension, and shock [22]. Despite the real risk of these events, existing evidence suggests that they are relatively uncommon. A 2006 systematic review of studies of patient outcomes during interfaculty transport found only one case of a patient dying during transport [23]. Subsequent studies confirmed that the risk of adverse events during inter-facility transport is low, with major adverse events occurring less than 5 % of the time [24] or not at all [25]. One important caveat of these studies is that they all were performed under the existing ad hoc system where patients are subjectively selected for transfer, and these analyses were of relatively mature transport systems which collect enough data to analyze. It is conceivable that under formal regionalization, in which more patients and sicker patients will undergo transfer, that adverse events may increase, particularly if regionalization is not accompanied by quality and access improvement in the transport system [26].

Throughput and Crowding

By definition, regionalization would involve a major reorganization of admission and discharge patterns within a region. Regional referral centers, which in many areas are already frequently operating at capacity, would see an increase in admissions with a concomitant increase in average ICU census. This change could result in several adverse effects. First, when ICUs are full there can be admission delays from the emergency department, ward or operating room. These delays are characterized by increased risks of mortality [27], and emergency department crowding in itself is associated with morbidity among patients seeking emergency care [28]. Second, when ICU beds are needed but not available, less sick patients may be prematurely discharged from the ICU to ward. These premature discharges are also associated with an increased risk of death [29]. Third, ICUs operating at capacity may be harmful to patients within the ICU, even if they are not prematurely discharged. Capacity strain can mean less attention paid to each individual patient with greater potential for errors. Countering this claim are data showing that ICU admission during times of high census is not associated with higher risk of death compared to times of low census [30]. However, census is a crude marker for overall strain, and novel methods that account for severity of illness may show different results [31].

To address concerns about overcrowding, any regionalization efforts must include sophisticated approaches to measure and manage bed census [32]. The need for an ICU bed in a hospital is not merely a function of the patient's physiology and the ICU; it also depends critically on the availability and capability of non-ICU floor beds. Improving the observation and rapid response capabilities of non-ICU beds may play an important role. Furthermore, regionalization must include evidence-based guidelines about which patients are eligible for ICU admission and which patients can be managed on appropriately staffed hospital wards. In many health systems ICU beds are over utilized with as many as half of ICU patients having an extremely low risk of death [33], suggesting that these beds are being used to substitute for unresponsive floor options. Efforts to reduce ICU utilization among low risk patients, and to facilitate the reverse triage of patients whose need for high level care is completed, may mitigate concerns about overcrowding as more high-risk patients are brought to referral centers.

Distance and Quality Tradeoffs

Inherent in any regionalization schema is the notion that patients, at least those triaged in the field, may need to bypass the closest hospital in favor of a more capable hospital. This creates a tradeoff between distance and quality, particularly for time sensitive conditions such as acute myocardial infarction, stroke, and severe sepsis. In these conditions it is not clear whether it is better to get some care as quickly as possible even if that care is not definitive, or to get definitive care first even if that care is delayed through longer transport times. In acute myocardial infarction, for example, percutaneous transluminal coronary angioplasty (PTCA) improves outcomes compared to intravenous thrombolysis [34]. However, early thrombolysis may be superior or at least equal to delayed PTCA [35], demonstrating a tension between early care and definitive care that is relevant to critical care regionalization as a whole.

Another more subtle tradeoff between distance and quality stems from patient preferences for care. To the degree that regionalization means centralization, it entails transporting patients some distance from their homes in order to receive the best quality critical care available. The implicit assumption here is that patients, and their families, are willing to travel large distances in exchange for an increased chance of survival. Critical illness is already a substantial strain on family members, with high rates of depression and post-traumatic stress disorder [36]. Sleeping in a hotel or hospital waiting room far from the support structures of friends and family members may exacerbate this strain. Although this issue has not been studied directly in critical care, evidence in other fields suggests that many patients prefer to have their care close to home even if it means a higher risk of bad outcomes [37]. Thus a major challenge to regionalization is keeping the system patient centered by focusing on all outcomes that are important to patients and designing systems that take seriously and mitigate these potential familial burdens.

Cascade Iatrogenesis

Another insidious risk of regionalization is the notion of cascade iatrogenesis, which occurs when early decisions to initiate seemingly minor therapies lead to the development of multiple adverse events [38]. In this case, the theoretically innocuous early decision is the transport to a regional referral center, particularly among lower risk patients who may not benefit from transfer. Since no triage scheme is perfectly specific, many low risk patients will ultimately receive care at regional centers [39]. Used to higher risk patients, these centers may routinely perform invasive procedures such as central venous catheter insertion and pulmonary artery catheter placement [40]. These therapies can cause harms such as infection and pulmonary embolus, which can in turn lead to greater harms. To mitigate this concern, regionalization should proceed only when triage is sufficiently specific prevent too many low risk patients being transferred to regional referral hospitals.

Loss of Skill at Referring Centers

If referring centers see fewer and fewer critically ill patients, they may become less and less able to care for those patients who do present to their facility with critical illness. Some residual undertriage—the failure to refer all patients who might benefit from regionalization—is very likely, given both the predictable imperfections of any EMS system and patients' decisions to self-transport to hospitals [9]. It is not clear to what extent such deskilling actually occurs and can be prevented. Of note, providers at community hospitals that frequently initiate referral note that the transport of high acuity patients frees them to focus on what they feel is their primary area of expertise, the care of the numerous other lower acuity, but still sick, patients [41].

The Evidence for Regionalization

There is little direct evidence that regionalization improves patient outcomes or reduces costs in medical critical care. However, indirect evidence is provided by regionalization in fields that are analogous to critical care and clinical trials of complex therapies that entail transfer to a regional referral center.

Analogous Clinical Fields

Trauma and neonatal care provide the best indirect evidence that critical care regionalization can improve intensive care quality. Trauma systems evolved out of triage lessons learned from mid-twentieth century military conflicts [42]. Although trauma systems vary from country to country, and indeed even within countries, evidence suggests that patients with severe traumatic injury receiving care at designated trauma centers experience lower mortality than those receiving care at other hospitals [14]. Similarly, high-risk neonatal care is highly regionalized in most developed nations, with the preponderance of evidence indicating that extremely small premature newborns experience increased survival when they receive care at a designated neonatology center [43].

These analogies are useful because of the many similarities between trauma, neonatal care, and general critical illness. All of these conditions are high-risk, have demonstrated volume-outcome relationships and require extensive expertise and infrastructure. However, there are many differences between these disease states and critical illness that should prevent us from making too direct a comparison [44]. In particular, triage is much easier in trauma and neonatal care than in critical illness, which occurs both in the field and within the hospital. General critical illness is also much more prevalent than trauma or high-risk neonatology, meaning that regionalization would be a much greater enterprise. Finally, and perhaps most importantly, critical illness is not a disease itself but is a syndrome, and a poorly defined syndrome at that. Perhaps the greatest limitation to the trauma and neonatal care analogies is that it is much harder to define the types of patients who may benefit from care in a regional center.

The CESAR Trial

To date there is only one clinical trial that involved any form of regionalization for general critical illness, the United Kingdom trial of conventional ventilator support versus ECMO for severe adult respiratory failure (CESAR) [45]. CESAR randomized 180 adults with severe hypoxemic respiratory failure to either conventional mechanical ventilation at their admission hospital or transfer to a regional referral hospital for ECMO. Patients randomized to transfer to the ECMO center were less likely to experience the combined endpoint of death or severe disability at 6 months (relative risk = 0.69, 95 % confidence intervals: 0.05–0.97, $p = 0.03$).

The CESAR trial was designed to study ECMO, not regionalization. Yet importantly for the issue of regionalization, only 75 % of patient transferred to the ECMO center actually received ECMO—the others continued to receive conventional ventilator support. And all patients in the ECMO group, regardless of whether they received ECMO, received more days of lung protective ventilation (23.9 days versus 15.0 days, $p < 0.001$). Thus, a reasonable interpretation of CESAR is that it was transfer to a regional referral hospital and receipt of lung protective ventilation, not ECMO, that led to the improvement in outcomes. Future research should evaluate whether transfer to a regional hospital improves outcomes independent of salvage therapies such as ECMO. Indeed even if ECMO itself was responsible for the improvement in outcomes, the CESAR trial provides conceptual support for regionalization, since ECMO is unlikely to be available at all hospitals.

Key Elements of a Regionalized System

An effective regionalized system of care requires both key technologies and the development of organizational practices to effectively utilize those technologies. We have elsewhere argued that an effective interhospital transfer system would function as an infrastructure, in the technical sense of that term—as a ubiquitous and invisible set of tools that allow ready movement of patients to where they would get the best care [46]. Here we summarize key pieces of that infrastructure.

Identification of Regional Centers

Regionalization requires selecting a subset of hospitals as centers for the care of some kinds of patients. Some system for selecting who is—and therefore who is *not*—a regional center is necessary. Self-designation, at least in the case of trauma centers, appears to lead to a system with simultaneously significant redundancy and also coverage gaps [47], diluting the potential benefits. However, self-designation, when based on objective organizational criteria, may seem fair and avoids having some particular individual "pick winners." Centers with high patient volumes might be selected, given relatively consistent volume-outcome literature, although this strategy risks excluding high-quality but low-volume centers [48]. If sufficiently high-quality risk-adjusted mortality data is available, those data could be used to select regional centers [5]. The preferences of political leaders might be used; if this led to increased funding, such a system might well offer similar or greater benefits to patients as one chosen exclusively from performance data.

Whatever system is used, institutional inertia is likely to prevent updating of center designation as technology, skills, and population distribution change. There have been few explicit studies of systems for updating and dynamically reallocating regional centers, despite the fact that this is likely a pressing problem.

Triage of Patients

As noted above, a sufficiently sensitive and specific system is necessary to identify the patients who will benefit from the move to a regionalized center without simply sending all patients—some of whom might suffer. The extensive focus on early detection of stroke, ST-elevation myocardial infarction, and significant trauma in the Advanced Cardiac and Trauma Life Support courses emphasize the inadequacy of common sense for determining who should be considered for regionalization. Similarly, the acute respiratory distress syndrome and severe sepsis appear to be frequently under-diagnosed in clinical practice [49]. Thus an effective regionalization system may require aggressive case-finding, which is becoming increasingly possible with the advance of electronic medical records and decision-support [50].

Strict triage criteria need to be balanced against the realities that the benefits of transfer to a regional center may include a reevaluation of the diagnosis and plan of care. Such benefits are emphasized by findings such as the CESAR trial, and similar results in myocardial infarction and stroke, that the benefits of transfer are often not fully explained by the particular procedure often used to justify the transfer [46]. Ideally, a system of regionalization would include not just forward triage of particularly critical patients, but "reverse triage" of patients no longer needing specialized care. There have been promising studies of this approach for percutaneous coronary intervention for myocardial infarction, but more work is needed in general critical care [51].

Table 14.2 Potential value of regionalization approaches[a]

Patients	Mechanical ventilation (non-post-operative)	Acute myocardial infarction who underwent a transfer
Originating hospitals	Lower than median volume hospitals	Non-revascularization hospitals
Mechanism for regional center designation	Nearest higher than median volume hospitals	Revascularization hospital with best 30-day risk-standardized mortality rate
Change to the system	New transfers	Rerouting existing transfers
Maximum transfer	100 miles	100 miles
Population studied	Inpatients in eight U.S. states	Medicare beneficiaries
Number of patients transferred in simulation	74,357	30,875
Potential lives saved acutely	4,720	834
Number needed to transfer to save 1 life	16	37

[a]Summarized are two simulations. One is of the potential benefits of transferring most mechanically ventilated patients from lower volume to higher volume hospitals; most of these patients had not actually been transferred [17]. The second is of the benefits of rerouting acute myocardial infarction transfers from non-revascularization hospitals; rather than go to where they actually went, this study simulated the incremental benefit of sending them to the nearby revascularization center with the best 30-day measured outcomes [12]. Note that these numbers needed to transfer compare favorably with numbers needed to treat for many accepted therapies

Observational work also suggests that careful attention needs to be paid to the incentives used to drive patient identification and transport. For example, Italian studies suggest that interhospital transfer of patients is primarily driven by interhospital business relationships, rather than patient-outcome focus [52]. U.S. data similarly show that a reorganization of the system to emphasize improved patient outcomes is possible; indeed, it might offer significant additional benefits for patients (Table 14.2) [12, 13]. These findings together remind us that patients are transferred, or not, for a complex set of reasons. In order to achieve patient-centered goals of regionalization, then it will be necessary to implement and monitor patient-centered incentives to insure optimal behavior.

Safe and Effective Interhospital Transport

Despite the numerous reports of safe and effective interhospital transport in the published literature, there is essentially no systematic data on the availability and quality of such transport. Some U.S. community hospitals report substantial difficulty in obtaining sufficient critical care transport even in the current, non-regionalized system [41]. Different parts of the developed world vary widely in the availability, training, and credentialing of providers for interhospital transport. Generalizable studies of the cost-effectiveness of different models are urgently needed. In the meantime, individual system planners and managers need to conduct individualized evaluations of their own transport system and whether it can meet the needs of their regionalization plans.

Ongoing Performance Monitoring

Regionalization by definition involves greater coordination of the care of more patients. With such increasing complexity, informal performance measurement should be replaced by greater explicit measurement and management. Indeed, the recent United States Institute of Medicine report that called for regionalized emergency care noted that these systems must accountable to their outcomes [53]. In a small hospital or ICU, implicit review by one's partners may offer reasonable ability to adjust to changes in capacity, patient need, and technology—and to provide focused formative feedback and remediation. It is implausible that such a system would work well on a metropolitan or provincial scale. Greater explicit measurement has been a central feature of organizational growth across a wide range of human endeavor, and regionalization of complexly ill patients seems no different.

Complementary Strategies

The core component of regionalized critical care is the systematic triage and transport of patients to regional referral centers. Yet there are other potentially important components to regionalization that might complement triage and transport, providing additional benefits above and beyond any quality gains that might be expected by concentrating care at regional centers of excellence.

ICU Telemedicine

ICU telemedicine uses audio-visual technology to provide critical care services from a distance [54]. Facilitated by the electronic health record and high-bandwidth internet connections, ICU telemedicine typically involves not only remote monitoring of critically ill patients and intervention when necessary, but also screening for routine evidenced based practices. Telemedicine is an attractive complementary approach to critical care regionalization because the expertise of a trained intensivists can be brought to any hospital, no matter how small or how far away from a regional referral center. Additionally, telemedicine can help reconcile the distance and quality tradeoffs inherent in regionalization achieved purely through triage and transport, as patients can potentially receive high quality care both quickly and close to home.

At this time there is little consensus about when and how telemedicine is best applied [55]. Existing programs use a variety of different commercial applications, monitoring strategies and approaches for engaging bedside clinicians. The evidence underlying ICU telemedicine is mixed, with many studies showing substantial improvements in outcome while others suggesting no benefit or even harm [56]. The strongest evidence comes from a recent multicenter study which combined remote monitoring with routine screening for evidence-based practices [57]. Additionally, the intervention in this study occurred in a setting in which the telemedicine physicians also worked in the target hospitals [58]. Unfortunately, this last component weakens the potential for telemedicine to truly improve care at the regional level, since large distances will preclude the telemedicine physicians from also providing bedside care. Thus the trust and effective communication that is essential for high quality critical care may not be possible with telemedicine, even as a complement to other forms of regionalized care.

Community Outreach

Community outreach refers to the systematic effort to standardize and improve the quality of critical care within a region. Under a community outreach model, not only are the sickest patients transferred to regional hospitals, but regional hospitals participate in a program of education designed to speed adoption of evidence-based practice and improve the quality of care. This model of regionalization, more aptly termed "regional" critical care rather than "regionalized" critical care, has been endorsed by several consensus groups in emergency medicine and critical care [59].

The benefits of these regional quality improvement networks, as well as their inherent challenges, are described in a detail in a separate chapter. Specific to regionalization, their benefits include the possibility of keeping some patients in their community, obviating the need for expensive and stressful transfers. Additionally, these networks can help maintain a baseline quality of care that mitigate the loss of experience that comes from routinely transferring out the sickest patients. For example, had all patients in the CESAR trial received consistent lung protective ventilation, even at the small community hospitals, survival may have increased in those hospitals both for patients eligible for ECMO and other patients with acute respiratory failure as well.

Conclusion

Regionalization is a theoretically powerful, conceptually sound approach to improving regional ICU quality. By taking advantage of clinical experience, increasing access to scarce expertise and creating economies of scale, regionalization could both improve outcomes and reduce costs. Yet at this time the evidentiary base for regionalization remains sparse. Indirect evidence from regionalization comes from successes in neonatal care, the volume-outcome relationship in critical care and CESAR, a clinical trial of ECMO that involved transfer to a regional referral hospital. However there is no direct evidence to date, let alone comparative effectiveness data on alternative organizational strategies. There are no current efforts to create a holistic regionalized system that spans disease states. Ultimately, demonstration projects will be required to determine if true regionalized care is superior to the existing ad hoc system of pre-hospital triage and interhospital transfers for patients with critical illness. As researchers, investigators and policy makers develop those demonstration projects, we should continue to work on alternative and complementary strategies to improve critical care quality at the regional level.

References

1. Shortell SM, Casalino LP. Health care reform requires accountable care systems. JAMA. 2008;300(1):95–7.
2. Iwashyna TJ, Christie JD, Kahn JM, Asch DA. Uncharted paths: hospital networks in critical care. Chest. 2009;135(3):827–33.
3. Davies A, Jones D, Bailey M, Beca J. Extracorporeal membrane oxygenation for 2009 influenza A (H1N1) acute respiratory distress syndrome. JAMA. 2009;302:1888–95.
4. Kumar A, Zarychanski R, Pinto R, et al. Critically ill patients with 2009 influenza A (H1N1) infection in Canada. JAMA. 2009;302(17):1872–9.
5. Iwashyna TJ, Courey AJ. Guided transfer of critically ill patients: where patients are transferred can be an informed choice. Curr Opin Crit Care. 2011;17(6):641–7.
6. Nathens AB, Jurkovich GJ, Cummings P. The effect of organized systems of trauma care on motor vehicle crash mortality. JAMA. 2000;283:1990–4.
7. Nguyen Y-L, Kahn JM, Angus DC. Reorganizing adult critical care delivery: the role of regionalization, telemedicine, and community outreach. Am J Respir Crit Care Med. 2010; 181(11):1164–9.
8. Angus DC, Shorr AF, White A, Dremsizov TT. Critical care delivery in the United States: Distribution of services and compliance with Leapfrog recommendations. Crit Care Med. 2006;34:1016–24.
9. Vassar MJ, Holcroft JJ, Knudson MM, Kizer KW. Fractures in access to and assessment of trauma systems. J Am Coll Surg. 2003;197(5):717–25.
10. Glickman SW, Kit Delgado M, Hirshon JM, et al. Defining and measuring successful emergency care networks: a research agenda. Acad Emerg Med. 2010;17(12):1297–305.
11. Iwashyna TJ, Christie JD, Moody J, Kahn JM, Asch DA. The structure of critical care transfer networks. Med Care. 2009;47(7):787–93.

12. Iwashyna TJ, Kahn JM, Hayward RA, Nallamothu BK. Interhospital transfers among Medicare beneficiaries admitted for acute myocardial infarction at nonrevascularization hospitals. Circ Cardiovasc Qual Outcomes. 2010;3(5):468–75.
13. Veinot TC, Bosk EA, Unnikrishnan KP, Iwashyna TJ. Revenue, relationships and routines: the social organization of acute myocardial infarction patient transfers in the United States. Soc Sci Med. 2012;75(10):1800–10.
14. MacKenzie EJ, Rivara FP, Jurkovich GJ. A national evaluation of the effect of trauma-center care on mortality. N Engl J Med. 2006;354:366–78.
15. Durham R, Pracht E, Orban B, Lottenburg L, Tepas J, Flint L. Evaluation of a mature trauma system. Ann Surg. 2006;243(6):775–83, discussion 783–5.
16. Kahn JM. Volume, outcome, and the organization of intensive care. Crit Care. 2007;11(3):129.
17. Kahn JM, Rubenfeld GD, Rohrbach J, Fuchs BD. Cost savings attributable to reductions in intensive care unit length of stay for mechanically ventilated patients. Med Care. 2008;46(12): 1226–33.
18. Jacobs P, Rapoport J, Edbrooke D. Economies of scale in British intensive care units and combined intensive care/high dependency units. Intensive Care Med. 2004;30:660–4.
19. Dunning D, Johnson K, Ehrlinger J. Why people fail to recognize their own incompetence. Curr Dir Psychol Sci. 2003;12:83–7.
20. Dawson NV, Connors AF, Speroff T, Kemka A, Shaw P, Arkes HR. Hemodynamic assessment in managing the critically ill: is physician confidence warranted? Med Decis Making. 1993; 13(3):258–66.
21. Iberti TJ, Fischer EP, Leibowitz AB, Panacek EA, Silverstein JH, Albertson TE. A multicenter study of physicians' knowledge of the pulmonary artery catheter. Pulmonary Artery Catheter Study Group. JAMA. 1990;264(22):2928–32.
22. Warren J, Fromm Jr RE, Orr RA, Rotello LC. Guidelines for the inter-and intrahospital transport of critically ill patients. Crit Care Med. 2004;32:256–62.
23. Fan E, MacDonald RD, Adhikari N, Scales DC. Outcomes of interfacility critical care adult patient transport: a systematic review. Crit Care. 2005;10:R6.
24. Ligtenberg JJ, Arnold LG, Stienstra Y. Quality of interhospital transport of critically ill patients: a prospective audit. Crit Care. 2005;9:R446–51.
25. Seymour CW, Kahn JM, Schwab CW, Fuchs BD. Adverse events during rotary-wing transport of mechanically ventilated patients: a retrospective cohort study. Crit Care. 2008;12:R71.
26. Gebremichael M, Borg U, Habashi NM, Cottingham C, Cunsolo L, McCunn M, Reynolds HN. Interhospital transport of the extremely ill patient: the mobile intensive care unit. Crit Care Med. 2000;28(1):79–85.
27. Chalfin DB, Trzeciak S, Likourezos A. Impact of delayed transfer of critically ill patients from the emergency department to the intensive care unit. Crit Care. 2007;35:1477–83.
28. McConnell KJ, Pines JM. The effect of emergency department crowding on clinically oriented outcomes. Acad Emerg Med. 2009;16:1–10.
29. Goldfrad C, Rowan K. Consequences of discharges from intensive care at night. Lancet. 2000;355(9210):1138–42.
30. Iwashyna TJ, Kramer AA, Kahn JM. Intensive care unit occupancy and patient outcomes. Crit Care Med. 2009;37(5):1545–57.
31. Gabler NB, Ratcliffe SJ, Strom BL, Angus DC, Rubenfeld GD, Halpern SD. ICU capacity strain on the day of admission increases the risk of in-hospital death. Am J Respir Crit Care Med. 2012;185:A5073.
32. Terwiesch C, Diwas KC, Kahn JM. Working with capacity limitations: operations management in critical care. Crit Care. 2011;15(4):308.
33. Chen LM, Render M, Sales A, Kennedy EH, Wiitala W, Hofer TP. Intensive care unit admitting patterns in the veterans affairs health care system. Arch Intern Med. 2012; 172(16):1220–6.

34. Keeley EC, Boura JA, Grines CL. Primary angioplasty versus intravenous thrombolytic therapy for acute myocardial infarction: a quantitative review of 23 randomised trials. Lancet. 2003;361(9351):13–20.
35. Bonnefoy E, Steg PG, Boutitie F, et al. Comparison of primary angioplasty and pre-hospital fibrinolysis in acute myocardial infarction (CAPTIM) trial: a 5-year follow-up. Eur Heart J. 2009;30(13):1598–606.
36. Azoulay E, Pochard F, Kentish-Barnes N, et al. Risk of post-traumatic stress symptoms in family members of intensive care unit patients. Am J Respir Crit Care Med. 2005;171(9): 987–94.
37. Liu JH, Zingmond DS, McGory ML, SooHoo NF, Ettner SL, Brook RH, Ko CY. Disparities in the utilization of high-volume hospitals for complex surgery. JAMA. 2006;296(16):1973–80.
38. Hofer TP, Hayward RA. Are bad outcomes from questionable clinical decisions preventable medical errors? A case of cascade iatrogenesis. Ann Intern Med. 2002;137(5 Part 1):327–33.
39. Seymour CW, Kahn JM, Cooke CR. Prediction of critical illness during out-of-hospital emergency care. JAMA. 2010;304:747–54.
40. Wiener RS, Welch HG. Trends in the use of the pulmonary artery catheter in the United States, 1993–2004. JAMA. 2007;298(4):423–9.
41. Bosk EA, Veinot T, Iwashyna TJ. Which patients and where: a qualitative study of patient transfers from community hospitals. Med Care. 2011;49(6):592–8.
42. Boyd DR. Trauma systems origins in the United States. J Trauma Nurs. 2010;17(3):126–34, quiz 135–6.
43. Lasswell SM, Barfield WD, Rochat RW, Blackmon L. Perinatal regionalization for very low-birth-weight and very preterm infants: a meta-analysis. JAMA. 2010;304(9):992–1000.
44. Kahn JM, Branas CC, Schwab CW. Regionalization of medical critical care: what can we learn from the trauma experience? Crit Care Med. 2008;36:3085–8.
45. Peek GJ, Mugford M, Tiruvoipati R, et al. Efficacy and economic assessment of conventional ventilatory support versus extracorporeal membrane oxygenation for severe adult respiratory failure (CESAR): a multicentre randomised controlled trial. Lancet. 2009;374(9698):1351–63.
46. Iwashyna TJ. The incomplete infrastructure for interhospital patient transfer. Crit Care Med. 2012;40(8):2470–8.
47. Branas CC, MacKenzie EJ, ReVelle CS. A trauma resource allocation model for ambulances and hospitals. Health Serv Res. 2000;35(2):489–507.
48. Glance LG, Osler TM, Mukamel DB, Dick AW. Estimating the potential impact of regionalizing health care delivery based on volume standards versus risk-adjusted mortality rate. Int J Qual Health Care. 2007;19:195–202.
49. Rubenfeld GD. Epidemiology of acute lung injury. Crit Care Med. 2003;31:S276–84.
50. Escobar GJ, LaGuardia JC, Turk BJ, Ragins A, Kipnis P, Draper D. Early detection of impending physiologic deterioration among patients who are not in intensive care: development of predictive models using data from an automated electronic medical record. J Hosp Med. 2012;7(5):388–95.
51. Estévez-Loureiro R, Calviño-Santos R, Vázquez JM, et al. Safety and feasibility of returning patients early to their originating centers after transfer for primary percutaneous coronary intervention. Rev Esp Cardiol. 2009;62(12):1356–64.
52. Lomi A, Pallotti F. Relational collaboration among spatial multipoint competitors. Soc Netw. 2012;34:101–11.
53. Institute of Medicine (U.S.). Committee on the future of emergency care in the United States health system. Hospital-Based Emergency Care. New York: National Academy Press; 2007.
54. Breslow MJ. Remote ICU care programs: current status. J Crit Care. 2007;22(1):66–76.
55. Kahn JM. The use and misuse of ICU telemedicine. JAMA. 2011;305(21):2227–8.
56. Young LB, Chan PS, Lu X, Nallamothu BK, Sasson C, Cram PM. Impact of telemedicine intensive care unit coverage on patient outcomes: a systematic review and meta-analysis. Arch Intern Med. 2011;171(6):498–506.

57. Lilly CM, Cody S, Zhao H, Landry K, Baker SP, McIlwaine J, Chandler MW, Irwin RS, University of Massachusetts Memorial Critical Care Operations Group. Hospital mortality, length of stay, and preventable complications among critically ill patients before and after tele-ICU reengineering of critical care processes. JAMA. 2011;305(21):2175–83.
58. Mullen-Fortino M, DiMartino J, Entrikin L, Mulliner S, Hanson CW, Kahn JM. Bedside nurses' perceptions of intensive care unit telemedicine. Am J Crit Care. 2012;21(1):24–31, quiz 32.
59. Rokos IC, Sanddal ND, Pancioli AM. Inter-hospital communications and transport: turning one-way funnels into two-way networks. Acad Emerg Med. 2010;17:1279–85.

Part IV
Critical Care: Global and Future Perspectives

Chapter 15
International Perspectives on Critical Care

Hannah Wunsch

Abstract Comparisons across countries of critical care provide important information on availability of critical care resources, implications of triage decisions, and delivery of care in the intensive care unit (ICU) for critically ill patients. The variety of populations, resources, care patterns, and cultures create an opportunity to understand the impact of different care choices, and potentially reveal areas for focus for quality improvement. Comparisons across countries highlight the lack of a standard definition of an ICU bed. Large differences also exist in length of hospital stay and discharge patterns, with variability in the use of support facilities, such as hospice care and skilled nursing facilities. These differences reveal the need for appropriate outcome measures that are not skewed by such variation. Knowledge of provision of critical care across regions and countries may improve networks and facilitate both daily care of patients and disaster planning.

Keywords Critical care • Intensive care unit • Beds • International health problems • Outcome measures • Triage • Patient discharge • Clinical practice variation

Healthcare is delivered in very different ways across the globe. As we continually seek to improve care and outcomes while minimizing costs, the breadth and depth of care delivery options practiced around the world can help us to understand the consequences of our care choices. International comparisons of critical care provide important information on use of intensive care unit (ICU) beds, and delivery of care for critically ill patients. Moreover, international data can elucidate clinical study data so that publications from other countries are interpreted appropriately. Finally,

H. Wunsch (✉)
Department of Anesthesiology, College of Physicians and Surgeons, Columbia University, 622 West 168th Street, PH5-527D, New York, NY, USA

Department of Epidemiology, Mailman School of Public Health, Columbia University, New York, NY, USA
e-mail: hw2125@cumc.columbia.edu

D.C. Scales and G.D. Rubenfeld (eds.), *The Organization of Critical Care*, Respiratory Medicine 18, DOI 10.1007/978-1-4939-0811-0_15,

in a world of potential global pandemics and natural disasters, the need for critical care services may not always adhere to borders. Therefore, information on critical care services worldwide is now essential to ensure appropriate planning. This chapter describes the challenges of international comparisons and emphasizes the areas where studies of international comparisons have provided important information relevant to the delivery of critical care.

Definitions

A key point highlighted by international comparisons is the very question of what constitutes a critically ill patient, or an ICU bed [1, 2]. For example, American definitions of ICU beds may focus on having specific nurse to patient ratios, while some European countries have definitions that focus on the type or severity of organ dysfunction that can be supported [3]. While some of these definitions may lead to common pathways and patients who are typical worldwide of critically ill patients, these differences may also lead to difficulty of comparisons if the underlying cohorts represent different types of patients with varying severity of illness. For example, in a study of medical patients admitted to ICUs in the USA and UK, 70 % of the patients admitted to the ICU in the UK were mechanically ventilated, while in the USA the number was 30 % [4]. Many of the patients admitted in the USA to ICUs were likely cared for in high-dependency (step-down) units in the UK, which still have a nurse to patient ratio of 1:2, and can provide some forms of organ support (except for mechanical ventilation) [5]. Such differences can lead to a mis-match in the comparison of patients, and also highlights the need to study these differences and explore ways to align definitions across regions and countries. Critical care as a specialty would benefit from adoption of internationally agreed upon definitions, specifically with regard to the definition of an ICU bed, as this would help facilitate appropriate comparisons as well as to allow for better understanding of available resources worldwide.

Regional Differences in Critical Care Availability

Despite the difficulty imposed by a lack of standardization of terminology, international studies of ICU beds demonstrate such a magnitude of variability of provision, as to overcome much of the uncertainty regarding definitions [3, 6, 7]. The largest extremes are international—from sub-Saharan Africa, where there are often few hospital beds capable of providing supplemental oxygen to countries such as Germany and the USA with 20–25 ICU beds per 100,000 population [3, 6, 7]. Even within the European Union, with substantially decreased heterogeneity in terms of gross domestic product and overall standard of living, the differences in provision of critical care are large, with a many-fold difference in overall provision of ICU beds for the population between the UK (3–7 ICU beds per 100,000 population) and Germany (25–30 ICU beds per 100,000 population) [3, 7].

The provision of critical care beds can be examined in many ways. The most common approach is to assess the ICU bed availability for a given population by examining ICU beds per capita in a specified region. Another is to examine ICU beds as a proportion of all hospital beds. The two do not necessarily yield the same results regarding provision; for example, the USA has a lot of critical care beds per capita, but relatively few hospital beds [3]. This leads to a very high ratio of ICU beds to hospital beds and changes the dynamic of care within hospitals [8]. In contrast, Germany has a similar number of ICU beds for the population as the USA, but also has many more hospital beds, so that only a small percentage of all the hospital beds are for critical care [3].

Differences in critical care delivery are not just limited to the country-level. Similar to a fractal, the same variation that is visible when comparing critical care internationally is often visible when the scope is narrowed to the national, regional, or local level [9]. This may be particularly true in countries where there are large differences in urban/rural provision of healthcare resources [1]. Even in a country such as the USA, the provision of ICU beds per capita varies from 10.1 to 59.5 per 100,000 population across regions [9].

Local variation can sometimes be driven by factors unrelated to variation seen on the larger scale. For example, a hospital that performs coronary artery bypass grafting, or liver transplantation, will have substantially different needs for intensive care compared with a community hospital that does very little surgery and mostly treats emergency medical cases. Moreover, at the local level, some of the variation in provision of services may be offset by the ability to make use of the inter-connectedness of ICU facilities, such that local variation can be overcome to some degree through the use of critical care transfer systems [10].

Regional Differences in Critical Care Outcomes

Trying to interpret differences in outcomes associated with critical illness is the biggest challenge in international studies. The problems of comparing outcomes can be divided into at least six areas (see Table 15.1): the denominator, patient selection, delayed admissions, discharge practice, other care locations, and end-of-life care. With attempts to assess differences in outcomes internationally, we have been able to begin to tease apart how all of these factors impact the type and quality of care delivered to critically ill patients. Due to the large differences across systems, studies often end up highlighting the differences in delivery rather than providing concrete conclusions regarding the outcomes.

Table 15.1 Challenges in the regional, national, or international comparisons of outcomes in critical care

Challenge	Description
Denominator	• Different age distributions • Genetic predispositions to critical illness • Underlying burden of comorbidity in the population • Rates of surgery and/or trauma in the population
Patient selection	• Admission dependent on availability of ICU beds • Severity of illness threshold for admission to ICU • Decision to perform a high-risk operation requiring intensive care
Delayed admissions	• Route for admission to ICU related to underlying availability of ICU beds • Tendency for stabilization on wards, or treatment in emergency department prior to transfer to ICU
Other care locations	• Availability of stepdown/intermediate care • Recovery room capable of providing ICU-level care • Protocols that allow for care of certain patients, or delivery of certain medications (such as vasopressors) on wards
Discharges	• Availability of skilled care or other intermediate care facility versus discharge home • Availability of ventilator weaning facilities
End-of-life	• Religious or cultural preferences for intensity of treatment • Expectations for intensive care • Legal framework for provision of care

Denominator

The "denominator" problem is due to the fact that one needs to compare similar populations with regard to age distribution, genetic predisposition to disease, underlying comorbidities, and also any instigating problems that may lead to critical illness (such as the rate of trauma), in order to fairly assess differences in outcomes for those patients [11]. One of the biggest factors that may impact who develops a critical illness may be the underlying health of a population. For example, comorbidities such as diabetes may predispose people to developing critical illnesses due to increased risk of infection and renal failure. In a comparison of two cohorts of middle-aged people in the USA and Great Britain, the Americans were twice as likely to have diabetes and a third more likely to have hypertension [12]. These increased comorbidities that may predispose to critical illness can also impact outcomes from critical illness itself. For example with diabetic patients important aspects of recovery, such as wound healing, may also be impaired.

Patient Selection

A related issue is one of patient selection. Along with differences in predisposition to critical illness are the many factors that lead to the decision to admit a patient to the ICU. One large difference may be in decisions regarding use of surgery that will change the likelihood of using intensive care services. For example, in a study comparing Alberta Canada and Western Massachusetts, the per capita rate of major reconstructive vascular procedures was 3.4 times higher in the US cohort compared with the Canadian cohort, leading to an overall greater use of critical care services, and a higher mortality rate in the USA, likely related to operating on sicker patients [13].

Outside of specific surgical procedures, admission decisions are notoriously hard to capture due to the fact that they are often emergent and occur prior to ICU admission [11]. Data collected, such as in the SOAP study, demonstrate that the percentage of patients with sepsis in the ICU varies dramatically across Europe, likely driven by the underlying differences in bed availability [3, 14]. A comparison of admissions to intensive care in New Zealand versus the USA noted the difference in ICU beds as a percentage of hospital beds (1.7 % of total beds in the New Zealand hospitals versus 5.6 % in the US hospitals). The average age of the patients admitted to intensive care was substantially lower in New Zealand (42 versus 55 in the USA), and fewer patients in New Zealand had severe chronic health conditions or were admitted after elective surgery [15].

Variation in admission practices is certainly not limited to differences between countries. For example, an analysis of the frequency of admission to ICU for patients admitted to the hospital with diabetic ketoacidosis in New York State found a range of ICU admission of 0 to 100 % across hospitals [16]. A study from the US Veterans Affairs hospitals also demonstrated large variation in admission practices for a relatively homogenous patient population [17]; for patients who were admitted directly from the emergency room to the ICU, 53.2 % had a 30-day predicted mortality at admission of 2 % or less. When examined by individual hospital, the rate of ICU admission for all emergency room admissions with this low predicted risk of death ranged from 1.2 to 38.9 %.

While this observed variation may be vexing, it brings up the important question of what constitutes appropriate admission policies for intensive care? This is an area with little guidance for practitioners. For example, the Society of Critical Care Medicine guidelines recommend only that "ICU admission criteria should select patients who are likely to benefit from ICU care," [18] without clear data to support which patients fall into this category. We may be able to begin to leverage the differences in decision-making between regions and countries to understand the consequences of more liberal or conservative admission patterns [19].

Delayed Admissions

The timing of admission to ICU may have a large impact on outcomes, and may be influenced by the overall provision of intensive care beds. In a study of medical ICU admissions in the USA and UK, patients in the USA were much more likely to be admitted directly from an emergency room to the ICU, whereas patients in the UK were more likely to receive care on a regular ward prior to ICU admission [4]. Hospital mortality for patients in the UK was much higher than in the USA; however when the analysis was restricted to patients who came directly from the emergency room, the outcomes were more similar, suggesting that the routing of patients to the ward first may be detrimental in some cases. In particular, patients with severe sepsis, or septic shock, may gain great benefit from early admission to ICU [20, 21]. A recent study from France found that patients who were initially denied admission to ICU, but then subsequently admitted, had higher mortality than patients who received intensive care immediately [22]. In a smaller study of emergency department (ED) patients with community-acquired pneumonia, patients who had delayed transfer to the ICU (defined as transfer to the wards and then the ICU on day 2 or 3 of the hospital stay versus directly from the ED), had substantially increased hospital mortality (odds ratio 2.07, 95 % CI 1.12–3.85) [23]. A similar study by Chalfin et al. of patients who stayed in the ED for more than 6 h versus those transferred to the ICU in under 6 h found both increased risk of hospital death and longer hospital stay for patients having a delayed admission [24].

Other Care Locations

As care of hospitalized patients has become more complex, there has been a growth of care options within many hospitals. The simple model of ICU beds and floor beds may now be complicated by intermediate (or high-dependency or stepdown) beds, recovery room beds, vent weaning beds, coronary care unit beds, telemetry beds, and short-stay "observation" beds that may all provide options for patients in and around their need for critical care. A survey of the use of "respiratory" intermediate care units across Europe found substantial heterogeneity in the availability of these units [25]. The role of these types of beds, in particular, remains unclear in comparisons across countries (or hospitals, for that matter). A few small studies suggest that having step-down beds may alter the length of stay and severity of illness of patients in the ICU, but this area has not been fully explored [25–27].

Discharges

International data highlight the ways in which hospital discharge patterns may vary. The driving factor appears to be the availability of alternate care options outside of the acute care hospital. Many countries have no alternatives to sending patients home, leading to patients staying in the hospital until physically well enough to be discharged home, which then translates into longer lengths of stay in the acute care hospital [4]. The USA, in particular, has a different model for care, with use of both sub-acute nursing facilities (SNF) and long-term acute care facilities (LTAC) as discharge options, particularly for chronically critically ill patients [28]. Currently, up to 33 % of Medicare patients cared for in ICUs in the USA are discharged to SNFs or LTACs, with projected growth in the coming years [29, 30]. Transferring patients to facilities who are not yet well enough to go home clearly alters average ICU and/or hospital length of stay and, perhaps more importantly, ICU and/or hospital mortality, thereby potentially altering the perceived efficacy of ICU-specific interventions [31]. Due to the use of these facilities, short-term outcomes after critical illness in the USA are particularly difficult to compare with other countries. For example, in a direct comparison of severely ill medical patients, 53.9 % of patients were discharged to a skilled care facility in the USA, with only 7.9 % discharged to similar facilities in the United Kingdom [4]. These data reinforce the importance of longer-term follow-up of critically ill patients to ensure valid, comprehensive estimates of outcomes. But, additional follow-up beyond acute care hospitalizations is often prohibitively expensive and time-consuming. One proposal is to use the measure of "discharge home," rather than hospital mortality as a more equivalent short-term comparator. However, some patients in the USA are able to go home after a short stay in another care facility, which may then create additional biases.

End-of-Life Choices

End-of-life cultural preferences and practices are also diverse. In ICUs in some regions in Europe physicians are two to three times as likely as in other regions to withdraw life-sustaining treatment [32–34]. Additionally, the defaults regarding cardio-pulmonary resuscitation may vary, even between regions in the same country [35–37]. International differences in the attitudes and care approaches at the end of life can have profound effects on study results, even in randomized-controlled trials. For example, a study of non-invasive ventilation in acute cardiogenic pulmonary edema in the UK demonstrated an intubation rate of 2–3 %, yet a 7-day mortality of 9 %, suggesting that many patients who died were never intubated [38]; this same pattern of care is unlikely to occur in places such as the USA. We know, for example, that approximately 20 % of people in the USA receive intensive care prior to death, whereas only 5 % do in the UK [39]. This raises the question of what is gained by the additional intensive care, and alternatively what opportunities to save lives may be lost by the lower use [19].

The religious and cultural differences that exist between individual physicians themselves have a large impact on end-of-life practices, with the median time from ICU admission to any limitation of therapy varying by as much as 6 days, depending upon physician religion [40]. Different societies also have varying perceptions of chronically critically ill patients. The preferences for dialysis, mechanical ventilation, artificial nutrition, etc. may differ and drive treatment choices. For example, in a study of home mechanical ventilation across European countries, the prevalence varied from 0.1 per 100,000 population up to 9.6, depending on the country [41].

Conclusions

The variety of populations, resources, care patterns, and cultures create an opportunity to learn from others. International data on critical care can elucidate care patterns and reveal areas for focus for quality improvement. The creation of a standard definition of an ICU bed would help to limit uncertainty and improve the quality of comparisons. Data from international comparisons highlighting the wide range of processes of care and patient flow patterns also underscore the need for appropriate outcome measures that are not skewed by such variation. Finally, we are beginning to gain a better understanding of the overall availability of resources across many countries. Such knowledge of provision of critical care may improve networks and facilitate both daily care of patients and disaster planning.

Sources of Support Award Number K08AG038477 from the National Institute on Aging.

References

1. Adhikari NK, Rubenfeld GD. Worldwide demand for critical care. Curr Opin Crit Care. 2011;17:620–5.
2. Murthy S, Wunsch H. Clinical review: international comparisons in critical care – lessons learned. Crit Care. 2012;16:218.
3. Wunsch H, Angus DC, Harrison DA, et al. Variation in critical care services across North America and Western Europe. Crit Care Med. 2008;36:2787–9.
4. Wunsch H, Angus DC, Harrison DA, Linde-Zwirble WT, Rowan KM. Comparison of medical admissions to intensive care units in the United States and United Kingdom. Am J Respir Crit Care Med. 2011;183:1666–73.
5. Audit Commission. Critical to success. London: Audit Commission; 1999.
6. Adhikari N, Fowler R, Bhagwanjee S, Rubenfeld G. Critical care and the global burden of critical illness in adults. Lancet. 2010;376:1339–46.
7. Rhodes A, Ferdinande P, Flaatten H, Guidet B, Metnitz PG, Moreno RP. The variability of critical care bed numbers in Europe. Intensive Care Med. 2012;38:1647–53.
8. Hall WB, Willis LE, Medvedev S, Carson SS. The implications of long-term acute care hospital transfer practices for measures of in-hospital mortality and length of stay. Am J Respir Crit Care Med. 2012;185:53–7.
9. Carr BG, Addyson DK, Kahn JM. Variation in critical care beds per capita in the United States: implications for pandemic and disaster planning. JAMA. 2010;303:1371–2.
10. Iwashyna TJ, Christie JD, Moody J, Kahn JM, Asch DA. The structure of critical care transfer networks. Med Care. 2009;47:787–93.
11. Wunsch H. A triage score for admission: a holy grail of intensive care. Crit Care Med. 2012;40:321–3.
12. Banks J, Marmot M, Oldfield Z, Smith JP. Disease and disadvantage in the United States and in England. JAMA. 2006;295:2037–45.
13. Rapoport J, Teres D, Barnett R, et al. A comparison of intensive care unit utilization in Alberta and western Massachusetts. Crit Care Med. 1995;23:1336–46.
14. Vincent JL, Sakr Y, Sprung CL, et al. Sepsis in European intensive care units: results of the SOAP study. Crit Care Med. 2006;34:344–53.

15. Zimmerman JE, Knaus WA, Judson JA, et al. Patient selection for intensive care: a comparison of New Zealand and United States hospitals. Crit Care Med. 1988;16:318–26.
16. Gershengorn HB, Iwashyna TJ, Cooke CR, Scales DC, Kahn JM, Wunsch H. Variation in use of intensive care for adults with diabetic ketoacidosis. Crit Care Med. 2012;40:2009–15.
17. Chen LM, Render M, Sales A, Kennedy EH, Wiitala W, Hofer TP. Intensive care unit admitting patterns in the veterans affairs health care system. Arch Intern Med. 2012;172:1220–6.
18. No authors listed. Guidelines for intensive care unit admission, discharge, and triage. Crit Care Med. 1999;27:633–8.
19. Wunsch H. Is there a starling curve for intensive care? Chest. 2012;141:1393–9.
20. Kumar A, Roberts D, Wood KE, et al. Duration of hypotension before initiation of effective antimicrobial therapy is the critical determinant of survival in human septic shock. Crit Care Med. 2006;34:1589–96.
21. Rivers E, Nguyen B, Havstad S, et al. Early goal-directed therapy in the treatment of severe sepsis and septic shock. N Engl J Med. 2001;345:1368–77.
22. Robert R, Reignier J, Tournoux-Facon C, et al. Refusal of ICU admission due to a full unit: impact on mortality. Am J Respir Crit Care Med. 2012;185(10):1081–7. doi:10.1164/rccm.201104-0729OC.
23. Renaud B, Santin A, Coma E, et al. Association between timing of intensive care unit admission and outcomes for emergency department patients with community-acquired pneumonia. Crit Care Med. 2009;37:2867–74.
24. Chalfin DB, Trzeciak S, Likourezos A, Baumann BM, Dellinger RP. Impact of delayed transfer of critically ill patients from the emergency department to the intensive care unit. Crit Care Med. 2007;35:1477–83.
25. Corrado A, Roussos C, Ambrosino N, et al. Respiratory intermediate care units: a European survey. Eur Respir J. 2002;20:1343–50.
26. Vincent JL, Burchardi H. Do we need intermediate care units? Intensive Care Med. 1999;25:1345–9.
27. Wagner DP, Knaus WA, Draper EA. Can intermediate care substitute for intensive care? Crit Care Med. 1988;16:361–2.
28. Kramer AA, Zimmerman JE. Institutional variations in frequency of discharge of elderly intensive care survivors to postacute care facilities. Crit Care Med. 2010;38:2319–28.
29. Wunsch H, Guerra C, Barnato AE, Angus DC, Li G, Linde-Zwirble WT. Three-year outcomes for Medicare beneficiaries who survive intensive care. JAMA. 2010;303:849–56.
30. Zilberberg MD, Shorr AF. Prolonged acute mechanical ventilation and hospital bed utilization in 2020 in the United States: implications for budgets, plant and personnel planning. BMC Health Serv Res. 2008;8:242.
31. Kahn JM, Kramer AA, Rubenfeld GD. Transferring critically ill patients out of hospital improves the standardized mortality ratio: a simulation study. Chest. 2007;131:68–75.
32. Sprung CL, Cohen SL, Sjokvist P, et al. End-of-life practices in European intensive care units: the Ethicus Study. JAMA. 2003;290:790–7.
33. Frost DW, Cook DJ, Heyland DK, Fowler RA. Patient and healthcare professional factors influencing end-of-life decision-making during critical illness: a systematic review. Crit Care Med. 2011;39:1174–89.
34. Ball CG, Navsaria P, Kirkpatrick AW, et al. The impact of country and culture on end-of-life care for injured patients: results from an international survey. J Trauma. 2010;69:1323–33. discussion 33–4.
35. Cook DJ, Guyatt G, Rocker G, et al. Cardiopulmonary resuscitation directives on admission to intensive-care unit: an international observational study. Lancet. 2001;358:1941–5.
36. Evans T, Nava S, Vazquez M, et al. Critical care rationing: international comparisons. Chest. 2011;140:1618–24.
37. Siegel MD, Stapleton R, Wunsch H. The ethical and economic impact of defaults. Semin Respir Crit Care Med. 2012;33:382–92.

38. Gray A, Goodacre S, Newby DE, Masson M, Sampson F, Nicholl J. Noninvasive ventilation in acute cardiogenic pulmonary edema. N Engl J Med. 2008;359:142–51.
39. Wunsch H, Linde-Zwirble WT, Harrison DA, Barnato AE, Rowan KM, Angus DC. Use of intensive care services during terminal hospitalizations in England and the United States. Am J Respir Crit Care Med. 2009;180:875–80.
40. Sprung CL, Maia P, Bulow HH, et al. The importance of religious affiliation and culture on end-of-life decisions in European intensive care units. Intensive Care Med. 2007;33:1732–9.
41. Lloyd-Owen SJ, Donaldson GC, Ambrosino N, et al. Patterns of home mechanical ventilation use in Europe: results from the Eurovent survey. Eur Respir J. 2005;25:1025–31.

Chapter 16
Critical Care in Low-Resource Settings

Srinivas Murthy, Sadath A. Sayeed, and Neill K.J. Adhikari

Abstract The care of critically ill patients is a global enterprise, regardless of the capacity of the specific healthcare system. In this chapter, we discuss the delivery of critical care in resource-limited settings with respect to the burden of critical illness, supply and costs of critical care resources, and ethical issues. We argue that the burden of critical illness in low-resource settings is substantial, increasing, and not met by current healthcare resources. Assuming an ethical framework of health as a human right, scale-up of critical care services must be considered along with more traditional public health interventions. Successful and cost-effective implementation of critical care in resource-limited settings will likely require local training of healthcare personnel and novel and domestically produced adaptation of existing technology, but the optimal approaches to organization of health services, knowledge translation, educational program design, and technology adaptation are largely unknown and will require additional research.

Keywords Global health • Critical care • Sepsis • Developing countries

Critical care has expanded tremendously, in terms of both clinical scope and global reach, over the past 60 years. Over that time, the integration of services to care for the sickest patients in the hospital has become a vital component of all health

S. Murthy (✉)
Department of Pediatrics, University of British Columbia, 4480 Oak Street, Vancouver, BC, Canada
e-mail: sgmurthy@gmail.com

S.A. Sayeed
Department of Global Health and Social Medicine, Boston Children's Hospital, Boston, MA, USA

N.K.J. Adhikari
Department of Critical Care Medicine, Sunnybrook Health Sciences Center and University of Toronto, Toronto, ON, Canada

D.C. Scales and G.D. Rubenfeld (eds.), *The Organization of Critical Care*, Respiratory Medicine 18, DOI 10.1007/978-1-4939-0811-0_16,

systems. Whether defined by the complexity of the interventions delivered or the training of the physicians involved, the organization and allocation of critical care resources is a vital consideration in all settings, including those with limited resources.

Health system design in resource-limited regions has traditionally focused on low-cost interventions, with more intensive resources restricted to referral hospitals in major cities. The provision of sanitation, immunizations, and adequate nutrition has long been established as a cost-effective path to public health when finances are constrained. India, for example, has made substantial regional improvements in health outcomes related to the expansion of immunization practices and the provision of clean water and sanitation in its rural regions [1, 2]. For common diseases such as HIV, malaria, and acute malnutrition, concerted global effort has produced feasible and inexpensive interventions for resource-limited countries [3–5]. This work has integrated high-income country interventions (primarily medications and vaccinations) into the resource-limited healthcare structure, with the ongoing challenges of limited diagnostic and therapeutic technology, and variable clinical training and experience. Although much global health work is focused on primary care, acute care is increasingly recognized as complementary and likely will help achieve the Millennium Development Goals of reducing acute illness, morbidity, and mortality in women and children, and has been endorsed by the World Health Organization [6, 7]. Accordingly, numerous middle-income countries have dramatically expanded the accessibility to intensive care units (ICUs), especially among the growing urban population [8–10].

This chapter will discuss issues pertaining to providing critical care resources in financially constrained regions, including formulating a research agenda for the future. Recently published reviews are available for further reading [11, 12].

The Global Burden of Treatable Critical Illness

There are a variety of approaches, all fraught with challenges, to defining the global burden of critical illness, defined as the number of patients that would potentially benefit from access to critical care resources [13]. One approach would be to count the patients admitted to ICUs around the world. However, this strategy would significantly underestimate the burden of critical illness in low-resource settings that lack the capacity to care for these patients in specialized units. For example, pneumonia is the leading cause of mortality in low-income countries globally [14]; proximal mechanisms of such deaths may have included critical care-specific syndromes such as respiratory failure, acute respiratory distress syndrome, or sepsis. Such syndromes are unique in that the definition depends on the availability of critical care interventions, such as mechanical ventilation and vasopressors. In contrast, most other acute conditions, such as myocardial infarction or trauma, are readily diagnosed and burden data therefore more easily determined.

A second approach would be to extrapolate high-income country epidemiology to low-resource settings. However, this is problematic for a variety of reasons. First, the diseases that lead to fatal outcomes differ, given the differing rates of co-morbidities related to lifestyle, such as obesity; genetic, such as sickle-cell disease; or environment, such as infectious diseases [15]. For example, data on sepsis incidence and prognosis from the USA or Europe would not be expected to apply to regions where malaria or dengue fever are endemic. Second, the demographic profile in low-resource settings is younger, and is mirrored by admission patterns to hospitals and ICUs, for whom the prognosis for recovery from critical illness may be better [20, 21]. Third, some critical illness also depends on the supply of other medical care; health systems that provide bone marrow transplantation for leukaemia and surgery for cardiovascular disease will generate more critical illness than those that do not.

A third approximation would assume that all deaths occurring in a region had critical illness at some stage of their illness. Adding these deaths to an estimate of the number of patients with critical illness who survive would produce a regional burden of critical illness. This approach may overestimate the burden of critical illness by including patients with terminal conditions for whom critical care would not be expected to help.

Observational studies of critical illness syndromes in the developing world are restricted to a few ICU-based studies that almost certainly underestimate the true population burden of these syndromes [15, 16]. Compared with developed world settings, which have some population-based epidemiologic data for critical illness syndromes such as ARDS, sepsis, and acute kidney injury, data for lower income countries are restricted to broad disease classifications, limiting inferences about critical illness prevalence or incidence [16–19].

Given the challenges in defining who will benefit from critical care, only rough estimates of the burden of critical illness can be extrapolated from mortality data, using the third approach outlined above. Patients with conditions such as malaria or pneumonia that respond to acute interventions such as fluids, mechanical ventilation, and antibiotics would likely have a lower risk of mortality with increased accessibility to critical care. In contrast, patients with chronic conditions that require a larger healthcare infrastructure to manage effectively, such as malignancy, would likely require investments in oncologic care to have any sustained benefit from access to episodic critical care. For this discussion, we assume that all acute conditions, including trauma, ischemic heart disease, pneumonia, and other acute infections that could lead to a fatal outcome are relevant for determining the global burden of critical illness. These conditions exclude chronic diseases such as neoplasms and hepatitis B infection for which the benefit of critical care is less clear. Using the number of deaths, based on Global Burden of Disease [14] data, to estimate the burden of critical illness and ignoring hospitalized survivors, the burden of critical illness is seen to be primarily in low- and middle-income settings (Table 16.1). It is evident that the global population that succumbs to critical illness is large, and assuming even partial mitigation by a modest expansion of critical care services, the potential lives saved are numerous [13].

Table 16.1 List of causes of death that would benefit from the availability of critical care services

Annual deaths by income group (in thousands)	High income	Upper middle income	Lower middle income	Low income
Population	977,189	579,621	2,464,976	2,412,669
Total deaths	8,144	5,556	18,793	26,251
Tuberculosis	15	98	444	907
Diarrhoeal diseases	14	35	308	1,806
Childhood diseases, i.e. pertussis, measles, tetanus	1	2	64	780
Meningitis	3	11	62	263
Malaria	0	2	30	857
Dengue	0	0	7	11
Japanese encephalitis	0	0	3	8
Lower respiratory infections	307	146	778	2,943
Upper respiratory infections	4	4	26	43
Maternal conditions	2	9	66	449
Perinatal conditions	37	95	650	2,397
Diabetes mellitus	224	142	381	393
Cardiovascular diseases	3,027	2,422	6,474	5,142
Respiratory diseases (COPD + Asthma)	476	219	2,012	1,328
Nephritis/nephrosis	127	59	254	298
Injuries (unintentional and intentional)	509	637	2,318	2,318
Deaths from conditions that would benefit from availability of critical care	*4,746*	*3,881*	*14,335*	*20,374*
Percentage of all deaths that would benefit from availability of critical care	**58.5**	**69.8**	**76.3**	**77.6**

Data are from Global Burden of Disease [14] and are based on official national data, disease modelling, or family recollection of the cause of death

Global Trends in Critical Illness

A number of social and economic trends will likely contribute to shifts in the burden of critical illness in low-resource settings. In high-income regions, the burden of critical illness is projected to rise considerably due to the aging population, their burden of co-morbid diseases, and broadly held expectations of the merits of life-sustaining interventions near the end-of-life. For the rest of the world, the crucial demographic trend is the rapidly urbanizing population, with more than half the world's population now living in cities with the proportion projected to rise further over coming decades [20]. This trend will locate a greater proportion of each country's population within reach of urban referral hospitals with ICUs (Fig. 16.1) [21]. Faster than the pace of urbanization, however, is the 10 % annual rate of rise of the slum-dwelling population, currently estimated as 33 % of the urban population in all developing regions globally and 62 % in sub-Saharan Africa [22]. This latter trend may increase the transmission of infectious diseases and thus the incidence of sepsis-related syndromes.

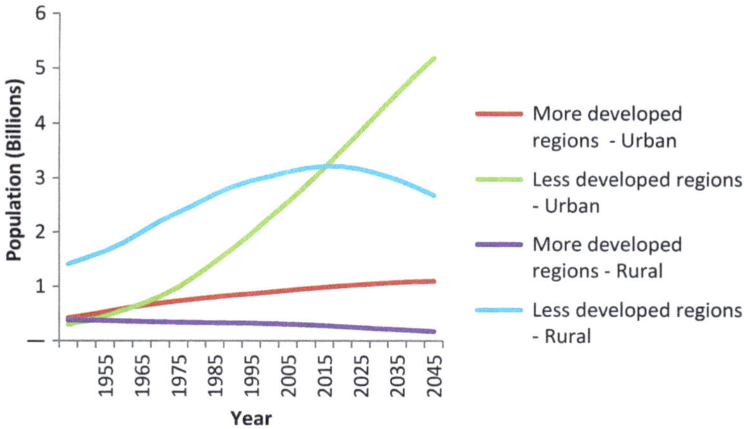

Fig. 16.1 Urban and rural population by development regions, 1950–2050 (projected). Data available from http://esa.un.org/unpd/wup/index.htm [21]

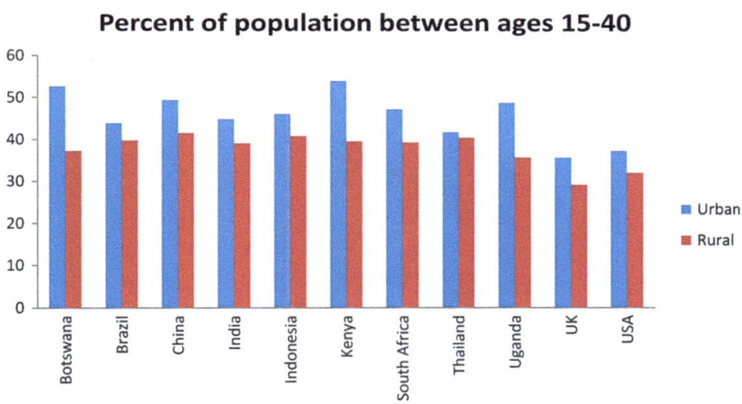

Fig. 16.2 Percent of population between ages 15–40 in urban and rural regions. *Source*: UNdata (data.un.org)

As SARS and the recent H1N1 influenza pandemic have clearly illustrated, critical care resources remain the last defense against large outbreaks of disease. With increasing rates of global urbanization and international migration, the potential risks of emerging and re-emerging infections rise as well, increasing the needs for critical care services to cope with large numbers of seriously ill patients [23]. The risks of bioterrorism and natural disasters will also remain, with more people affected, given population clustering. Cities are becoming younger as migrating labour shifts from rural to urban areas (Fig. 16.2) [20]. Therefore, urbanization is also associated with economic development, with poverty rates

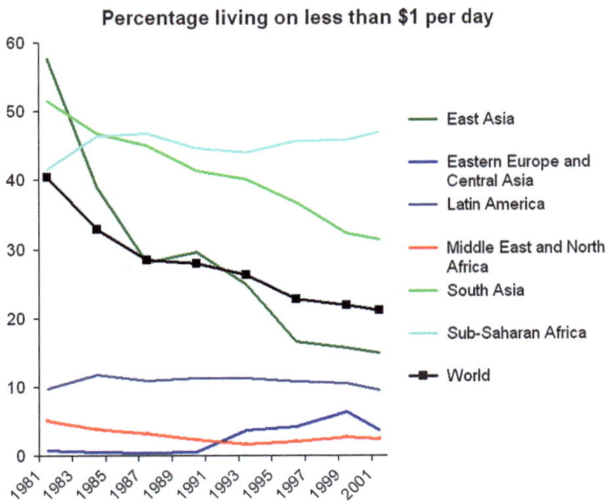

Fig. 16.3 Percentage living on less than $1 per day. *Source*: UNdata (data.un.org)

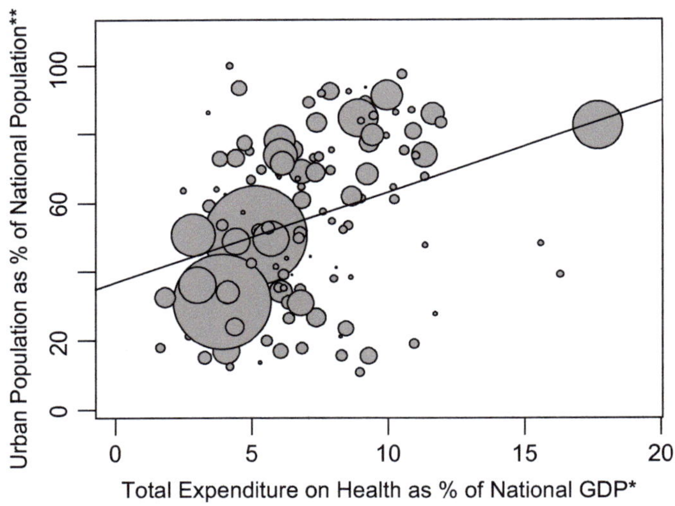

Fig. 16.4 Percentage of population living in urban settings compared with total expenditure on health as percentage of total GDP. Circle size represents population **Source*: WHO National Health Accounts Country Database, 2011. Available at www.who.int/nha ***Source*: World Urbanization Prospectus, 2011. Available at esa.un.org/unpd/wup/index.html

declining in many regions (Fig. 16.3). As economies develop, more income is available for healthcare, including potentially for critical care (Fig. 16.4).

Costs and Resources for Critical Care

There is no debate that critical care is expensive, even outside of high-income countries. For example, the daily ICU cost in a private hospital in India may be up to US$2,400 [24], similar to high-income settings. These costs include not only ICU costs (namely capital equipment, personnel, consumables) but also long-term survivor costs. Especially in severely cost-constrained environments, each of these cost categories must be minimized to deliver affordable, yet effective, intensive care. For example, although ensuring a constant power supply, acquiring ventilators, and scaling up infrastructure to supply oxygen are expensive, various adaptations may reduce costs. Examples include simplified oxygen systems using oxygen concentrators [25], refurbished incubators for infants [26], and inexpensive mechanical ventilators [27, 28]. Ultrasound and point-of care laboratory testing may reduce costs related to radiology and centralized laboratories. Domestic production of healthcare technology, as being developed in China and India, is another method to reduce costs and avoid importation from the USA or Europe [29]. Funders are likely to hesitate when extending the costly Western form of critical care to low-resource regions, and hence novel adaptations of existing technologies or new technologies must be developed.

In addition, a paramount concern is the dearth of appropriately trained personnel to deliver critical care in resource-limited settings. Given the sharp inequality in the distribution of academic ICUs and the specialized knowledge required, training opportunities in resource-poor regions remain sparse. In Nigeria, for example, there are only 380 critical care trained nurses for a population of over 140 million [30]. Existing ICUs are often staffed by providers who have partially trained in high-income regions and are at high risk of emigrating to these settings, further depleting personnel. Solutions to this "brain drain" are complex [31, 32]. In addition to imposing limitations on active poaching by high-income countries, resource-limited settings must increase the appeal for personnel to remain. Promising strategies include founding and recognition of national critical care societies [10], increasing domestic training programs for healthcare staff [8, 33], and utilizing physician extenders [34], all of which could help facilitate staff training and retention. Domestic training has proven successful, for example through programmes focused upon the retention of physicians in Ethiopia [35] and broad dissemination of short courses in intensive care [35, 36].

Consumables such as blood products and drugs are another area of substantial ongoing costs. Antibiotics comprise approximately 50 % of all drug and nutrition costs in Indian ICUs [37], with the need for more expensive drugs driven by antibiotic resistance [38]. Mitigating this, many countries have drug cost agreements with generic and brand-name pharmaceutical companies to reduce costs, but these typically are restricted to common outpatient drugs and should be extended to all drugs used in hospitals. Blood products, especially platelets [39] or leukoreduced blood [40], pose a particular challenge due to substantial fixed infrastructure costs to maintain a safe blood transfusion system.

There is substantial long-term morbidity for survivors of critical illness, even in young patients who were healthy prior to critical illness [41]. Long-term health-system utilization and costs of survivors of critical illness are difficult to estimate and likely context-dependent, given that costs for caring for survivors will be absorbed by families in many health systems [42, 43]. These significant down-stream costs of improved survival after critical illness should be anticipated as critical care resources expand.

Critical care medicine is an especially cost-intensive field, with its ratio of cost per life saved among the highest in healthcare [44], being focused on reversing acute organ dysfunction in individuals rather than preventing acute illness in populations. In developed settings, the cost-effectiveness of critical care, studied 5 years after admission, has been found to fall within acceptable ranges [45–47], defined by the World Health Organization as interventions costing up to three times the per capita gross domestic product of the region [48–50]. Hence, cost-effectiveness will depend on the baseline economic indicators of the region. Critical care interventions vary greatly in cost, and as noted above, even advanced technologies like ventilators can be manufactured more cheaply than in high-income countries. Therefore, regions must tailor the extent of their interventions to their economic situation [51].

The Supply of Critical Care Resources

The current distribution of critical care resources is unclear, given the lack of standardized definitions [52]. In high-income countries, variable definitions challenge international resource comparisons [53]. In many low- and middle-income countries, critical care is a private industry and not measured in national statistics [54]; in others, beds are misclassified as critical care even though they have no more resources than standard. Referral hospitals in major cities are the primary locales for intensive care, ideally centred within a regional transport infrastructure [55]. In general, however, access to critical care resources in developing regions remains sparse (Table 16.2) [56, 57]. This phenomenon extends from ICU infrastructure to processes of care; for example, the ability to implement recommended management strategies for sepsis, even those that are relatively inexpensive, is low across Africa [58] and parts of Asia [59].

The Ethics of Cost-Intensive Care in Cost-Limited Settings

Substantial ethical challenges emerge when considering the incorporation of critical care into financially disadvantaged regions, both in terms of its distribution and its practice. The argument for its provision in cost-limited settings rests primarily upon healthcare being accepted as a fundamental and universal human right. However, it is important to recognize the stakes when we insist that a right to health care is *universal*. If we accept the metaphor of rights as trump cards, we are

Table 16.2 Availability of intensive care resources by country

	Number of ICUs	Number of ICU beds per 100 hospital beds	Number of ICU beds per 100,000 population
North America			
Canada	319	3.4	13.5
USA	5,980	9	20
Caribbean and South America			
Colombia	89	3.5	–
Trinidad & Tobago	6		2.1
Europe			
Belgium	135	4.4	21.9
Croatia	123	3.3	20.3
France	550	2.5	9.3
Germany	–	4.1	24.6
Netherlands	115	2.8	8.4
Spain	258	2.5	8.2
Sweden	89	–	8.7
UK	268	1.2	3.5
Africa			
South Africa	308	1.7/8.9[a]	8.9
Zambia	29	0.2	–
Australasia			
Australia	160	–	8.0
New Zealand	26	0.9	4.8
China	–	1.8, 1.3–2.1	3.9, 2.8–4.6
Sri Lanka	52	–	1.6

Data are adapted from [13] and are estimates
[a]Public/private

imbuing them with a special normative force, and as such, they compel us to act in certain ways [60]. To give a common example, the right to free speech in the USA trumps many other important social aims. In general, someone can say offensive things in public places and cannot be legally stopped from doing so, because the right to free speech trumps other legitimate concerns. Similarly, but more controversially, we can insist that a right to health care *trumps* other legitimate aims, such as the accumulation of vast personal wealth [61]. Of course, we do not actually live in a world that treats access to adequate health care as a right with such a broad power to trump, despite declarations claiming otherwise [62]. In the hierarchy of human rights, we certainly do not prioritize it over many others. We also lack any tangible enforcement mechanisms because access to health care depends on a remarkably complex set of highly contextualized, economic, social, and political factors that defies the simple assertion of individual moral claims.

Thus, the contemplation of universal human rights, including even a "basic" right to health care [62], presents a formidable challenge for anyone seriously concerned with the just distribution of health care services across all human populations [63]. For example, this claim could appear to demand that if intensive care services are available to any, they must be available to all, a rarely acknowledged point.

As Thomas Pogge argues: "Our world is arranged to keep us far away from massive and severe poverty and surrounds us with affluent, civilized people for whom the poor abroad are a remote good cause alongside the spotted owl. In such a world, the thought we are involved in a monumental crime against these people...will appear so cold, so strained and ridiculous, that we cannot find it in our heart to reflect on it any farther" [64]. When high-income country citizens consider their moral obligations to those in living in poverty, basic health care services are generally favoured over intensive care medicine. To the extent that any services beyond basic health care are made available, they are often understood as generous gifts from donors. Even if we can appreciate the injustice of unequal access to intensive care, we accept practical ethical trade-offs—for example, vaccination programs vs. intensive care—which naturally follow from an economics-driven, rather than a rights-driven approach to healthcare.

Beyond dissemination, the administration of critical care resources in financially limited settings poses ethical challenges. As private hospitals currently supply most critical care in some regions, issues of distribution and accessibility inevitably arise [8, 54, 65]. Varying thresholds for end-of-life decisions in low-income settings have been clearly demonstrated to relate to the patient's economic status, and guidelines are lacking [66]. Finally, given the mismatch between critical care demand and supply in low-income settings, rationing is certain, especially in the absence of an evidence base to guide appropriate decisions [67].

A Research Agenda to Improve Critical Care Delivery and Future Directions

Given the knowledge gaps in critical care delivery in low-resource settings, and the potential for substantial improvements in health outcomes, there is a dire need for research on critical illness systems in resource-poor regions to better guide policymakers. First, cost-effectiveness analyses of current and proposed practices, from the societal perspective of various regions, need to be emphasized. Examples of practices include local training of nurses and physicians, regionalized care models with transport systems, and specific medical interventions such as mechanical ventilation or medications.

Second, technologies and interventions must be adapted to these settings, including sepsis management guidelines [57, 68], quick check emergency triage algorithms [69], and low-cost mechanical ventilators [28]. The recent example of the FEAST randomized trial, which unexpectedly found harm when fluid boluses were administered to febrile African children, illustrates the hazards of uncritical adoption in low-resource settings of resuscitation strategies that are generally accepted in high-income settings [70]. Clinical research and patient triage would benefit from adapted scoring systems that include easily measured parameters [71]. Similarly, while the clinical use of biomarkers in sepsis is controversial [72], a rapid point-of-care test to identify septic patients in community settings to expedite referral to higher level care centers is an area of focus for large funding organizations.

Third, population-based epidemiologic studies of the burden of critical illness, with definitions of critical illness syndromes adapted to decrease reliance on technology [73], are required for evidence-based policy creation and implementation. A more accurate estimate of the potential lives saved through critical care resource dissemination will serve to cement its role in the healthcare system, and ensure its expansion proceeds through an evidence-based trajectory.

Health services research is underemphasized in the developing world, as many health systems have scaled up simply through market demand. However, it is vital to determine how best to treat patients with critical illness based on need rather than financial considerations. Most importantly, patients who would benefit from a modest expansion of critical care capacity must be identified and offered treatment; in particular, those with a low burden of co-morbidity or reversible organ failure may be candidates for critical care, while those with severe underlying disease may be excluded [74]. Although the creation of ICU admission guidelines for low-resource settings is bound to be controversial, healthcare funders are likely to see them as integral to the success of a relatively limited investment in critical care. Other questions include the appropriate balance of private and public healthcare delivery, integration of pre-hospital, clinic, emergency, and transport systems, and regionalization of ICUs and ancillary hospital resources.

Conclusions

The scaling up of intensive care resources in lower income regions is under way because of growing national income and citizen expectations of healthcare. Questions regarding accessibility, distribution, and capabilities of ICUs are currently largely unanswered. As the field strives to answer these questions, there exists the possibility to save many lives in all global regions.

References

1. Mohanty S, Ram F. State of human development in states and districts of India. Mumbai: International Institute for Population Sciences; 2005.
2. Ram F, Shekhar C. Ranking and mapping of districts: based on socio-economic and demographic indicators. Mumbai: International Institute for Population Science; 2006.
3. Gilks CF, Crowley S, Ekpini R, et al. The WHO public-health approach to antiretroviral treatment against HIV in resource-limited settings. Lancet. 2006;368:505–10.

4. Arrow KJ, Gelband H, Jamison DT. Making antimalarial agents available in Africa. N Engl J Med. 2005;353:333–5.
5. Tectonidis M. Crisis in Niger – outpatient care for severe acute malnutrition. N Engl J Med. 2006;354:224–7.
6. Razzak JA, Kellermann AL. Emergency medical care in developing countries: is it worthwhile? Bull World Health Organ. 2002;80:900–5.
7. Weiser TG, Regenbogen SE, Thompson KD, et al. An estimation of the global volume of surgery: a modelling strategy based on available data. Lancet. 2008;372:139–44.
8. Prayag S. ICUs worldwide: critical care in India. Crit Care. 2002;6:479–80.
9. Ruangnapa K, Samransamruajkit R, Namchaisiri J, et al. The long duration of extracorporeal membrane oxygenation in a child with acute severe hypoxic respiratory failure treated in a resource-limited center. Perfusion. 2012;27:547–9.
10. Du B, Xi X, Chen D, Peng J. Clinical review: critical care medicine in mainland China. Crit Care. 2010;14:206.
11. Riviello ED, Letchford S, Achieng L, Newton MW. Critical care in resource-poor settings: Lessons learned and future directions. Crit Care Med. 2011;39:860–7.
12. Fowler RA, Adhikari NK, Bhagwanjee S. Clinical review: critical care in the global context–disparities in burden of illness, access, and economics. Crit Care. 2008;12:225.
13. Adhikari NK, Fowler RA, Bhagwanjee S, Rubenfeld GD. Critical care and the global burden of critical illness in adults. Lancet. 2010;376:1339–46.
14. Mathers C, Fat DM, Boerma JT. World Health Organization. The global burden of disease : 2004 update. Geneva: World Health Organization; 2008.
15. Lopez AD, Mathers CD, Ezzati M, Jamison DT, Murray CJL. Measuring the global burden of disease and risk factors. Disease Control Priorities Project. Washington DC: World Bank; 2006.
16. Li G, Malinchoc M, Cartin-Ceba R, et al. Eight-year trend of acute respiratory distress syndrome: a population-based study in Olmsted County, Minnesota. Am J Respir Crit Care Med. 2011;183:59–66.
17. Ali T, Khan I, Simpson W, et al. Incidence and outcomes in acute kidney injury: a comprehensive population-based study. J Am Soc Nephrol. 2007;18:1292–8.
18. Martin GS, Mannino DM, Eaton S, Moss M. The epidemiology of sepsis in the United States from 1979 through 2000. N Engl J Med. 2003;348:1546–54.
19. Rubenfeld GD, Caldwell E, Peabody E, et al. Incidence and outcomes of acute lung injury. N Engl J Med. 2005;353:1685–93.
20. The world goes to town: a survey of cities. The Economist, 3 May 2007. Retrieved from economist.com. 21 April 2014.
21. World Urbanization Prospects: The 2009 revision. United Nations, Department of Economic and Social Affairs. http://esa.un.org/unpd/wup/index.htm (2011). Accessed 30 Mar 2011.
22. UN-HABITAT. State of the world's cities 2010/2011 – cities for all: bridging the urban divide. New York: United Nations; 2011.
23. Alirol E, Getaz L, Stoll B, Chappuis F, Loutan L. Urbanisation and infectious diseases in a globalised world. Lancet Infect Dis. 2011;11:131–41.
24. Syed F. India's critical care facilities at critical juncture. Express Healthc Manag. 2005;6(8):1–9.
25. Matai S, Peel D, Wandi F, Jonathan M, Subhi R, Duke T. Implementing an oxygen programme in hospitals in Papua New Guinea. Ann Trop Paediatr. 2008;28:71–8.
26. Drexler M. Looking under the hood and seeing an incubator. The New York Times, 15 December 2008.
27. Williams D, Flory S, King R, Thornton M, Dingley J. A low oxygen consumption pneumatic ventilator for emergency construction during a respiratory failure pandemic. Anaesthesia. 2010;65:235–42.
28. Beringer RM, Eltringham RJ. The Glostavent: evolution of an anaesthetic machine for developing countries. Anaesth Intensive Care. 2008;36:442–8.

29. Parikh CR, Karnad DR. Quality, cost, and outcome of intensive care in a public hospital in Bombay, India. Crit Care Med. 1999;27:1754–9.
30. Okafor UV. Challenges in critical care services in sub-Saharan Africa: perspectives from Nigeria. Indian J Crit Care Med. 2009;13:25–7.
31. Mullan F. The metrics of the physician brain drain. N Engl J Med. 2005;353:1810–8.
32. Friedman E. An action plan to prevent brain drain: building equitable health systems in Africa. Boston: Physicians for Human Rights; 2004.
33. Ministry of Health of the People's Republic of China. 2011. http://www.moh.gov.cn/publicfiles/business/htmlfiles/mohyzs/s3577/200902/38935.htm. Accessed 31 Mar 2011.
34. Mustafa I. Intensive care in developing countries in the Western Pacific. Curr Opin Crit Care. 2004;10:304–9.
35. Alem A, Pain C, Araya M, Hodges BD. Co-creating a psychiatric resident program with Ethiopians, for Ethiopians, in Ethiopia: the Toronto Addis Ababa Psychiatry Project (TAAPP). Acad Psychiatry. 2010;34:424–32.
36. Joynt GM, Zimmerman J, Li TS, Gomersall CD. A systematic review of short courses for nonspecialist education in intensive care. J Crit Care. 2011;26:533 e1–10.
37. Biswal S, Mishra P, Malhotra S, Puri GD, Pandhi P. Drug utilization pattern in the intensive care unit of a tertiary care hospital. J Clin Pharmacol. 2006;46:945–51.
38. Gaur AH, English BK. The judicious use of antibiotics – an investment towards optimized health care. Indian J Pediatr. 2006;73:343–50.
39. Verma A, Agarwal P. Platelet utilization in the developing world: strategies to optimize platelet transfusion practices. Transfus Apher Sci. 2009;41:145–9.
40. Sharma RR, Marwaha N. Leukoreduced blood components: advantages and strategies for its implementation in developing countries. Asian J Transfus Sci. 2010;4:3–8.
41. Herridge MS, Tansey CM, Matte A, et al. Functional disability 5 years after acute respiratory distress syndrome. N Engl J Med. 2011;364:1293–304.
42. Kahn JM, Benson NM, Appleby D, Carson SS, Iwashyna TJ. Long-term acute care hospital utilization after critical illness. JAMA. 2010;303:2253–9.
43. Kahn JM, Angus DC. Health policy and future planning for survivors of critical illness. Curr Opin Crit Care. 2007;13:514–8.
44. Graf J, Wagner J, Graf C, Koch KC, Janssens U. Five-year survival, quality of life, and individual costs of 303 consecutive medical intensive care patients – a cost-utility analysis. Crit Care Med. 2005;33:547–55.
45. Lantos JD, Mokalla M, Meadow W. Resource allocation in neonatal and medical ICUs. Epidemiology and rationing at the extremes of life. Am J Respir Crit Care Med. 1997;156:185–9.
46. No authors listed. Understanding costs and cost-effectiveness in critical care: report from the second American Thoracic Society workshop on outcomes research. Am J Respir Crit Care Med. 2002;165:540–50.
47. Linko R, Suojaranta-Ylinen R, Karlsson S, Ruokonen E, Varpula T, Pettila V. One-year mortality, quality of life and predicted life-time cost-utility in critically ill patients with acute respiratory failure. Crit Care. 2010;14:R60.
48. Edejer TT-T. World Health Organization. Making choices in health : WHO guide to cost-effectiveness analysis. Geneva: World Health Organization; 2003.
49. CHOosing Interventions that are Cost Effective (WHO-CHOICE). World Health Organization, 2011. http://www.who.int/choice/en/. Accessed 30 Mar 2011.
50. Chisholm D, Evans D. Economic evaluation in health: saving money or improving care? J Med Econ. 2007;10:325–37.
51. Sachdeva RC. Intensive care – a cost effective option for developing countries? Indian J Pediatr. 2001;68:339–42.
52. Divatia JVBA, Bhagwati A, Chawla R, Iyer S, Jani CK, Joad S, Kamat V, Kapadia F, Mehta Y, Myatra SN, Nagarkar S, Nayyar V, Padhy S, Rajagopalan R, Ramakrishnan N, Ray B, Sahu S, Sampath S, Todi S. Critical care delivery in intensive care units in India: defining the

functions, roles and responsibilities of a consultant intensivist. Indian J Crit Care Med. 2006;10:53–63.
53. Wunsch H, Angus DC, Harrison DA, et al. Variation in critical care services across North America and Western Europe. Crit Care Med. 2008;36(2787–93):e1–9.
54. Jayaram R, Ramakrishnan N. Cost of intensive care in India. Indian J Crit Care Med. 2008;12 (2):55–61.
55. Hensher M, Price M, Adomakoh S. Referral hospitals. In: Disease control priorities in developing countries. 2nd ed. New York: Oxford University Press; 2006. p. 1229–44.
56. Becker JU, Theodosis C, Jacob ST, Wira CR, Groce NE. Surviving sepsis in low-income and middle-income countries: new directions for care and research. Lancet Infect Dis. 2009;9:577–82.
57. Cheng AC, West TE, Limmathurotsakul D, Peacock SJ. Strategies to reduce mortality from bacterial sepsis in adults in developing countries. PLoS Med. 2008;5:e175.
58. Baelani I, Jochberger S, Laimer T, et al. Availability of critical care resources to treat patients with severe sepsis or septic shock in Africa: a self-reported, continent-wide survey of anaesthesia providers. Crit Care. 2011;15:R10.
59. Phua J, Koh Y, Du B, et al. Management of severe sepsis in patients admitted to Asian intensive care units: prospective cohort study. BMJ. 2011;342:d3245.
60. Dworkin R. In: Waldron J, editor. Theories of rights. Oxford: Oxford University Press; 1984.
61. Pogge T. Relational conceptions of justice: responsibilities for health outcomes. In: Anand S, Sen A, Peter F, editors. Public health, ethics, and equity. Oxford: Oxford University Press; 2004.
62. Universal Declaration of Human Rights. United Nations. http://www.un.org/en/documents/udhr/index.shtml. Accessed 6 Feb 2012.
63. Engelhardt Jr HT. Critical care: why there is no global bioethics. J Med Philos. 1998;23:643–51.
64. Pogge T. World Poverty and Human Rights. 1st ed. London: Polity Press; 2002.
65. Narayana Hrudayalaya Hospitals. 2011. http://www.narayanahospitals.com/. Accessed 2 Apr 2011.
66. Miljeteig I, Sayeed SA, Jesani A, Johansson KA, Norheim OF. Impact of ethics and economics on end-of-life decisions in an Indian neonatal unit. Pediatrics. 2009;124:e322–8.
67. Truog RD, Brock DW, Cook DJ, et al. Rationing in the intensive care unit. Crit Care Med. 2006;34:958–63. quiz 71.
68. Dunser MW, Festic E, Dondorp A, et al. Recommendations for sepsis management in resource-limited settings. Intensive Care Med. 2012;38:557–74.
69. IMAI District Clinician Manual: Hospital Care for Adolescents and Adults. Package Vol 1 & 2. Geneva: World Health Organization; 2011.
70. Maitland K, Kiguli S, Opoka RO, et al. Mortality after fluid bolus in African children with severe infection. N Engl J Med. 2011;364:2483–95.
71. Watters DA, Wilson IH, Sinclair JR, Ngandu N. A clinical sickness score for the critically ill in Central Africa. Intensive Care Med. 1989;15:467–70.
72. Pierrakos C, Vincent JL. Sepsis biomarkers: a review. Crit Care. 2010;14:R15.
73. Ranieri VM, Rubenfeld GD, Thompson BT, et al. Acute respiratory distress syndrome: the Berlin definition. JAMA. 2012;307:2526–33.
74. Argent AC. Managing HIV, in the PICU – the experience at the Red Cross War Memorial Children's Hospital in Cape Town. Indian J Pediatr. 2008;75:615–20.

Chapter 17
Disaster Planning for the Intensive Care Unit: A Critical Framework

Daniel Ballard Jamieson and Elizabeth Lee Daugherty Biddison

Abstract Safe and efficient delivery of critical care during disasters is a complex endeavor that requires meticulous planning. Development of an initial plan should take an "all-hazards" approach, building a basic plan that covers all disaster types. Planners can then use a hazard-vulnerability analysis (HVA) to focus more specific planning on those disaster types for which a given health system, hospital, or intensive care unit is at greatest risk. Plans should incorporate three equally important areas: the availability and use of physical space, hospital resources (supplies and equipment) both on site and readily available, and staffing concerns. Potential need for evacuation should also be addressed. Horizontal (within hospital) and vertical (complete) evacuation planning should also be undertaken. Finally, disaster plans should include guidance for the allocation of scarce healthcare resources if all surge capacity is exhausted and evacuation is not possible. Scarce resource allocation planning is essential to maximizing the likelihood that limited resources will be distributed in a fair and transparent way during a crisis. Disasters create a myriad of challenges for healthcare delivery. Careful planning can mitigate the potential harms to patients in such situations and provide a structure for delivering safe, efficient care in spite of those challenges.

Keywords Intensive care unit • Disaster planning • All-hazards planning • Hazard vulnerability • Evacuation

D.B. Jamieson (✉)
Division of Pulmonary, Critical Care and Sleep Medicine, Medstar Georgetown University Hospital, 3800 Reservoir Road, Suite M4200, Washington, DC, USA
e-mail: Daniel.b.jamieson@gunet.georgetown.edu

E.L.D. Biddison
Department of Medicine, Johns Hopkins School of Medicine, Baltimore, MD, USA

Division of Pulmonary and Critical Care, Johns Hopkins School of Medicine, Baltimore, MD, USA

D.C. Scales and G.D. Rubenfeld (eds.), *The Organization of Critical Care*, Respiratory Medicine 18, DOI 10.1007/978-1-4939-0811-0_17,

Introduction

Healthcare disaster preparedness is a rapidly expanding field. Much thought and funding has been dedicated to healthcare disaster planning, both at the individual hospital level and through various government entities and university-based centers [1, 2]. The evidence base needed to guide healthcare disaster planning, however, remains limited. Most available critical care disaster planning guidance is based on expert consensus on best practices [3]. In 2007 a task force was convened by the American College of Chest Physicians, which produced the most comprehensive summary of best practices in the field at that time. These recommendations were first summarized in 2008 by the Task Force for Mass Critical Care of the American College of Chest Physicians Critical Care Collaborative Initiative and are currently undergoing revision [4–8] (Devereaux A, 13 July 2013, Personal Communication).

Healthcare disaster planning is complex and can be daunting. Here we argue that the foundation of all disaster planning should involve an all-hazards approach and should be based on a carefully executed hazard vulnerability analysis (HVA). We then address planning for surge capacity, focusing on three major planning areas identified by the Working group on Emergency Mass Critical Care: Increase in critical care space, equipment availability, and personnel [6]. Finally we address the logistics of the evacuation of the critically ill, and we explore life-saving resource allocation when all surge options have been exhausted and evacuation is not possible. Although we limit our focus here to the intensive care unit (ICU), we believe successful planning requires coordination across hospital units and departments and between regional and, at times, national organizations.

All-Hazards Planning and the Hazard Vulnerability Analysis

When initiating disaster planning, hospitals should adopt an all-hazards approach. This approach focuses initial, core planning efforts on response needs common to all disasters, simplifying both planning and implementation [9]. For example, all disaster responses should be carried out using an incident command system, with a clear hierarchical structure. Likewise, all responses require a communications plan, both within the hospital and with regional and national agencies. Given the variety and scale of many potential disasters, planning for all disaster types is an enormous undertaking; focusing on the capabilities common to all responses creates a foundation which can be augmented with additional detail to enable swift, efficient response to a broad range of disaster types, from a catastrophic weather event to an earthquake or a nuclear detonation.

Specific planning efforts beyond the all-hazards model should be focused on those disasters for which a given institution is most at risk. Those disasters are best identified through a systematic HVA [10]. An HVA may be undertaken at regional, hospital-wide, and unit levels to identify hazards that are most likely to occur in that area, hospital, or unit, so that plans can be tailored appropriately.

Disasters are inherently unpredictable. In recent years, the USA has experienced a large series of "never" events. These include an earthquake on the East Coast during the summer of 2011 [11], and the "super storm" hurricane Sandy impacting New York City and much of the mid-Atlantic in late 2012. Damage from the super storm necessitated evacuation of three hospitals with costs into the billions of dollars [12]. Although pre-event planning within a defined framework is essential for preparing an ICU to face disaster, planners must be aware that disaster response requires flexibility and learning in real time.

Planning for Surge Capability

Surges in critical care occur along a continuum of scale, and, as such, surge capability plans should be scalable. Conventional capability must be scalable to have contingency capability and even expand with the largest of disasters to "crisis" capability. Conventional capability refers to disasters in which medical care can be provided without disruption of services at the receiving hospital. Contingency capability refers to the ability to provide usual care, but only after modifications are made to standard utilization of space, supplies and staff, described below. Crisis capability represents the extreme situation in which the ability to provide usual care may be limited, even with implementation of all resources available for surge capacity [13].

Space

In a disaster, ICUs may face an influx of patients either immediately or over a period of weeks. Defining a hospitals specific surge capability (resources available above those used routinely) begins with identifying what physical locations (capacity) are available to care for the critically ill. There are nearly 94,000 ICU beds (nonfederal) in the USA. On average, 68 % of these beds are filled, although many hospitals have much higher average ICU occupancy [14, 15]. In an era of rising healthcare costs, it is rare for hospitals to maintain reserve critical care beds to manage surges in patient flow, simply because the cost of doing so is high. Thus, in the event of a surge of patients, many will likely need to be cared for outside of traditional ICUs. Post-anesthesia care units (PACU), emergency department critical care areas, and procedural areas equipped with oxygen and suction equipment should be evaluated and inventoried for surge capability. A preliminary estimate of surge capacity may be calculated taking into account these areas and the number of traditional critical care beds a given hospital typically has available. Planners must be aware that usual hospital operations and associated revenue are likely to be significantly hampered if areas such as PACUs and ORs are removed from normal use and elective surgeries are cancelled in order to provide surge capability. Depending on the duration of the disaster, cost considerations may become extremely important and may need to be addressed on a state or federal level. Of note, during a response, use of non-traditional patient care areas for delivery of critical care should only be undertaken after all patients that may be safely cared for outside of ICUs have been transferred to lower levels of care and others that may be safely evacuated elsewhere have been moved.

Additionally, hospital-wide bed management and patient tracking will increase in complexity, resulting in more opportunity for error. For this reason, early involvement of hospital information technology teams is recommended to optimize tracking of admissions, transfers, and discharges. For example, in some electronic medical records (EMRs), virtual patient beds will need to be created in areas not traditionally used to house in-patients.

Given the complexity of care for the critically ill and need for hospital resources such as oxygen, medical air, suction and monitoring equipment, these patients should remain in hospital areas, while other, non-critically ill patients may more safely be transferred out of the hospital setting. As a general rule, care should be provided in the area that care would be provided if no emergency existed, (i.e., initially the ICU). When that space fills, then the next most equipped space should be mobilized. This would likely be the PACU and emergency department followed by procedural areas. Monitored acute care wards and non-monitored wards may then be mobilized. All of these areas have the benefit of existing within the hospital structure. Only if the hospital is at capacity or has been structurally compromised should care of the critically ill outside of the hospital be considered.

Equipment

As healthcare delivery has become more sophisticated, the amount of equipment required to provide care for critically ill patients has increased dramatically. Although the number of ventilators is often thought of first when planning for increased capability, medical gas, pharmaceuticals and equipment for appropriate infection control practices are equally important. Before consideration of stockpiling equipment in preparation for an emergency, an evaluation of the hospital physical plant is appropriate. Do the beds identified as available for surge each have the electrical and medical gas infrastructure to support a ventilator? These questions are critical, as the capability of a hospital's physical plant may be the true "rate-limiting step" for increasing numbers of available critical care beds.

Sufficient amounts of medical grade oxygen must be available, ideally through the existing hospital infrastructure. Replacement or supplemental oxygen supplies may be obtained including compressed gas cylinders and oxygen concentrators, but liquid systems are the best option given the ability to store in bulk and provide oxygen to the greatest number of patients. Compressed oxygen tanks are acceptable for short-term use but are not feasible for long-term supply, given cost and storage constraints. Oxygen concentrators are generally not acceptable except for use in non-ventilated patients requiring supplemental oxygen, because most are unable to deliver the high flows needed to power positive pressure ventilation [16].

Numerous epidemics result in respiratory failure, and the need for respiratory support should be expected to increase in any mass casualty event. Without planning for increases in the need for ventilator support, many patients will likely die. Planners should work with facility managers at their institutions to quantify the number of ventilators a hospital's physical plant can support, as well as the number of ventilators available. Machines capable of providing positive pressure ventilation for mass casualty care include not just full-featured mechanical ventilators, but also anesthesia machines, portable (both pneumatically powered and internal gas source) as well as EMS transport ventilators. Although manual ventilation is acceptable for transport, it is not feasible from a staffing, infection control, or oxygen conservation standpoint and should not be considered a significant option for long-term ventilation. Options to rapidly increase the overall number of available ventilators for a national response has been assessed and was found to be lacking [16, 17].

It is estimated that there are approximately 62,118 full feature mechanical ventilators nationwide (median of 19 per 100,000 people) [18]. Relocation of these ventilators in the event of a disaster presents a considerable logistical challenge [6]. Strategies to increase ventilator supply in a given institution or region include renting, accessing the Strategic National Stockpile (SNS), or repurposing anesthesia units. Rental supplies may be helpful but cannot be expected to adequately meet demand. A regional drill of a respiratory failure epidemic affecting a 27-hospital network revealed 16 ventilators available to meet surge demand capable of handling 2,500–3,500 beds [19]. The SNS is maintained by the US Centers for Disease Control and Prevention. This stockpile initially consisted of approximately 4,400 ventilators. An additional 4,500 ventilators were added to the SNS in 2009–2010. Each state designates an SNS official to maintain their allocation policy, which is organized by region [20]. Institutions can request stockpile ventilators during a disaster through their state's designated official [21–24].

Pharmaceutical supply is also an important area of concern and focus, and pharmacists should be included in preparedness planning efforts. Most hospitals rely on lean inventory and frequent restocking, given the cost of storing medications and their limited shelf life. Pharmaceutical shortages occur nationwide even in the absence of a disaster, secondary to the supply chain and possible over-reliance on individual manufacturers for some of our most frequently utilized medications [25]. Given the realities of the current healthcare funding environment, processes for rapid procurement of essential medications should be established and evaluated. Utilizing knowledgeable pharmacists will also be paramount, given the need to employ alternative medications when supplies of first-line medications run low. In a pandemic, specific supplies of certain medications (antibiotics, antivirals) may become dangerously low. As with ventilators, the federal government through the SNS maintains a stockpile of medications that can be distributed in an emergency

[26]. Planners should be aware that accessing stockpiled medications is likely to take at least several days and should prepare accordingly.

Additional preparedness activities should include careful estimation of ancillary equipment needs, including ventilator supplies (extra circuits, pulse oximetry probes, humidification devices), monitoring supplies (EKG leads, temperature probes), and infection control equipment (masks, gowns, gloves). Determining the amount of supplies necessary for a fully functional ICU bed and then determining multiples to equal the number of critical care surge beds will provide an estimate for the amount of supplies needed. Depending on the type of disaster, these supplies may be available from stockpiles in other areas of the hospital. Table 17.1 details the nonrespiratory medical equipment that is essential for emergency mass critical care. The Mass Critical Care Task Force project, Definitive care for the Critically Ill During a Disaster, has also published guidance on ancillary equipment planning for surge positive pressure ventilation.

Personnel

Staffing of ICUs during an emergency is an additional challenge. There are shortages of fully trained critical care staff (nurses, respiratory therapists, pharmacists, intensivists) even at baseline [27–29]. Some studies have shown that 10–60 % of staff may not report for work in the event of a disaster. More staff may be absent if the disaster is an epidemic, or if the disaster impacts family life, including closure of schools, daycare, etc. [30]. These concerns suggest that staffing for a significant critical care surge will require modification of existing staffing models. Off-duty staff may be recalled to the hospital to properly care for a surge of patients. Staff trained in anesthesia, either anesthesiologists or other ancillary staff, will likely possess airway and ventilator management skills that could make them a reasonable source of supplementary critical care personnel. Transferring individual staff within and throughout local hospitals will minimize the chance that one particular unit or hospital may become overwhelmed. Identifying which hospitals may be able to share staff will enable credentialing and training to occur prior to a disaster.

If recalling off-duty staff or utilizing staff from other units or hospitals does not meet staffing needs in a disaster, "tiered staffing" has been recommended. A tiered staffing model has been described by the Working Group on Emergency Mass Critical Care and the Mass Critical Care Task Force [3, 7]. These team-based models incorporate non-critical care trained clinicians and nurses to provide the general medical management of the patients, allowing intensivists to focus on airway and ventilator management as well as other critical care related issues. The working group recommends that when tiered staffing is implemented, each non-critical care clinician should be responsible for up to six patients, and each intensivist should be able to oversee four non-intensivists. Each intensivist would thus be able to care for 24 patients [3]. When utilizing tiered staffing, expectations of staff brought from other clinical areas should be clearly delineated.

Table 17.1 Suggested nonrespiratory medical equipment for emergency mass critical care[a]

Devices	Reusable/consumable	Duration of use	Minimum number per 10 treatment spaces for 10 day[b]	Comments
Hemodynamic support				
CVC	Consumable	Duration of need	13	Multilumen percutaneously inserted, nontunneled CVCs or PICCs (with skilled operators) are acceptable; assumption: average of 1 CVC per patient; some patients many not require CVCs and some may require multiple CVCs during a 10-day period
CVC ancillary supplies (e.g., administration sets, insertion site dressings, flush)	Consumable	Per institutional preference	Sustained-use equipment: 13 × units of equipment per patient × 10/duration of use (d); daily consumable equipment: 13 × units of equipment per patient per day × 10 day	
Peripheral IV equipment	Consumable	4 day	65	
IV crystalloid solution	N/A	4–5 L on day 1, 2–3 L on days 2 and 3; 1–2 L/day thereafter	200 L	Crystalloid choice is dependent on institutional practice; volume may be reduced if institution prefers hypertonic saline solution
IV pump (multilumen)	Reusable	Duration of need	10	Patients requiring additional pumps may be too ill to support during extreme shortages
Miscellaneous equipment				
Disposable bath package	Consumable	2–3 day	35	
Nasogastric/orogastric tubes	Consumable	Duration of need	13	Route for enteral nutrition and medications in ventilated patients; if there are insufficient enteral

(continued)

Table 17.1 (continued)

Devices	Reusable/ consumable	Duration of use	Minimum number per 10 treatment spaces for 10 day[b]	Comments
				feeding pumps, bolus feeding by gravity is an acceptable alternative
Nasogastric/orogastric tube ancillary supplies (e.g., securing tape, syringe, ophthalmic lubricating ointment)	Consumable	Per institutional preference	Sustained-use equipment: 13 × units of equipment per patient × 10/ duration of use (d); daily consumable equipment: 13 × units of equipment per patient per day × 10 day	
Optional equipment				
Continuous heart rate and rhythm monitor	Reusable	Duration of need	10	May consider at least one device capable of cardioversion (for nonpulseless but unstable arrhythmias)
ECG cable/leads	Reusable	(consumable)	Duration of need	10 or 13
ECG patches	Consumable	Duration of need	100	
Sequential compression device	Reusable	Duration of need	10	Dependent on institutional practice and patient VTE risk and risk of adverse event from chemical VTE prophylaxis
Sequential compression boots	Consumable	Duration of need	13	
Patient monitoring				

Noninvasive BP cuff	Consumable	Duration of patient stay	1 small; 10 standard; 3 large adult; 1 thigh	Consumable cuff or cuff cover is acceptable; proportions of sizes may vary based on anticipated patient sizes
Thermometer	Reusable or	consumable	Duration of patient stay	I:3 disposable probes
Temperature measurement site based on institutional preference				
Urinary catheter with collection bag	Consumable	Duration of need	13	

Reproduced with permission: [7]

[a]Pediatric-specific equipment, while not presented to limit the complexity of the suggestions, should be considered. Some devices may be used interchangeably for adults and most pediatrics (e.g., mechanical ventilators approved for adult and pediatric use). Amounts of pediatric-specific equipment should be determined by regional analysis of need in consultation with pediatric experts. *N/A* not applicable, *CVC* central venous catheter, *PICC* peripherally-inserted central venous catheter, *VTE* venous thromboembolism

[b]Equipment for ten patient care spaces for 10 days assumes: 30 % patient turnover (clinical improvement and deaths)

A final issue related to staffing is that of navigating the EMR. Systems and order sets often differ both between and within hospital, and staff may be very familiar with EMR functionality in their home hospital or unit but not in the ICU to which they are reassigned. Identification and EMR-specific training of non-critical care staff who may be re-assigned to ICUs in the event of a disaster is imperative to avoid medical errors related to the EMR.

Evacuation

Although planning for surge critical care within conventional hospital space presents real challenges, an even more complex task is the planning and execution of an evacuation of critically ill patients. An evacuation may take place either horizontally or vertically. A horizontal evacuation refers to the removal of patients and staff from an *area* of the hospital that is no longer safe, either because of structural damage, security concerns or loss of hospital resources (electricity, medical gases, etc.) A vertical evacuation refers to removal of staff and patients from the entire hospital in the event that the entire hospital is no longer safe. The patient, equipment, and patient records must be transported in unusual conditions from the hospital, to transport, and then into another care environment, likely with a different set of clinicians. The hazards and opportunities for error inherent in this required sequence of events are numerous.

During the 1990s as many as 20 hospitals were evacuated each year in the USA [31]. In May of 2011, a tornado in Joplin, Missouri struck St. John's Regional Medical Center, killing four people in the hospital and on the hospital grounds. The hospital was evacuated in the immediate aftermath of the storm and subsequently demolished because it was structurally unsound [32]. More recently, two major hospitals in New York City were evacuated during and after hurricane Sandy after power was lost and back-up generators were compromised. No one was injured during these evacuations, even though they took place at night, without power, and during a hurricane. The Veterans Affairs Hospital in New York City was also evacuated because of Hurricane Sandy, although the decision to evacuate was made prior to the storm's arrival. These examples and others suggest that hospital evacuation can occur safely with appropriate planning [33, 34].

In general, evacuation will be necessary if significant damage has occurred to the hospital building or if conditions at or near the hospital are expected to worsen to the point that damage is likely. In either event, an evacuation decision is made based on an assessment of the risk associated with sheltering in place versus the risk associated with moving complex critically ill patients [35]. The difficulty of determining when to evacuate was illustrated clearly during and after Hurricane Sandy, when three hospitals required evacuation, but only one evacuated prior to the storm [33, 34].

Evacuation planning requires addressing two major sets of issues: those related to the disaster itself and those related to the patients who need to be evacuated. With regard to the disaster itself, planning and decision-making will vary based on whether it is a one-time event, such as a power-outage or tornado, or an ongoing event, such as an earthquake with aftershocks. The urgency of the evacuation will also impact planning and implementation. Will the event require immediate, rapid response to an immediate threat or can the evacuation be done in a more controlled fashion as with a predicted storm or dwindling resources without ability to re-supply? The care needs and stability of the patients for transport must also be assessed. Appropriate portable equipment must be assigned to each patient along with skilled staff to accompany the patient during transport [36].

When evacuating a large facility, both portable equipment and staff will likely be in short supply. Critical care transport teams, who often transfer critically ill patients in routine situations, may be of some help if the disaster is limited geographically, but they are also likely to be overwhelmed by high demand. Equipment and staff initially assigned to the evacuating hospital will need to return to the hospital after successful transport of one patient, to prepare the next patient and care for those who remain.

Transport of the critically ill has grown more complex as the amount of equipment routinely used to care for them has increased. In a disaster, the complexity may be compounded by damage to the hospital physical plant, necessitating alternative routes of egress or traversing of stairs. To accomplish transport safely, use of specially designed evacuation litters or sleds is recommended. Each hospital should determine the number of evacuation sleds needed to evacuate their facility in a timely fashion and should facilitate acquisition and storage of these key items. Guidelines have been published to assist hospitals in determining their needs [37]. Finally, the importance of drills cannot be overemphasized. Practicing evacuations prior to an actual emergency, even on a limited scale, provides real-time experience to hospital staff and helps identify areas of concern to be addressed in an organized fashion.

Resource Allocation

Even with the most comprehensive response plans, during a disaster demand for critical care services and equipment may significantly exceed supply. If patients cannot be transferred to other facilities with additional critical care capability, and alternate equipment is not available, hospitals should have in place a mechanism for the fair allocation of limited resources. Absolute scarcity of resources necessitates a shift in the providers' focus from the need of the individual patient to optimizing the survival of the greatest number of individuals. It is essential that all options for expanding existing resources be exhausted before implementing a scarce resource allocation plan, given the significant ethical concerns associated with any deviation from usual standards of care. As would be expected, planning for the allocation of scarce critical care resources in this context is extremely challenging, as it opens the possibility of withholding critical care treatment from patients who might receive it under usual circumstances.

Several authors have published guidelines that focus on resource allocation [5, 38–41]. These guidelines attempt to answer whether it is ethically permissible to withhold or withdraw treatment from one patient to allocate that resource to another patient who may be more likely to survive. The published protocols [5, 40] have different strengths and weaknesses. Each addresses what criteria may be used to allocate ventilators or other similar resources, but they vary in complexity and associated efficiency. Choosing a protocol to implement in advance of a mass casualty event may reassure those involved in triage decision-making that every effort has been made to provide efficient, fair use of critical care resources. Although several allocation strategies may be ethically and morally permissible, the Institute of Medicine has outlined basic norms and processes that should be adhered to in developing a protocol for a given institution or community [42].

In general, a resource allocation plan should specify inclusion criteria, a prioritization tool, and a description of the triage team structure [40]. The inclusion criteria are designed as criteria for admission to a critical care unit. Respiratory failure will likely be the most common criteria used, however hemodynamic collapse and need for vasopressors could also be a criteria, if support cannot be provided in other areas of the hospital.

If exclusion criteria are utilized, categories related to the severity of illness or injury and the patients overall prognosis may be included. Those who support using exclusion criteria suggest that if patients are severely injured and not expected to survive, they may be excluded from admission to the ICU, as resources provided to support them prior to death would be better utilized for patients who are expected to survive but require critical care support to do so. Some suggest that severe co-morbidities may also be taken into account when developing exclusion criteria, although this category may be more problematic than others.

A triage tool should be applied to all patients regardless of their reason for requiring critical care, and is helpful to not only exclude patients from the ICU, but also prioritize patients for care. One option is to use an illness severity score such as the Sequential Organ Failure Assessment (SOFA) score, and categorize patients according to their score. A SOFA score >11 has been associated with >90 % mortality in some contexts and has been suggested by some to be an acceptable criterion for withholding critical care [43]. An important caveat to the use of SOFA scores is that the mortality associated with a particular score may vary depending on the type of disease process. This fact was illustrated during the H1N1 influenza outbreak, during which a SOFA score of 11 only resulted in a mortality rate of 59 %, not the predicted 90 % mortality [44].

Finally, when an allocation system is in place, it is important to continually reassess patients, as their status for inclusion or exclusion may change given underlying co-morbidities and response to treatment. Reassessment may suggest that resources should be re-allocated to ensure that the greatest number of victims be given the highest chance for survival. Equally important in the triage process is the need for transparency and accountability for triage teams. The difficult process of resource allocation must take place openly and via protocol to relieve the pressure felt by individuals tasked with making these difficult decisions and to ensure that all involved understand the process as it unfolds.

Conclusion

Provision of critical care in a disaster is a complex enterprise. Although daunting, the successful development and testing of a disaster plan for each ICU is necessary given the possibility of disaster occurring at any time. Planning should begin with a hazard vulnerability analysis and should follow an all-hazards model. This approach will allow the majority of resources to be focused on those disasters that are most likely to occur, while ensuring that all major concerns are addressed. The disaster plan should focus on the increased use of physical space, increased staffing and hospital resources available, and input should be sought from all units and staff that will be involved in a disaster response. The possibility of evacuation must be considered, both horizontal (from one unit or hospital wing to another) and vertical (out of a hospital building completely). Evacuation of critically ill patients is a complex enterprise, but recent history suggests it can be done without significant increase in morbidity or mortality. Finally, although priority should be placed on expanding capacity, planners must also develop structures for allocation of resources when surge capacity is exhausted and evacuation is not possible.

References

1. US department of health and human services. HHS grants to bolster disaster planning for health care, public health. http://www.hhs.gov/news/press/2013pres/07/20130703a.html (2013). Accessed 10 Oct 2013.
2. UPMC center for health security annual report. http://www.upmchealthsecurity.org/about-the-center/annual_report/archive/annual_report_2013.html(2013). Accessed 24 Apr 2014.
3. Rubinson L, Nuzzo JB, Talmor DS, O'Toole T, Kramer BR, Inglesby TV. Augmentation of hospital critical care capacity after bioterrorist attacks or epidemics: Recommendations of the working group on emergency mass critical care. Crit Care Med. 2005;33(10):2393–403.
4. Devereaux A, Christian MD, Dichter JR, Geiling JA, Rubinson L. Task force for mass critical care. Summary of suggestions from the task force for mass critical care summit, January 26–27, 2007. Chest. 2008;133(5 Suppl):1S–7.
5. Devereaux AV, Dichter JR, Christian MD, et al. Definitive care for the critically ill during a disaster: a framework for allocation of scarce resources in mass critical care: from a task force for mass critical care summit meeting, January 26–27, 2007, Chicago, IL. Chest. 2008;133 (5 Suppl):51S–66.
6. Christian MD, Devereaux AV, Dichter JR, Geiling JA, Rubinson L. Definitive care for the critically ill during a disaster: current capabilities and limitations: from a task force for mass critical care summit meeting, January 26–27, 2007, Chicago, IL. Chest. 2008;133(5 Suppl):8S–17.

7. Rubinson L, Hick JL, Curtis JR, et al. Definitive care for the critically ill during a disaster: medical resources for surge capacity: from a task force for mass critical care summit meeting, January 26–27, 2007, Chicago, IL. Chest. 2008;133(5 Suppl):32S–50.
8. Rubinson L, Hick JL, Hanfling DG, et al. Definitive care for the critically ill during a disaster: a framework for optimizing critical care surge capacity: From a task force for mass critical care summit meeting, January 26–27, 2007, Chicago, IL. Chest. 2008;133(5 Suppl):18S–31.
9. Bayntun C. A health system approach to all-hazards disaster management: a systematic review. PLoS Curr. 2012;4:e50081cad5861d.
10. Schultz CH, Mothershead JL, Field M. Bioterrorism preparedness. I: the emergency department and hospital. Emerg Med Clin North Am. 2002;20(2):437–55.
11. Calvert S, Walker C. Earthquake in Virginia rattles Baltimore and the east coast. The Baltimore Sun, 8 August 2012.
12. Bernstein N, Hartcollis A. Bellevue hospital evacuates patients after backup power fails. The New York Times, 1 November 2012.
13. Hick JL, Barbera JA, Kelen GD. Refining surge capacity: conventional, contingency, and crisis capacity. Disaster Med Public Health Prep. 2009;3(2 Suppl):S59–67.
14. Groeger JS, Guntupalli KK, Strosberg M, et al. Descriptive analysis of critical care units in the United States: patient characteristics and intensive care unit utilization. Crit Care Med. 1993;21(2):279–91.
15. Halpern NA, Pastores SM. Critical care medicine in the United States 2000–2005: an analysis of bed numbers, occupancy rates, payer mix, and costs. Crit Care Med. 2010;38(1):65–71.
16. Daugherty EL, Branson R, Rubinson L. Mass casualty respiratory failure. Curr Opin Crit Care. 2007;13(1):51–6.
17. Osterholm MT. Preparing for the next pandemic. N Engl J Med. 2005;352(18):1839–42.
18. Rubinson LF, Vaughn FF, Nelson SF, et al. Mechanical ventilators in US acute care hospitals. Disaster Med Public Health Prep JID – 101297401. 0821(1938–744).
19. Hick JL, O'Laughlin DT. Concept of operations for triage of mechanical ventilation in an epidemic. Acad Emerg Med. 2006;13(2):223–9.
20. Center for disease control office of public health preparedness and response. http://www.cdc.gov/phpr/(2014). Accessed 24 Apr 2014
21. Esbitt D. The strategic national stockpile: roles and responsibilities of health care professionals for receiving the stockpile assets. Disaster Manag Response. 2003;1(3):68–70.
22. Malatino EM. Strategic national stockpile: overview and ventilator assets. Respir Care. 2008;53(1):91–5. discussion 95.
23. The strategic national stockpile – the LTV-1200 ventilator. https://www.aarc.org/education/webcast_central/archives/2009/09_22_2009_ltv_1200.asp(2009). Accessed 10 Oct 2009.
24. CareFusion shipping ventilators to CDC for national emergency preparedness. http://www.infectioncontroltoday.com/news/2009/10/carefusion-shipping-ventilators-to-cdc-for-nation.aspx(2009). Accessed 10 Oct 2009.
25. U.S. department of health and human services: drug shortages. http://www.fda.gov/drugs/DrugSafety/DrugShortages/default.htm(2014). Accessed 24 Apr 2014.
26. Office of public health preparedness and response. strategic national stockpile. http://Www.cdc.gov/phpr/stockpile/stockpile.htm. 10 October 2013.
27. Stechmiller JK. The nursing shortage in acute and critical care settings. AACN Clin Issues. 2002;13(4):577–84.
28. Knapp KK, Quist RM, Walton SM, Miller LM. Update on the pharmacist shortage: national and state data through 2003. Am J Health Syst Pharm. 2005;62(5):492–9.
29. Angus DC, Kelley MA, Schmitz RJ, White A, Popovich Jr J. Committee on Manpower for Pulmonary and Critical Care Societies (COMPACCS). Caring for the critically ill patient current and projected workforce requirements for care of the critically ill and patients with pulmonary disease: can we meet the requirements of an aging population? JAMA. 2000;284(21):2762–70.

30. Wise RA. The creation of emergency health care standards for catastrophic events. Acad Emerg Med. 2006;13(11):1150–2.
31. Sternberg E, Lee GC, Huard D. Counting crises: US hospital evacuations, 1971–1999. Prehosp Disaster Med. 2004;19(2):150–7.
32. Livingston I. A year after the Joplin tornado disaster. The Washington Post, 21 May 2012.
33. Hartocollis A. New York health chief defends decision not to evacuate hospitals. The New York Times, 24 January 2013.
34. Bernstein N, Hartocollis A. Bellvue hospital evacuates patients after backup power fails. The New York Times, 31 October 2012.
35. Downey EL, Andress K, Schultz CH. Initial management of hospital evacuations caused by Hurricane Rita: a systematic investigation. Prehosp Disaster Med. 2013;28(3):257–63.
36. Daugherty EL, Rubinson L. Preparing your intensive care unit to respond in crisis: considerations for critical care clinicians. Crit Care Med. 2011;39(11):2534–9.
37. Massachusetts department of public health hospital evacuation toolkit. http://www.mass.gov/eohhs/gov/departments/dph/programs/emergency-prep/hospital-and-ems/mdph-hospital-evacuation-toolkit.html(2014). Accessed 24 Apr 2014.
38. Powell T, Christ KC, Birkhead GS. Allocation of ventilators in a public health disaster. Disaster Med Public Health Prep. 2008;2(1):20–6.
39. White DB, Katz MH, Luce JM, Lo B. Who should receive life support during a public health emergency? Using ethical principles to improve allocation decisions. Ann Intern Med. 2009;150(2):132–8.
40. Christian MD, Hawryluck L, Wax RS, et al. Development of a triage protocol for critical care during an influenza pandemic. CMAJ. 2006;175(11):1377–81.
41. Chapman KR, Mannino DM, Soriano JB, et al. Epidemiology and costs of chronic obstructive pulmonary disease. Eur Respir J. 2006;27(1):188–207.
42. Altevogt BM, Stroud C, Hanson SL, Hanfling D, Gostin LO, editors. Guidance for establishing crisis standards of care for use in disaster situations: a letter report. United States: The National Academies Press; 2009.
43. Ferreira FL, Bota DP, Bross A, Melot C, Vincent JL. Serial evaluation of the SOFA score to predict outcome in critically ill patients. JAMA. 2001;286(14):1754–8.
44. Shahpori R, Stelfox HT, Doig CJ, Boiteau PJ, Zygun DA. Sequential organ failure assessment in H1N1 pandemic planning. Crit Care Med. 2011;39(4):827–32.

Index

D.C. Scales and G.D. Rubenfeld (eds.), *The Organization of Critical Care*, Respiratory Medicine 18, DOI 10.1007/978-1-4939-0811-0,

MIX
Papier aus verantwortungsvollen Quellen
Paper from responsible sources
FSC® C105338

If you have any concerns about our products, you can contact us on
ProductSafety@springernature.com

In case Publisher is established outside the EU, the EU authorized representative is:
Springer Nature Customer Service Center GmbH
Europaplatz 3, 69115 Heidelberg, Germany

Printed by Libri Plureos GmbH
in Hamburg, Germany